Legal Issues in
Emergency Medicine

Legal Issues in Emergency Medicine

Rade B. Vukmir MD, JD
Critical Care Medicine Associates

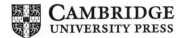

CAMBRIDGE
UNIVERSITY PRESS

University Printing House, Cambridge CB2 8BS, United Kingdom

One Liberty Plaza, 20th Floor, New York, NY 10006, USA

477 Williamstown Road, Port Melbourne, VIC 3207, Australia

314–321, 3rd Floor, Plot 3, Splendor Forum, Jasola District Centre, New Delhi – 110025, India

79 Anson Road, #06-04/06, Singapore 079906

Cambridge University Press is part of the University of Cambridge.

It furthers the University's mission by disseminating knowledge in the pursuit of education, learning, and research at the highest international levels of excellence.

www.cambridge.org
Information on this title: www.cambridge.org/9781107499379
DOI: 10.1017/9781316182192

First published 2018

Printed in the United States of America by Sheridan Books, Inc.

A catalogue record for this publication is available from the British Library.

Library of Congress Cataloging-in-Publication Data
Names: Vukmir, Rade B., author.
Title: Legal issues in emergency medicine / Rade B. Vukmir.
Description: Cambridge, United Kingdom ; New York, NY : Cambridge University Press, 2018. | Includes bibliographical references and index.
Identifiers: LCCN 2017049400 | ISBN 9781107499379 (hardback)
Subjects: | MESH: Emergency Medical Services – legislation & jurisprudence | United States | Legal Cases
Classification: LCC RA975.5.E5 | NLM WB 33 AA1 | DDC 362.18–dc23
LC record available at https://lccn.loc.gov/2017049400

ISBN 978-1-107-49937-9 Hardback

Contents

Contents

Disclaimer

The information contained herein is not meant to be relied on as legal advice in an actual legal issue or conflict. One should seek appropriate legal assistance in the specific area of concern if it is felt to be warranted.

The case studies present fictionalized hypothetical health-care events, and are not representative of any individual encounters.

Likewise, the legal case explanations provided were abstracted from the public record information, and no further accuracy is assured, or liability assumed.

Foreword

Physicians prefer when the practice of medicine is based upon science, and the art of using the patient–physician relationship to benefit the patient with a positive therapeutic outcome.

Most physicians like to think that if they are doing the best they can for their patients, they should not need to worry about the legal implications of each interaction, and each decision. This naïve approach simply does not work in the real-world practice of emergency medicine.

In the US, there are now over 150 million visits to emergency departments each year. The unique aspects of the clinical practice of emergency medicine make medical and legal dilemmas a daily unavoidable reality.

Each of the 106 chapters in *Legal Issues in Emergency Medicine* represents realistic, common practical issues that every emergency medicine physician and emergency department will face. Many of these issues occur multiple times in each shift. Often, these situations leave the emergency physician searching for an approach without having the formal legal and ethical basis necessary to make a legally wise and low-risk decision.

Legal Issues in Emergency Medicine is an invaluable resource for medical practitioners, legal experts and administrative professionals in practice and in training. It is practical, concise, and well organized.

The style of *Legal Issues in Emergency Medicine* is exactly what a busy practitioner would want as a reference or what emergency department leaders, hospital administrators or residents would desire as a training text. Each topic includes a clinical vignette, a review of the legal controversy, current medical scientific evidence, legal precedent, caselaw generating solutions and potential risk reduction programs.

The book covers key topics that have direct relevance in day-to-day acute patient care practice.

This approach allows practitioner exposure to a wide variety of medico-legal problems, allowing a pre-emptive, informed approach to problem-solving. One of the remarkable features of this valuable text is the ability to take extraordinarily complex issues such as advance directives, against medical advice (AMA), the Emergency Medical Treatment and Labor Act (EMTALA), involuntary commitment, and dozens of other issues and distill them into brief digestible summaries.

Few authors would be able to compile a text that is so informative, well organized and authoritative. Rade B Vukmir not only talks the talk but has walked the walk for decades. Dr. Vukmir has been trained in Emergency Medicine and Critical Care and has decades of clinical care experience. In addition, Dr. Vukmir has completed a degree in law with health-care certification. He has analyzed medico-legal issues involving patients, physicians, medical groups, and hospitals in every imaginable situation.

He has focused on providing guidelines to improve patient safety as well as decreasing both clinical and legal risk. This text is simply a must-have addition to any emergency department, reference library, legal office, and quality and risk management department.

Paul M Paris MD, FACEP, LLD(hon)
Professor of Emergency Medicine, University
of Pittsburgh School of Medicine, Emergency
Medicine Chair in Healthcare Quality

Preface

The case study format used in this book is grounded in both medical and legal disciplines, and provides an effective instructional tool to facilitate understanding for the members of both professions.

As physicians, we try to learn from every patient encounter. In the complex world of acute care medicine, the potential for a legal question to arise is becoming more common every day. Likewise, legal practitioners can benefit from a better understanding of the complexity of common medical dilemmas that may exist. Last but not least, the case studies will allow medical administrative professionals to appreciate the balance between the medical and legal disciplines and how they both impact the health care provided to patients.

Introduction

As a health-care provider, how often have you found yourself with a complex legal dilemma that requires a clear, concise response in the midst of a critical patient care event?

As a legal professional, how often have you been left to confront a complex medical decision-making process, when the legal direction may be clear?

As an administrator or management professional, how often have you had to balance the medical and legal aspects of a health-care situation that requires a nuanced outcome, focused on patient care?

This book is designed for medical providers, legal practitioners, and administrators both in practice and in training. The complexity of practice in emergency medicine requires a readily accessible source of complete and comprehensive information. This will allow medical practitioners first to prevent and then to address any legal risk that occurs. In addition, it will encourage legal professionals and medical administrators to participate in mitigation, prevention, and education programs.

The complexity of medical and legal dilemmas grows greater every day. Yet, no clear, concise, up-to-date book or data compilation is readily available to practitioners of all disciplines. Of course we have the internet, but a typical search has no filter to ensure that it delivers the highest-quality evidence or authoritative information.

My three decades of experience in emergency and critical care practice has made the need for a book such as this very clear to me. Its aim is to offer a clear pathway through some of the common, yet complex legal dilemmas encountered in day-to-day practice in emergency and acute care.

One important aspect of this book is the standardized presentation of problem, analysis, and problem-solving. First, the simple alphabetical listing of common medicolegal topics allows ease of access. Second, the case study format of each chapter facilitates understanding of difficult health-care concepts. Third, the review of the relevant medical literature provides an analysis of evidence-based practice. Fourth, the legal literature review and caselaw analysis allows practical understanding of the medico-legal decision-making interface. Lastly, each chapter concludes with clear guidelines on how to deal with complicated health-care issues.

This book is meant to inform readers of the complex legal issues that are likely to be encountered in an emergency, critical care, and acute care practice. However, it is not meant to be a comprehensive analysis of the specific legal issues discussed, nor is it meant to be relied upon for legal decision-making. Certainly, actual situations will require the kind of individualized analysis offered by an attorney or counselor.

The subject areas discussed in this book are familiar in emergency medicine, but they are also topical. They include protective care issues such as abandonment, competence, confidentiality, domestic violence, geriatric protection, indigent care, pediatric care, pregnancy, and suicide prevention. Operational issues such as the admission process, bed boarding, frequent users, guidelines and protocols, overcrowding, telephone advice, and triage are also considered. Legal issues discussed include adverse event disclosure, civil commitment, duty to warn, emergency consent, malpractice claims, research consent, and subpoena. Public protection topics such as controlled substance use, driver impairment, and criminal acts are explored. Regulatory matters such as the Emergency Medical Treatment and Labor Act (EMTALA), Health Insurance Portability and Accountability Act (HIPAA), and Protected Health Information (PHI) are discussed in depth. Critical illness topics such as brain death certification, code response, resuscitation, and unanticipated death are reviewed. Lastly, problematic management areas such as the disruptive provider, difficult patient encounters, professional boundary issues, and violence in the emergency department are examined.

To conclude, this work provides a unique and innovative examination of the complex interface of medical and legal principles in emergency, critical, and acute care medicine.

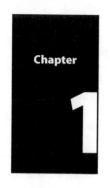

Abandonment in the Emergency Department

Case

The patient was an elderly woman, brought to the emergency department (ED) by emergency medical services (EMS) for difficulty walking. The paramedics said that she was unable to get around any more at home. When asked, they said the family was on their way and would follow the ambulance to the hospital. But no family members came. When the admitting physician asked the patient how she was, she said "I'm OK," in a frail, delicate voice, with just a hint of a smile. She said she had difficulty walking, and her appetite had been poor over the last few weeks. When asked, she stated that she was cared for by a daughter and granddaughter who both worked hard jobs and had families of their own.

The history did not reveal any acute medical issues. She was quite aware of her circumstances, and she added that her primary care physician had discussed "putting her in a nursing home." A physical exam found that she was weak, with poor muscle tone, but with no specific focus. The conventional laboratory and radiographic screening tests were all normal in relation to her age.

When ED staff eventually managed to contact the family, the local caregiver's phone was disconnected and an out-of-state relative gave the ED another local phone number. The ED staff finally contacted a granddaughter, who tearfully stated she was at work at a new job and couldn't come to the hospital.

Medical Approach

An all-too-common scenario in the ED is a family member or family unit that can no longer effectively care for an elderly relative. Typically, there are financial or psychosocial stressors that cause the home care system to falter so that families feel they have no other choice but to turn to the hospital facility for help.

Often, our role in the ED is to help both patients and families.

Patient abandonment has been labeled "granny dumping" in the popular media.[1] The American Association of Retired Persons notes that patient abandonment is a small but growing problem in the health-care industry. According to the Centers for Disease Control (CDC), in the United States it tends to be more common in sunbelt retirement community areas such as Florida, California, Texas, and Arizona.[2]

The typical approach is that EMS are summoned for transport for a pretext illness and then a request for admission follows, or else there is no family response for a request to discharge the patient.

Most practitioners in this situation would turn to the Area Agency on Aging or the National Adult Protective Services Association for an objective analysis of the patient's living circumstances. The Elder Justice Act, Title VI was included as part of the 2010 Patient Protection and Affordable Care Act.[3] This defined neglect as "the failure of a caregiver or fiduciary to provide the goods or services that are necessary to maintain the health or safety of an elder." The behavior can be either active or passive, e.g., not providing access to nourishment, hydration, environmental protection, or economic self-determination.

Lachs et al. performed a nine-year observational cohort study of 2812 community-dwelling older adults linked with the elderly protective service records.[4] Protective services evaluated 6.5% (184) of the individuals, and found that one quarter, or 47 (1.6% of the total, 95% CI 1.0–2.1%) had corroborated abuse or neglect. A pooled logistic regression model found age, race, poverty, functional disability, and cognitive impairment to be associated risk factors. The study found the nature of social welfare screening overestimates the influence of race and poverty as risk factors.

Remember, there is an obligatory requirement to report neglect of the elderly to authorities in all states, based on individual state statutes. The "mandated reporter," often a medical professional who has an obligation to report, can be cited and subject to a fine of up $1000 or 6 months incarceration, as well as incurring civil liability for not reporting in states such as California.[5] Penalties may be harsher if there is willful concealment or if this action results in a patient's death.

Legal Analysis

Abandonment issues are often centered around caring for people who are dependent, including those at age extremes both young and old.

For the Young

In *In re: Matter of Patricia Dubreuil*, the pregnant patient presented through the ED, signed a general consent, and required an emergency cesarean section.[6] However, she did not sign a blood transfusion consent form, as this would have violated her religious beliefs. As she was married but separated, the facility attempted to compel this lifesaving intervention, citing a theory of abandonment affecting her four children who were under her care. The district court held that in the absence of demonstrating the existence of a proper child care and custody plan, the state's interest in prolonging her life outweighed her right to individual wishes regarding her medical care. The circuit court affirmed and she sought discretionary review, arguing her rights to privacy, bodily self-determination, and religious freedom had been infringed. The Supreme Court of Florida quashed the district court decision, finding that there was no evidence that her children would be abandoned.

In *Sacks* v. *Thomas Jefferson University Hospital*, a child was brought to the ED, requiring stitches on her forehead.[7] Her mother was permitted to remain during the procedure. The mother was asked to help hold the child but she felt faint, left the treatment room and fell, sustaining injury. The hospital moved for dismissal, alleging they owed no duty to the mother, who was not a patient. The district court affirmed this decision.

The Restatement (Second) of Torts (1965) provides:

§323 Negligent Performance of Undertaking to Render Services. One who undertakes, gratuitously, or for consideration, to render services to another which

they should recognize as necessary for the protection of other person or things is subject to liability to the other for physical harm resulting from their failure to exercise reasonable care to perform his undertaking, if (a) their failure to exercise such care increases the risk of harm, or (b) the harm is suffered because of the other's reliance upon that undertaking.[8]

Liability under §323 can only be imposed only upon "one who undertakes ... to render service to another" according to *Fabian* v. *Matzko*, 236 Pa. Super. 267, 270–271, 344 A.2d 569 (1975), as offered by the district court.[9] They held that the hospital cannot be held liable for causing the fainting episode or preventing the fall as no physician–patient relationship was ever established. They concluded the mother voluntarily entered the treatment area, was not required to help hold the patient, and "abandoned" her daughter when she felt faint and left the room. The defendant acquired no special duty to protect, or duty to direct family in an unpleasant medical circumstance.

For Older Patients

In *Carter* v. *Prime Healthcare Paradise Valley*, the elderly patient underwent hip surgery, presented to the ED with chest pain, and was transferred to a skilled care facility.[10] His condition gradually declined, with pneumonia and pressure ulcers, and he eventually died after a hospital visit. The family filed suit against the hospital and skilled care facility for violation of the Elder Abuse and Dependent Adult Civil Protection Act, alleging willful misconduct and wrongful death.[11] Here, abuse was defined as physical abuse, neglect, financial abuse, abandonment, isolation, abduction, or other treatment with resulting physical harm, pain, or mental suffering. The trial court sustained the defense demurrer without leave to amend as they held that the criteria required by the elder abuse statute such as abandonment were not met. The Court of Appeals of California, Fourth District, Division One affirmed the judgment, noting that alleged negligence is not the same as abandonment.

Conclusion

The ED is often the center of controversy regarding neglect or abandonment of patients who may present in a poor health condition. The emergency medicine community has always attempted to err on the side of caution, relying on a strategy of hospital admission where uncertainty exists.

References

1. Emergency rooms bearing the burden of abandoned elderly. Deseret News. November 29, 1991.

2. Arias E. United States life tables, 2009. *National Vital Statistics Reports* 2014;62(7):1–63.

3. Patient Protection and Affordable Care Act (Public Act 111–148), 42 U.S.C. & 18001 et seq. (2010).

4. Lachs MS, Williams CS, O'Brien S, Pillemer KA. Adult protective service use and nursing home placement. *Gerontol.* 2002;42(6):734–739.

5. California Welfare and Institutions Code §15630–15632.

6. In re Matter of Dubreuil, 629 So. 2d 819 (1993).

7. *Sacks* v. *Thomas Jefferson Hospital*, 684 F. Supp. 858 (1988).

8. Restatement of Torts Second §323 Negligent Performance of Undertaking to Render Services.

9. *Fabian* v. *Matzko*, 344 A.2d 569 (1975).

10. *Carter* v. *Prime Healthcare Paradise Valley*, 129 Cal. Rptr.3d 895 (2011).

11. Welfare and Institutions Code (WIC). Chapter 11. Elder Abuse and Dependent Adult Civil Protection Act [15600–15675].

Chapter 2

Abandonment of Patient by Treating Physician

Case

The patient presented to the emergency department (ED) with chest pain. He was 55 years of age, but looked much older. He was slight in build, with hair thinning at the temples. He complained of substernal chest pain with radiation to the arm, and dyspnea on exertion. He improved with aspirin and nitroglycerin.

The ED physician attempted to admit him, but there seemed to be an issue. His attending physician stated that the patient could not be admitted to their service. They explained that the patient had recently been "fired from the practice" for ongoing non-compliance with treatment recommendations. When this issue was presented to the patient, he said that it was news to him. The patient stated that during an office visit last week his doctor had "got a little testy" with him. However, his current physician said the new doctor could have his records when they notified the new doctor's office.

Once again, his primary care physician (PCP) was asked about the patient's admission. "Just admit him to the on-call physician," was the response. The PCP was asked if the patient had been properly notified of the ending of the relationship, and if a care transition plan had been put in place. The question was not answered, as he seemed perturbed, and replied "just notify the on-call physician to get him admitted." The admitting physician for unassigned patients was contacted for the admission, but the case was referred to the medical staff office for an opinion as well.

Medical Approach

There is a clear obligation to provide ongoing care when a physician–patient relationship is established. The patient is entitled to expect that care will be provided until suitable arrangements can be made to transfer care to another health-care provider. Sometimes the care relationship can be terminated abruptly, leaving an ED physician to intervene.

Although a patient is free to leave a physician at any time, the physician has an obligation to provide a care transition plan. Abandonment may occur if an existing patient–physician relationship is unilaterally terminated by the health-care provider when the patient has ongoing health-care needs and there is no adequate care transition plan (Table 2.1).

Five elements are required to support a cause of action for the tort of health-care abandonment.[1] First, the health-care treatment was unreasonably discontinued. Second, the termination of the health-care relationship occurred without the patient's knowledge. Third, the health-care provider failed to enact an acceptable care transition plan. Fourth, the provider should have reasonably foreseen the hazards arising from this premature termination; this firmly establishes the proximate cause relationship. Fifth, the patient suffered harm as a direct result of this termination (Table 2.2).

The Healthcare District of Palm Beach County has promulgated the following five-step program to avoid patient abandonment accusations.[2] First, they suggest providing written notice by certified mail with return receipt. Second, the health-care professional should provide a succinct explanation for the change, such as therapeutic non-compliance or appointment cancellation. Third, a transition timeframe of 30 days of ongoing care appears to be the standard. Fourth, the provider should help to recommend or facilitate the transfer to another provider. Fifth, the patient should be asked for a signed consent to facilitate the medical record transfer to another health-care professional (Table 2.3).

Table 2.1 Patient–physician abandonment criteria

1. Pre-existing relationship
2. Unilateral termination by physician
3. Ongoing health-care need
4. No transition plan provided

Table 2.2 Five elements of abandonment cause of action

1. Treatment unreasonably discontinued
2. Termination of health care without the patient's knowledge
3. Failure to arrange for follow-up care
4. Reasonably foreseeable consequences of termination
5. Patient suffered harm or loss

Reference: Indest.[1]

Table 2.3 Five-step program to avoid an abandonment allegation

1. Provide written notice by certified mail
2. Provide brief explanation
3. Provide service for a 30 day transition period
4. Provide a referral recommendation
5. Facilitate record transfer with signed consent

Reference: Wiewora.[2]

Legal Analysis

In *Mack* v. *Soung*, the patient was placed in a nursing facility during her final days. She developed a decubitus ulcer that was treated on site, after which her physician allegedly refused to transfer her to the hospital.[3] She died a few days after the physician gave written notice of his withdrawal from her care, mailed to the patient's former residence, but did not contact her family directly. The family alleged "willful and abrupt abandonment," and brought suit alleging multiple legal theories and submissions. They cited the Elder Abuse and Dependent Adult Civil Protection Act §15600 et seq., which states that:

> Any person who has assumed full or intermittent responsibility for the care or custody of an elder or dependent adult, whether or not that person receives compensation, including … any elder or dependent adult care custodian, health practitioner … is a mandated reporter;

and a complaint of intentional infliction of emotional distress.[4] The trial court sustained demurrers to both causes of action without leave to amend. The appellate court affirmed in part, holding that this behavior did not fulfill the criteria for intentional infliction, and reversed the decision in that health-care professionals who assume care are liable for neglect, abuse, or abandonment.

In *Elder* v. *Sutter Medical Foundation*, an unpublished opinion refers to a lawsuit filed concerning the care continuum from the facility to the convalescent care center and managed care provider.[5] The patient fell, injuring her lower leg, progressed from the hospital to the convalescent care center, and was discharged home. There was allegedly an issue with authorization for an outpatient anticoagulant for management of a thromboembolism to which she eventually succumbed. The patient's family filed suit alleging elderly abuse, wrongful death, and abandonment, citing failures of continuing duty of care relating to the referral, communication, and medication certification. The trial court sustained the demurrers of the care center and foundation and entered judgment in their favor, holding there was no evidence of abandonment. Abandonment was defined as "the unilateral severance by the physician of the professional relationship with the patient without reasonable notice at a time when there is still the necessity of continuing attention."[6] The appellate court affirmed the decision that the essentials of abandonment were not pled successfully by the plaintiff. However, the state department of health found violation of a state regulation requiring established procedures to handle medical emergencies with deviation from admission criteria and process policy. "Home health providers are required to have in place written policies and procedures that include a plan to handle medical emergencies."[7]

Conclusion

There are clear, well-established guidelines regarding the unilateral severing of the patient–physician relationship that must be followed in order to avoid ethical and legal violations. Obviously, this provision is only available in the context of non-emergent patient care.

References

1. Indest GF. Patient Abandonment. *Home Health Care Law Manual* (Gaithersburg, MD: Aspen Publishers, 1996).

2. Wiewora RJ. Ending the patient/physician relationship. Access 2012;143:2.

3. *Mack* v. *Soung*, 95 Cal. Rptr.2d 830 (2000).

4. Welfare and Institutions Code (WIC). Chapter 11. Elder Abuse and Dependent Adult Civil Protection Act [15600–15675].

5. *Elder* v. *Sutter Medical Foundation*, No. C077380, January 12, 2016.

6. *James* v. *Board of Dental Examiners*, 172 Cal. App.3d 1096 (1985).

7. California Code of Regulations 22 CA ADC §74721: Written Administrative Policies, subd (c) (1).

Chapter 3

Admission

Case

The patient had presented with a "blister" on the bottom of her foot. That was her only complaint, and she had no fever or other systemic illness. Her hygiene was poor and her appearance gave rise to concerns about her living circumstances. Her medical history did not reveal diabetes or vascular insufficiency. She declined an offer of social service evaluation to potentially assist.

On completion of the physical exam, it was noted there was no redness or drainage at the site: just a single, apparently chronic, dense callus located at the base of her first metatarsal. The physician attempted to reassure her that everything was fine, and the callus could be followed on an outpatient basis by the podiatry service. The patient voiced her disapproval of this plan. Another attempt at reassurance failed, so she was offered some additional testing. The complete blood count, basic metabolic panel (BMP), C-reactive protein, and plain radiograph of the foot were normal. These results were discussed with the patient, without achieving better insight, but in other respects her decision-making was normal.

She then stated that she "knew her rights," and that the medical staff were obligated to admit her to the hospital according to the "Hill–Burton Act." Further consultation with mental health found she was indeed competent. The patient advocate concurred with the discharge plan, but felt that the offer of services was required and courtesies should be extended. A follow-up appointment was made and transportation home was offered, which the patient accepted.

Medical Approach

It is important to recognize that hospitals are not required to admit patients. This assumes a reasonable medical evaluation, performed by the person qualified to do so at that institution. If this person concludes that the patient is not experiencing an acute medical condition, the patient can be directed to care delivered in the outpatient setting, as was done in this case.

Since 2010, the Patient Protection and Affordable Care Act (ACA) has invoked the "prudent layperson, acting reasonably" standard for determining a medical emergency that would compel payment by the insurer.[1] For Medicare hospitals the Centers for Medicare & Medicaid Services (CMS) requires that inpatient admissions be supported by the clinical documentation and supplemented by a specific diagnosis and treatment plan.[2] They recommend that screening tools should be used, not exclusively, but as part of the overall evaluation process. In addition, they state that inpatient care be "necessary, reasonable and appropriate" for that specific patient, in that particular set of circumstances.

The Hospital Survey and Construction Act (Hill–Burton Act) was enacted in 1946/7 awarding grants and loans to hospitals for postwar construction and modernization.[3] The community service obligation mandates that the facility should provide emergency service to people within its catchment area as long as they operate with a not-for-profit (NFP) status. The uncompensated care provision provides free or reduced-cost care for 20 years after project completion, and is means tested and time limited. According to the Department of Health and Human Services, in 2015 only 152 hospital facilities nationwide had a remaining free or reduced-cost health-care obligation.[4] Clearly, a significant amount of uncompensated or reduced-fee care is provided by most facilities, but only a minority is related to this particular law.

Legal Analysis

In *Richard* v. *Adair Hospital Foundation*, the family alleged their child was denied admission to the emergency department (ED) on two occasions.[5] The limited proof in the record comes from the family depositions. They allege they drove their sick child to the door of the ED. Mother and baby remained in the vehicle, where the appellant claimed the nurse refused to examine the child or call the doctor. The family left, and could not find their own doctor. They returned to the ED 2 hours later with the same request, and were met in the driveway by the nurse, who allegedly stated the child did not have a fever. The child was transported to another facility about 9 hours later, was admitted with pneumonia described as critical, and died.

A physician testified that the child's survival chances would have been greater if admitted at the earlier visit. The trial court awarded the defense's summary judgment motion as there was no genuine issue in fact as causation could not be established. The Court of Appeals of Kentucky reversed the decision, holding that the hospital twice refusing admission, when an unmistakable emergency situation may have existed, was an issue of fact and the summary judgment for the defense was premature.

In *Hunt* v. *Palm Springs General Hospital*, the patient presented with seizure after taking his chronic medications, was seen by an "unlicensed resident physician," who then contacted his physician, and was subsequently discharged home.[6] He returned to the ED about 10 hours later and was seen by his physician. An admission inquiry found there were previous unpaid bills. This admission decision could have been overridden by the attending physician if an emergency condition existed, but it allegedly was not. The patient was then moved from the ED room to the adjacent hall, and transferred to another hospital 4 hours later, where he died the next day. The trial court awarded a directed verdict to the facility holding there was no duty, as he was seen by his physician and not admitted. The District Court of Appeal of Florida, Third District reversed and remanded for a new trial, holding that the duty to a non-admitted patient was a question for the jury. As well, they erred in a hypothetical distinction between the resident, attending physician, and hospital in assigning responsibility.

Conclusion

The obligation to evaluate and treat patients has a legal basis in common law, case precedent, and statutory regulation. Most physicians have the capability of entering into a care contract with mutual consent to exercise their skill in caring for the patient. The duty to treat is self-evident in emergency medicine, with all patients encountered at least being screened for additional care needs.

References

1. Patient Protection and Affordable Care Act (Public Act 111–148), 42 U.S.C. & 18001 et seq. (2010).

2. Medicare Program Integrity Manual, Chapter 6, Section 6.5.1, www.cms.gov/manuals/downloads/pim83c06.pdf.

3. Hospital Survey and Construction Act of 1946 (Hill-Burton Act), Title VI of Public Health Services Act. 42 C.F.R. §53.111–113.

4. Health Resources and Services Administration (HRSA), Department of Health and Human Services, Hill-Burton Free and Reduced-Cost Health Care, www.hhs.gov.

5. *Richard* v. *Adair Hospital Foundation Corporation*, 566 S.W.2d 791 (1978).

6. *Hunt* v. *Palm Springs General Hospital*, 352 So. 2d 582 (1977).

Advance Directives

Case

The emergency medical services (EMS) squad called with a familiar radio message – it was a cardiac arrest. The patient had been down for 15 minutes, and the EMS paramedics had performed the usual resuscitative interventions. The patient had received numerous rounds of defibrillation, epinephrine, and amiodarone without success. After another 15 minutes of resuscitative efforts in the emergency department (ED), the patient responded and there was a resumption of heartbeat.

As the medical staff began the remainder of the post-resuscitative interventions, the patient was clearly unresponsive, which was not unexpected in this situation. The patient would be admitted to the intensive care unit (ICU) to evaluate his likelihood of post-resuscitative recovery, which was recognized as likely to be poor at this point. During the call for admission, the ICU physician requested clarification of the patient's advance directive status.

The family now began to arrive: a son and daughter, in some distress, as might be expected. However, they said their dad had been sick recently, and not capable of doing the things that he had done previously or enjoyed. The daughter said that a couple of weeks ago her father had stated that he was tiring from his illness and felt poorly a lot of the time. At this point the patient's current significant other arrived in the ED lobby. She was distraught as well. When questioned about the patient's advance directive, she stated that he had none that she knew of. He had been doing a lot better recently. In fact, they were thinking about going on a vacation cruise. There was a clear discrepancy in related history here. With the help of social work, the physician took the family to the counseling room to discuss the current advance directive. The children spoke first. They stated there had been some animosity

in this second relationship and they felt they should be the decision-makers here. The significant other then pointed out that although she and the patient were not married they had lived together for the last 5 years. She felt that he would have wanted her to make the decision regarding his ultimate care course.

The patient's brother arrived in the hospital waiting room and asked to see his brother. He then produced his brother's last will and testament, which had an advance directive within the document itself. It offered little clarity, but stated that he did not want to be preserved on life support for an extended period of time. The significant other said that meant that he wanted to be resuscitated and give it a chance, whereas his children suggested it meant that he did not want to continue in this fashion.

His significant other stated that they had lived together and she knew the patient's desires best. The children said that they were his closest living relatives and they should make the decision. The brother said he had known him the longest and he had filed an advance directive with the attorney and that should be followed.

The ICU physician was advised that there was a family disagreement over resuscitation efforts. The existing advance directive dictated additional care, at least at this point. The patient was then transferred to the ICU.

Medical Approach

This is not an uncommon scenario in the ED. A sudden catastrophic event occurs, and multiple family members are involved with different opinions about their loved one's care. The first issue to be resolved here is the viability of the advance directive. This dictates care clearly: as long as a valid advance directive is signed by a competent patient, it is followed explicitly.

If there are questions concerning the advance directive, the family is consulted to comment and give an opinion. This is a "substituted judgment" argument for the patient, in which the family members give an opinion on resuscitation. Here, additional care efforts are dictated by what the patient would want, not what the family would want.

The second issue is who should make the decision in cases like this, which is often a matter of controversy. The typical hierarchy in an adult relationship would be spouse, children, parents, and siblings, in that order.[1]

The third issue is often the nature of the "significant other" relationship, whether it is a legal marriage, a common-law marriage arrangement, or a live-in situation. This often turns on state-based guidelines concerning the requirements for a common-law relationship. Typically, this requires cohabitation to have existed for a period of time such as 5 or 10 years, as well as the capacity of presenting oneself outwardly as a married couple. This typically goes beyond just managing living expenses and daily life events.

A study by Emanuel et al. found advance directives are desired by 89% of the general public and 93% of outpatients.[2] Life-sustaining treatment was decided against in 71% of poor-outcome scenarios such as dementia, coma, and vegetative state. The American College of Emergency Physicians (ACEP) Ethics Committee have explored the Physician Orders for Life-Sustaining Treatment (POLST) approach in attempts to make decision-making clearer and improve remaining quality of life compared to using "do not resuscitate" (DNR) or advance directive documents.[3]

Legal Analysis

Patients have a definite preference for deciding their own care and course. In *Anderson* v. *St Francis-St George*, the patient would have died and not suffered any subsequent medical conditions, except for the defibrillation against his instructions.[4] The issue of first impression for the court is whether life-prolonging treatment provided against the patient's instructions makes the provider responsible for all foreseeable consequences under the claim of "wrongful living." Whether intentional or negligent, interference with the person's legal right to die would constitute a breach of the duty to honor the wishes of the patient. Thus, once it is established that "but for" the conduct of the

medical professional, death would have resulted, the causation element of the "wrongful living" claim is satisfied. The trial court and appellate court held there was no evidence for an action for "wrongful living." However, the appellate court held that damages could be recovered under a negligence or battery theory. The Supreme Court of Ohio found this argument without merit, that there was no causation between the defibrillation and the subsequent medical conditions. As well, they concluded there was no evidence of damage or injury from the defibrillation, such as tissue burns or broken bones. They reversed the appellate court decision and entered judgment for the appellant.

In *Wright* v. *Johns Hopkins Health Systems Corporation*, the family of the decedent sued based on wrongful prolongation of his life, by resuscitating him from cardiac arrest, allegedly contrary to his advance directive and expressed intent.[5] The Life Sustaining Procedures Act allowed one to execute an "advance directive" directing the withholding or withdrawal of life-sustaining procedures in the event that two physicians certified the individual to be in a terminal condition.[6] The Health Care Decisions Act eliminates the preterminal requirement and overlies the common-law right to refuse life-sustaining medical procedures.[7] The circuit court entered judgment for the defendants, as the patient was not in a preterminal condition, nor were the defendants at that time, "required to delay resuscitation, even for the minutes required to seek and obtain either consent of a health-care agent or formal medical certification of the decedent's pre-arrest medical condition as might warrant a declination to resuscitate." The Court of Appeals of Maryland affirmed the circuit court decision, holding that cardiopulmonary resuscitation (CPR) was authorized. The individual does have a cause of action for a health-care provider's failure to comply with the individual's advance directive. However, the facts were not sufficient to conclude the causes of action for negligence, wrongful death, battery, and lack of informed consent. In this particular situation, because the significant other's relationship with the patient did not satisfy the criteria for common-law marriage, the children made the decisions regarding their father's care.

Conclusion

Clearly as patient and family understanding advances in this area, the medical community must adapt to a more sophisticated and individualized approach to end-of-life care. This care should optimize patient autonomy in direct and indirect decision-making.

References

1. American Medical Directors Association: Society for Post-Acute and Long-Term Care Medicine. White paper on surrogate decision-making and advance care planning in long-term care, The Hierarchy of Medical Decision-Making for Incapacitated Nursing Home Residents, Columbia, MD, 2003. www.paltc.org/amda-white-papers-and-resolution-position-statements/white-paper-surrogate-decision-making-and.

2. Emanuel LL, Barry MJ, Stoeckle JD, Ettelson LM, Emanuel EJ. Advance directives for medical care – a case for greater use. *N Engl J Med.* 1991;324(13):889–895.

3. Jesus JE, Geiderman JM, Venkat A, Limehouse WE Jr, Derse AR, Larkin GL, Henrichs CW 3rd, ACEP Ethics Committee. Physician orders for life-sustaining treatment, and emergency medicine: ethical considerations, legal issues, and emerging trends. *Ann Emerg Med.* 2014;64(2):140–144. DOI:10.1016/j.annemergmed.2014.03.014.

4. *Anderson* v. *St Francis-St George Hospital*, 77 Ohio St.3d 82 (1996).

5. *Wright* v. *Johns Hopkins Health Systems*, 728 A.2d 166 (1999).

6. Life Sustaining Procedures Act. Maryland Code §§5-601-5-614 (1982, 1990).

7. Health Care Decisions Act. Maryland Code §§5-601-5-618 (1982, 1994, 1998).

Advanced Practice Providers

Case

A physician worked in a busy emergency department (ED) that used advanced practice providers (APP) as part of the patient care team. The physicians worked in a separate geographic area, but were available to the APPs if they had a question about care. Typically, at the end of the shift they would have signed the charts of all the patients they had seen, including those they did not see specifically and merely cosigned the documentation for their care.

The APP had presented several cases that evening, including a family of three. She told the physician they all had colds, and she had already discharged them. She said, "Please just sign the charts, they were fine." The physician was a little concerned and asked if he needed to see any of them, and again the APP replied no, they just had colds. The mother had to leave to pick up another child. The charts were cosigned, and the physician went on to the next case.

Nine months later, hospital counsel notified the physician they were in receipt of a summons. The complaint alleged medical malpractice involving the youngest of those children seen that evening by the APP. It alleged a failure to diagnose a serious infectious disease with both the APP and the physician listed as defendants, as well as the pediatrician. Hospital counsel were informed that the physician did not see the patient, and that by the time the physician was made aware, the APP had already seen the family, evaluated them, and discharged them. The physician had no chance to be involved with the patients or interact with them. The hospital counsel asked how the physician was involved in this case: "the record was attested to, correct?" The ED physician acknowledged he had cosigned the documentation, but that was standard protocol in place at the time.

Medical Approach

The world of medical malpractice as it applies to APPs, and their interface with the supervisory physician, can be nuanced. Liability typically depends on the manner of supervision – whether this is true administrative supervision by a physician, or a coworker or clinical supervisor arrangement.

The next issue is the type of care provided – whether the physician sees the patient at all. Obviously when the physician sees the patient, there is more attendant responsibility than if they just sign off on the chart. In addition, it is site specific with guidelines based on state law precedents. When the signature is purely administrative and the patient is not seen, the duty is more tenuous. This situation, in which a physician who sees a patient assumes more risk than a physician who does not, seems almost contrary to the social good.

The American College of Emergency Physicians (ACEP) evaluated the practice of physician assistants (PAs) in an emergency medicine survey with a 50% (351/700) response rate.[1] First, patient assignment to PA care was most commonly random (80%), followed a triage process (38%), by physician (21%), assigned to the observation unit (1%), or other (1%). Second, the patient management approach finds a little more than half (52%) of patients being seen by the physician as well. Third, the ED physician does not evaluate, or rarely sees, 28% of the patients. Fourth, a significant proportion of PAs perform complex procedures, such as endotracheal intubation or fracture reduction.

The PA contributes to the ED patient care mission in a significant way. Brook et al. evaluated 160 PA shifts ranging from 4 to 13 hours, with mean productivity 1.16 patients per hour (95% CI 1.12–1.20) and generated 2.35 relative value units per hour (95% CI 1.97–2.72).[2] There was no correlation with shift length or department census. This contribution to the ED is

Table 5.1 Addressing physician-assistant physician supervisory risk

1. Careful selection, hiring, and credentialing process
2. Patient care protocols and practice policies
3. Patients seen independently or conjointly
4. Care records, oversight, and review program
5. Culture of collaboration
6. Proper documentation of consultations
7. Continuing education
8. Malpractice separate and joint liability

Reference: Victoroff.[3]

invaluable, as those who work in this environment can attest.

Although PAs have a significantly lower rate of malpractice claims than physicians do, physicians are often concerned about their involvement in supervision-related litigation, according to a survey by Victoroff and Ledges.[3] The key to avoiding the allegation of negligent PA supervision by the physician is a defined management approach, as summarized in Table 5.1.

First, the process of PA selection, hiring, and credentialing is a crucial step. Second, protocols and practice policies directing PA care optimize patient outcomes. Third, the crucial decision is what patients are seen independently by a PA, compared to those seen in conjunction with the physician. Fourth, maintenance of comprehensive care records, and an oversight and review program, are crucial. Fifth, the culture of collaboration is crucial to success. The physician should reach out in the care event and offer assistance, rather than waiting to be asked for input. Sixth, proper documentation of all consultations with the acknowledgment of conjoint care is perhaps the most important risk tool. Seventh, to further reduce the risk of vicarious liability, providing continuing education to all involved is helpful. Eighth, since litigation is inevitable, policies must address both separate and joint liability for maximal protection.

An analysis of the National Practitioner Data Bank (NPDB) Report from 2003 to 2012 identified 147,870 claims and found that the majority of medical malpractice claims involved physicians (89.6%, 132,513) followed by professional nurses including nurse

practitioners (NPs; 4.1%, 6167), and other practitioners including PAs (6.2%, 9190).[4]

Perhaps the most comprehensive analysis was performed in 2009 by CNA HealthPro and the Nurses Service Organization (NSO) analyzing data from 3000 NPs, expanding on their previous 1994–2004 study.[5] They found the average claim indemnity was $189,300 and legal expense cost $42,900. Those NPs who were employed in family medicine or geriatrics accounted for the majority of claims (84.3%), while the pediatric/neonatal claims were the most expensive ($318,150). The most expensive negligence claims were for providing service outside of the scope of their practice ($450,000), found in only 1% of cases. The most common allegations in NP litigation were errors in diagnosis ($186,168), medication errors ($147,554), and errors in treatment ($111,971).

Legal Analysis

The most common question asked is, what is the physician liability for APP supervision?

In *Rubin* v. *USA*, the complainant alleged failure to adhere to standards and improper medical care resulting in the death of the decedent after outpatient care provided at the Veterans Administration Medical Center.[6] The family alleged that the patient was overmedicated with narcotic analgesics, to his detriment. The court found that the plaintiff failed to prove by a preponderance of evidence that the method of care or treatment deviated from that of standard practice for this condition. As well, the use of the PA to assist the physician in the care plan was not negligent, and the care provided by the designate was appropriate.

In *Bowie Memorial Hospital* v. *Wright*, the patient presented to the ED after a car accident and was evaluated by an employed PA.[7] The patient had a knee fracture diagnosed, but the foot radiograph was allegedly misplaced, or the fracture was missed during the reading. The patient was transferred to another facility and underwent knee surgery. The patient allegedly had two subsequent surgeries for the missed foot fracture. The plaintiff alleged there were no PA supervision protocols in the ED, and no protocol to review radiographs within 24 hours.

The facility moved to dismiss the claim, alleging the expert report "failed to establish how any act or omission of employees of the hospital caused or contributed to the patient's injuries," according to the Medical Liability and Insurance Improvement Act medical expert requirements.[8] The trial court dismissed the plaintiff's claim, apparently feeling the receiving orthopedist could as well have made the diagnosis. The appeal court reversed and remanded, holding that the trial court abused its discretion when it dismissed the plaintiff's claim. This appeal court decision was reversed by the Supreme Court of Texas, which dismissed the plaintiff's claim with prejudice, acknowledging the medical expert's good-faith effort to comply with the Act.

In *Benish* v. *Grotte*, the family alleged their daughter was negligently evaluated in the ED, and died 12 hours after discharge.[9] This was an interlocutory appeal challenging the court order denying motions to dismiss filed by the nurse, NP, and physician. They alleged the expert reports were "inadequate" since they did not utilize the "willful and wanton negligence" required by the Texas Civil Practice and Remedies Code §74.153.[10] The trial court denied the appellants' motion to dismiss, and this decision was upheld by the appeal court.

However, recent court decisions have raised concerns about additional oversight liability of physicians for APPs. In *Watkins* v. *Affiliated Internists*, the estate of the deceased patient filed suit against the PA, who prescribed narcotics, and the supervising physician.[11] The state board entered into a consent order, where the physician acknowledged a lack of written PA oversight protocol, and failed to review the medical record within 10 days as required. The trial court denied a motion to amend the complaint as negligence per se, acknowledging this board ruling as administrative and not establishing a standard of care. The Tennessee Court of Appeals reversed, concluding the administrative ruling indeed "established a minimum standard of care" for the physician that needed to be followed, and remanded to the trial court to decide causality of this deviation.

In *Cox* v. *M.A. Primary and Urgent Care Clinic*, the patient sued the clinic and supervising physician, alleging the PA failed to diagnose her condition correctly.[12] The patient presented four times to the clinic allegedly with "respiratory problems and fatigue," and had multiple visits to other facilities before the diagnosis of cardiomyopathy was ultimately made. The plaintiff cardiology expert suggested that the PA was in violation of care standards, but was not familiar with PA care or supervisory standards. The trial court granted the defendant's motion for summary judgment, since the expert did not prove the medical standard as it applies to a PA. This decision was reversed by the appeal court, stating the care standard was the same for both the PA and the physician. The Supreme Court of Tennessee reversed, concluding the care standard for PA and physician was indeed different, reinstating the summary judgment for the defendants and dismissing the case.

Conclusion

The complexity and sophistication of the litigation process involving APP care has increased both in care standards and in physician supervisory requirements. All providers should be familiar with the provisions set out in federal guidelines, state medical licensure directives, and bylaws.

References

1. Physician Assistants in Emergency Medicine. Issue Brief. American Academy of Physician Assistants Department of Government & Professional Affairs. Alexandria, VA, September 2004:1–4.

2. Brook C, Chomut A, Jeanmonod RK. Physician assistants contribution to emergency department productivity. *West J. Emerg Med*. 2012;13(2):181–185. DOI:10.5811/Westmeath.2011.6.6746.

3. Victoroff M, Ledges M. PAs and malpractice. *Med Econ*. 2011;88(19):34–36, 41–42.

4. National Practitioner Data Bank 2012 Annual Report. US Department of Health and Human Services, Health Resources and Services Administration, Bureau of Health Professions, Division of Practitioner Data Banks. February 2014.

5. Understanding Nurse Practitioner Liability: CNA HealthPro Nurse Practitioner Claims Analysis 1998–2008. Risk Management Strategies and Highlights of the 2009 NSO Survey. CNA Chicago, IL, NSO Hatboro, PA:1–4.

6. *Rubin* v. *United States*, 88 F. Supp.2d 581 (1999).

7. *Bowie Memorial Hospital* v. *Wright*, 79 S.W.3d 48 (2002).

8. Texas Revised Civil Statutes. Article 4590i S 13.01.

9. *Benish* v. *Grottie*, 281 S.W.3d 184 (2009).

10. Texas Civil Practice & Remedy Code Annals S 74.153.

11. *Watkins* v. *Affiliated Internists*, No. M2008-01205-COA-R3-CV (Tenn. Ct. App. December 29, 2009).

12. *Cox* v. *Primary and Urgent Care Clinics*, No. M2007-01840-COA-R3-CV (Tenn. App.1-30-2009).

Adverse Event Disclosure

Case

The patient presented to the emergency department (ED) in full cardiac arrest. The radio message from the emergency medical services (EMS) medics stated that he had been cutting the grass and was found on the ground by his wife after about 10 minutes. They performed the usual cardiac arrest interventions, but to no avail. The patient was initially refractory to all resuscitative efforts provided by EMS. He then lost pulses and another round of resuscitation was begun. The paramedics had not intubated the patient in the field and were bagging upon arrival at the ED. He was quickly and successfully intubated by the physician. The successful intubation was confirmed with end-tidal CO_2 and chest radiograph. The patient then had a return of spontaneous circulation. One of the nurses was having difficulty placing the nasogastric tube and the physician offered to help. The nasogastric tube was placed and the nurse was asked to auscultate gastric sounds. She said the tube was in the proper position and "sounded good." The physician asked for another chest radiograph to verify placement. This indicated that the nasogastric tube was in the left mainstem bronchus, and it was then removed by the nursing staff without further incident.

The patient then lost spontaneous circulation again and rearrested. At this point he was unable to be resuscitated successfully. The family was ushered into the counseling area for a discussion with the physician and social worker concerning the patient's outcome. The family said that he had been sick for a long time, although he was still living at home. The physician suggested to the family that the present outcome was better than some alternatives for patients who lingered in a more debilitated state. She reported to the family that the paramedics had done everything they could and that resuscitative efforts had been continued in the ED. She suggested that although everything

possible had been done, the patient's disease burden was insurmountable.

There remained the issue of the potential misadventure that had occurred with the nasogastric tube. Although it was unlikely significant, or correlated to any adverse outcome, the issue was inadvertently revealed to the family. It was suggested that although a minor adverse event had occurred, it did not contribute to the patient's death. The family was obviously distraught about their loved one's demise. One son asked how they could be sure the malpositioned nasogastric tube did not cause his father's death. He was reassured that the events were unrelated: nothing was administered and nothing removed from the tube. It was unlikely the nasogastric tube had made any contribution whatsoever. The physician left the room, after asking the social worker to assist the family with final preparations.

The next day the physician received an inquiry from the quality improvement committee, questioning the placement of the nasogastric tube. On preliminary review they were comfortable with the care and course concerning immediate removal and recommended no further evaluation. Later that week the physician was contacted by the hospital attorney, who requested a meeting. The attorney was concerned the physician had revealed an adverse event to the patient's family without prior discussion with the risk management department and the hospital's legal office.

Medical Approach

Each institution has its own way of dealing with the disclosure of an adverse event to the patient or family. Some institutions prefer not to disclose until the issue has been discussed with quality improvement and hospital legal counsel, in order to put forward a unified explanation of any incident to the family or patient. Other facilities have a standardized early

Table 6.1 Requirements for disclosure of adverse events

1.	Perceptible effect not discussed in advance as known risk
2.	Necessitates a change in patient care
3.	Significant risk to future health, even if small
4.	Treatment or procedure provided without consent

Reference: National Center for Ethics in Health Care.[1]

Table 6.2 Adverse event disclosure

1.	Notification of adverse event
2.	Face-to-face meeting offered
3.	Assistance in filing a legal claim

Reference: Kraman and Hamm.[2]

Table 6.3 Benefits of the adverse event disclosure program

1.	Enhanced patient satisfaction
2.	Strengthened physician–patient relationship
3.	Reduced physician stress
4.	Promotion of safe and high-quality health care

Reference: ACOG.[3]

Table 6.4 Adverse event disclosure guidelines

1.	Share only accurate facts concerning the event
2.	Disclose as soon as possible
3.	Confidentiality and privacy should be preserved
4.	Disclosure by treating or trusted physician
5.	Focus on patient condition and treatment plan
6.	Use easy-to-understand terms
7.	Describe investigation and future mitigation
8.	Express regret and concern

Reference: Pelt and Faldmo.[4]

disclosure process for revealing an adverse event to a patient. The former group feels that early disclosure encourages medicolegal adverse activity. The latter group feels that although this may occur, the honest approach is better accepted by families, resulting in less overall litigation.

The Veterans Health Administration, through its National Center of Ethics in Health Care, was one of the first organized medical groups to advance the doctrine of early disclosure of adverse medical events.[1] They concluded that routine disclosure is ethically obligatory if any of the preconditions summarized in Table 6.1 are met.

First, the adverse effect had not been discussed as a potential risk to be encountered, while the patient suffered perceptible harm. Second, the adverse effect necessitated a change in the patient's care. Third, the event posed a significant risk to the patient's future health, even if the likelihood of risk was small. Fourth, there was a treatment or procedure that was provided without the patient's consent. This strategy was tested by Kraman and Hamm in an "extreme honesty is the best policy" risk management approach within the Veterans Affairs Health System.[2] The system provided notification of the adverse patient care event and offered a face-to-face meeting and assistance in filing a legal claim if requested (Table 6.2). These authors reported an increase in the total number of claims filed, but the actual financial outlay was 50% less, resulting in an overall saving in litigation costs.

The American College of Obstetricians and Gynecologists (ACOG) Committees on Patient Safety and Quality Improvement and Professional Liability have also commented on adverse event disclosure.[3] They suggest that disclosure and discussion of adverse events with the patient are morally and ethically necessary to achieve patient autonomy. The disclosure process is improved by education, policies, programmatic training, and resources accessible to the staff. The benefits of this program are enhanced patient satisfaction, strengthened physician–patient relationships, reduced patient stress, and promotion of safe, high-quality health care (Table 6.3).

The ACOG suggest general guidelines that should be followed in the adverse event disclosure process (Table 6.4).[4] First, the facts should be gathered beforehand, so that only accurate information is shared with the patient. Second, disclosure should occur as soon as possible, especially when the event is serious. Third, confidentiality should be preserved, meeting in a private area, but inquiring whether administrative support is required. Fourth, the disclosure should be made by the treating or trusted physician, although additional support from nursing staff, risk management, or a hospital attorney may be necessary. Fifth, the discussion should focus on the patient's condition and treatment plan. Sixth, the information should be conveyed in a way that is easy to understand. Seventh, the patient and family should be informed that the

Table 6.5 Adverse event disclosure: corrective action plan

1.	Addressing the consequences of the event	59%
2.	Practice improvements	28%
3.	Patient disclosure	9%
4.	Hospital-wide corrective action plan	9%
5.	Personal practice changes	7%

Reference: Lander et al.[5]

issue is being investigated and a plan generated to prevent this problem in the future. Eighth, and most importantly, the physician should express regret and concern for the family.

A survey study of 2500 otolaryngologists with an 18.6% response rate was performed by Lander et al.[5] They reported that 45% (210) of physician respondents reported experiencing an adverse patient care event, with 10% (22) experiencing emotional distress, and 2% (5) were the subject of a legal action. The corrective actions included addressing the event consequences in 59% (107), practice improvements in 28% (60), patient disclosure in 9% (19), hospital-wide corrective action in 9% (19), and personal practice changes in 7% (14) (Table 6.5).

Legal Analysis

Interestingly, the Supreme Court of the United States has rejected a bright-line rule on the disclosure of adverse event reports. In *Matrixx Initiatives, Inc.* v. *Siracusano*, adverse statements made concerning an over-the-counter cold medicine were suggested to be the subject of a disclosure mandate.[6] Investors filed suit against the pharmaceutical company for not disclosing issues compelled by the Securities Exchange Act of 1934 and the Securities and Exchange Commission Rule 10b-5.[7,8] The district court held that the mere existence of adverse event reports does not satisfy the "materiality" standard, as results were not statistically significant. The United States Court of Appeals, Ninth Circuit reversed, holding that the complaints had pled sufficiently to avoid a dismissal motion. The "total mix" information standard to determine materiality carries the day, and does not require the information to attain statistical significance. Here, they rejected a bright line rule that only "statistically significant" information would be included. Rather, they favored the premise that all relevant information might be considered. The Supreme Court affirmed 9–0 that the materiality of the pharmaceutical company's non-disclosure of adverse events reports does not depend on the lack of statistically significant health risk.

In *Wyeth* v. *Levine*, the use of an anti-nausea medicine was occasionally associated with catastrophic consequences when inadvertently administered by an inter-arterial route.[9] The warnings, which were appropriate when first approved by the US Food and Drug Administration (FDA) in 1955, were subsequently modified with a labeling change warning. The plaintiff filed a "failure to warn" claim. The defendant claimed that the FDA approval preempted the state claim. The district court denied the company's summary judgment motion, which was also affirmed by the Vermont Supreme Court. The question raised was whether the FDA drug labeling judgments were a complete defense of the tort claim. Subsequently, the United States Supreme Court held that they were not an adequate defense, and did not preempt state law product liability claims.

Conclusion

Another school of thought analyzes if an adverse event truly correlates with patient care quality or subsequent malpractice action, or has no effect at all. Whatever approach is adopted, it is important for medical staff to be aware of the care and disclosure protocol involved in an adverse event at their facility, and comply with both the quality initiatives and medical malpractice protective interventions.

References

1. National Center for Ethics in Health Care, Veterans Health Administration, Department of Veterans Affairs. Disclosing adverse events to patients: a report by the National Ethics Committee of the Veterans Health Administration. 2003; March:1–15.

2. Kraman SS, Hamm G. Risk management: extreme honesty may be the best policy. *Ann Intern Med.* 1999;131(12):963–967.

3. American College of Obstetricians and Gynecologists Committees on Patient Safety and Quality Improvement, and Professional Liability. Disclosure and Discussion of Adverse Events. Number 520, March 2012.

4. Pelt JL, Faldmo LP. Physician error and disclosure. *Clin Obstet Gynecol.* 2008;51(4):700–708.

5. Lander L, Connor JA, Shah RK, Kentala E, Healy GB, Roberson DW. Otolaryngologists's responses to errors and adverse events. *Laryngoscope*. 2006;116(7):1114–1120. DOI:10.1097/01.mlg.0000224493.81115.57.

6. *Matrixx Initiatives, Inc* v. *James Siracusano*, 131 S. Ct. 1309 (2011).

7. Securities Exchange Act of 1934, 15 U.S.C. §78a et seq.

8. Securities and Exchange Commission, 17 C.F.R. §240. 10b-5 (2010).

9. *Wyeth* v. *Levine*, 129 S.Ct. 1187 (2009).

Against Medical Advice

Case

A patient presented at the emergency department (ED) stating she had a terrible headache. The pain had started in the back of her head, and had come on quite suddenly. She looked uncomfortable and the physician was concerned. The treatment plan offered a comprehensive workup that included a head CT scan, as well as CT angiography to define her intracerebral blood vessels, to make sure she did not have an aneurysm.

After these tests were done, it was suggested she would require a lumbar puncture to completely exclude an intracranial hemorrhage. The patient was concerned about this as she had a previous epidural procedure when she was pregnant, and did not want to undergo it again. It was suggested she should await the results of the current testing and then talk about it later. The hope was that she would acquiesce to the further testing over time.

As expected, her CT scan and CT angiogram were negative for aneurysm and once again the subject of the lumbar puncture was approached. The patient still had concerns and refused consent because she did not want to go through the process again. After another extensive discussion she was offered admission as the next safe alternative, in the hope that she might change her mind during that process, but again she declined. She said she had responsibilities at home to take care of and declined any social service assistance.

The medical staff still had concerns, but after a lot of thought they recognized the patient would have to sign out against medical advice (AMA). She signed the AMA form and proceeded on her way. The next day the physician received a call from risk management questioning the care, as described on the AMA form, and asking if they were comfortable with the outcome of the care event.

Medical Approach

The Discharge Against Medical Advice embodied in the AMA form is an additional contract, in which the patient accepts they will contravene a recommended medical decision and take responsibility for their own actions and medical outcome. The common-law premise is that the AMA form protects the physicians and the health-care facility from liability if the patient has an untoward outcome, but it seems that the AMA form is only partially successful in avoiding litigation. The allegation is that the patient and family do not truly understand the repercussions of their decision, and there is actually a failure of communication. Normally, as "reasonable" decision-makers, they would not have made such an irrational decision "but for" the "negligent" communication.

The estimate is that 0.83–1.53%, or 1 in every 65–120, discharges from a general hospital are AMA, with potential for adverse consequences and subsequent litigation.[1] In the same study Devitt et al. identified eight cases in the LexisNexis and WestLaw databases and conclude that in no case was the AMA form entirely protective. The proper understanding is that the AMA form is merely a "withdrawal of the original informed consent," and does not provide complete indemnity for the provider.

The most commonly asked question is, "What happens to patients who leave against medical advice?" Hwang et al. studied 97 patients who left AMA from an urban hospital general medicine teaching service.[2] Those patients who left AMA were more likely to be readmitted within 15 days (21% vs. 3%, $P < 0.001$) and were more likely to be male and to have history of alcohol abuse. Therefore, AMA was a significant predictor of readmission, analyzed by a Cox proportional hazard model (adjusted hazard ratio 2.5, 95% CI 1.4–4.4).

Table 7.1 Predictors of AMA Discharge: incidence 0.83–1.53%

1. Younger age
2. Medicaid or uninsured
3. Male
4. Current or past alcohol or drug abuse

Reference: Alfandre.[3]

Table 7.2 Elements of an informed refusal

1. Patient or decision-maker is competent
2. Decision is voluntary
3. Risks were discussed
4. Discuss specific risks, benefits, and alternatives
5. List refusal complications to health and life

References: Tanner and Safranek,[7] Moskop.[8]

Table 7.3 Essential elements of the AMA process

1. Enlist another health-care provider witness
2. Involve family in the discussion when appropriate
3. Revisit the issue more than once
4. Use all reasonable means to alter decision
5. Address outpatient follow-up issues
6. Discharge instructions (site dependent)
7. Attending physician and resident perform discharge procedure
8. Involve staff physician or charge nurse to ensure accountability
9. Encourage return

Similar survey data was reported by Alfandre, citing a 1–2% AMA discharge rate.[3] Predictors of AMA discharge included younger age, with Medicaid insurance or uninsured, male, with current or previous alcohol or drug abuse (Table 7.1).

Is it an urban myth that if a patient signs out AMA, their insurance company may not pay for service? Schaefer et al. evaluated 46,319 patients admitted from 2001 to 2010 to an internal medicine practice at a single academic center.[4] The overall AMA rate was 1.1% (536), and payment was declined in only 4.1% of cases. These declinations were largely administrative, due to incorrect demographic information, and none of them were related to the AMA discharge status. Most residents (68.6%) and almost half of the attending physicians (43.9%) believed that payment for care would be declined. The attending physicians, but not residents, were more likely to have informed the patients that they would be likely held "financially responsible," measured on the Likert scale (most 4.2 vs. least 1.7, $P < 0.001$). However, the motivation for this practice was well intended, "so the patient will reconsider staying in the hospital," as practiced by 84.8% of residents and 66.7% of attending physicians ($P = 0.008$).

Legal Analysis

An important consideration is the cost of care. Naderi et al. evaluated 1854 patients in a private hospital in India and found that 3.8% (55) signed out AMA.[5] The patients' rationale for leaving was financial in 83% of cases, time constraints in 9%, emotional stress in 4%, and "other" in 4%.

The sympathy factor often figures prominently in the available caselaw. In *Lyons* v. *Walker Regional Medical Center*, an incarcerated patient presented to the ED with abdominal pain.[6] After arrival, he refused further evaluation, suffered a critical bout of diabetic ketoacidosis (DKA), and died. The Alabama Supreme Court discounted the hospital's contributory

negligence defense, citing the patient's decision-making. They supported the plaintiff's contention that poor communication by the health-care providers worsened the patient's condition and resulted in the subsequent poor outcome.

Perhaps more importantly, we should reconsider our own terminology. The AMA concept is more accurately referred to as an "informed refusal of care," which procedurally is a revocation of a previous voluntary, informed consent. First, the "informed refusal" must establish that the patient or decision-maker is competent. Second, that the patient's decision is truly voluntary. Third, that the risks of the choice were genuinely discussed with the patient. Fourth, that the risks, benefits, and alternatives of treatment were specifically discussed. Fifth, the consequences of treatment refusal, including the jeopardy to health and life, must be listed,[7,8] as summarized in Table 7.2.

Proper use of the AMA form requires, first, that there be a witness to the discussion, usually another health-care provider involved in the patient's care (Table 7.3). Second, ideally the patient's family should be involved in the discussion, to counter any allegation that the patient was not competent to make that decision based on their level of illness, or other miscommunication. Third, revisiting the issue on more than one occasion should be attempted, to give the patient and their family a chance to reconsider an AMA decision. Fourth, all means available should be used to try to change the patient's decision. Family members, other primary care physicians (PCP), or specialty physicians or consultants should be enlisted to participate in the decision-making. Fifth, if the decision is made to sign out AMA then it is important to attempt to address as many of the patient's issues as possible on an outpatient basis. This may include prescribing home medications, arranging consultations, referrals, and arranging outpatient testing. It is helpful to add a check status phone call the next day to ask about the patient's circumstances and condition. Sixth, there is an area of controversy regarding discharge instructions. Many discharge instructions are preprogrammed to suggest that any disease treated on an outpatient basis is benign and warrants discharge. This is often confusing to the patient, and to sign someone out AMA and give a discharge instruction that endorses a low-risk condition may pose a medicolegal predicament. It is therefore crucial to consider either not providing discharge instructions at all or using a template discharge instruction that gives general recommendations and indicates when to return, but does not provide support for benign diagnoses that can be managed on an outpatient basis. Seventh, in teaching institutions it is important to have the AMA discharge process performed by the attending physician in conjunction with any resident involved in the care process, to ensure accurate information. Often this process is left to nursing staff, although it is not appropriate for them to be the primary discussants. Eighth, in a non-teaching center, it is often helpful to use the staff physician and charge nurse to ensure accountability for the same purpose. Lastly, before the patient truly sets foot outside the door, it is desirable to make one final impassioned plea for the patient to remain under a physician's care until their medical conditions are diagnosed and stable.

The experienced provider recognizes the AMA premise does not provide complete immunity from legal liability, or from moral liability for that matter. In *Brownsville Medical Center* v. *Garcia*, a pediatric patient was allegedly kicked in the abdomen. The next day he was taken to a hospital outside of the United States and admitted for 4 days. He then left the hospital AMA with his parents, who stated, "There was never any change – he didn't get any better."[9] The family took him to another ED. When he was examined there he was apparently jaundiced, diagnosed with hepatitis and anemia, and discharged home to see his pediatrician in the morning. The pediatrician diagnosed an acute abdominal injury and the child was referred to yet another ED for surgical evaluation, transferred by air allegedly for payment issues, and died 8 days later. The family filed suit for medical negligence against numerous providers, prevailing in trial court with the decision affirmed by the Court of Appeals of Texas, Corpus Christi. The established facts, as testified to by social services, reflected the parent's behavior when he failed to improve, remaining in the waiting room, with "a very high degree of concern," and were "completely distraught about his condition." They held that the transfer ostensibly for better care did not appear to be in the child's best interest.

In *Kelly* v. *St Luke's Hospital of Kansas City*, a patient presented to the ED and was evaluated. Tests were performed and his private physician was consulted by the ED physician.[10] He had visited his PCP earlier in the day with the same complaint. His PCP had performed similar testing in the past, which was negative. The ED physician and resident postulated a gastrointestinal etiology, although cardiac was considered. Nonetheless he was offered admission, but allegedly declined, and was told to follow up with his PCP. He did not keep the follow-up appointment, but was seen three times over the next week. He was seen in another ED and diagnosed with gastrointestinal issues and pneumonia, but he allegedly declined admission again, saw his PCP again, and subsequently succumbed to a cardiac illness.

The trial court held there was no evidence that the practice of emergency medicine involves inherently dangerous activities, or other circumstances necessary to invoke the "non-delegable duty doctrine." Here, the employer would not be able to completely delegate all responsibility to a contracted third party for essential responsibilities, such as safety. The jury returned a unanimous verdict in favor of the hospital and the patient, finding no fault. The Missouri Court of Appeals, Western District affirmed, holding the appellants were not the subject of any discriminatory exclusion of evidence that could be interpreted as not providing an essential non-delegable service.

Conclusion

The most crucial issue is to let the patient know that this is not an adversarial process and they should be encouraged to come back at any step in the process if they are uncertain, or concerned. Most importantly, for every AMA discharge, physicians should feel they have done their utmost to provide the appropriate level of care direction to the patient, even when it is difficult, or when circumstances may not allow sufficient time for discussion.

References

1. Devitt PJ, Devitt AC, Dewan M. Does identifying a discharge as "against medical advice" confer legal protection? *J Fam Pract.* 2000;49(3):224–227.

2. Hwang SW, Li J, Gupta R, Chien V, Martin RE. What happens to patients who leave hospital against medical advice? *CMAJ.* 2003;168(4):417–420.

3. Alfandre DJ. "I'm going home": discharges against medical advice. *Mayo Clin Proc.* 2009;84(3):255–260.

4. Schaefer GR, Matus H, Schumann JH, Sauter K, Vekhter B, Meltzer DO, Arora VM. Financial responsibility of hospitalized patients who left against medical advice: medical urban legend? *J Gen Intern Med.* 2012;27(7):825–830. DOI:10.1007/s11606-012-1984-x.

5. Naderi S, Acerra JR, Bailey K, Mukherji P, Taraphdar T, Mukherjee T, et al. Patients in a private hospital in India leave the emergency department against medical advice for financial reasons. *Int J Emerg Med.* 2014;7:13–18. DOI:10.1186/1865-1380-7-13.

6. *Lyons* v. *Walker Regional Medical Center*, 791 So. 2d 937 (2000).

7. Tanner C, Safranek S. How should you document a patient's refusal to undergo a necessary intervention. *J Fam Pract.* 2007;56(12):1048–1049.

8. Moskop JC. Informed consent and refusal of treatment: challenges for emergency physicians. *Emerg Med Clin North Am.* 2006;24:605–618.

9. *Brownsville Medical Center* v. *Garcia*, 704 S.W.2d 68 (1985).

10. *Kelly* v. *St Luke's Hospital of Kansas City*, 826 S.W.2d 391 (1992).

Americans with Disabilities Act and Education

Case

The medical student was struggling through most of the clinical rotation. This was a standard emergency medicine rotation, a block lasting 4 weeks. This rotation typically occurs in the fourth year of medical school for trainees who are hoping to go into emergency medicine. The program director is in charge of the medical student rotation, as well as being responsible for the emergency medicine training program.

This particular candidate seemed to struggle with the academic aspects of medical education, both during the clinical didactic sessions and in clinical rotation time. He had difficulties with formulating a clinical diagnosis and treatment that was both efficient and effective in the emergency department (ED) setting. More than one of the attending staff physicians had commented on the suboptimal performance of this trainee. At the end of the rotational block, the program offered a small emergency medicine exit exam, for which this student did not attain a passing grade. After discussion with the educational working group, they offered a second version of that exam, which the student also failed.

In conjunction with the preceptor and clinicians, the student was given a failing grade for his fourth-year emergency medicine clinical elective. After that the student contacted the dean of the medical school, suggesting that he had actually performed admirably in the clinical rotation and had difficulty with the exam based on a learning condition that required accommodation to retake the test. The dean of students contacted the residency office for an inquiry and remedy plan for the issue that was raised by the medical student. The response was that the exam had been given twice in two different versions, as an accommodation to the trainee, but in conjunction with the clinical rotation recommendations, a failing grade was still warranted. The student had then subsequently requested a testing strategy to accommodate his learning disability requirements.

Medical Approach

Most clinicians may have never encountered this complex scenario. The educators may have felt they had been more than fair, with extra remedial education time and two attempts to allow the student to pass a test. However, the Americans with Disabilities Act (ADA) requires reasonable accommodation for any and all disabilities, including learning disorders. This requirement is in place unless an "undue hardship" exists, defined by extraordinary difficulty or expense in achieving the accommodation. The accommodation should apply to testing circumstances that may assist the trainee in passing a test that they normally would be capable of doing, "but for" their specific disability. However, it does not allow them to pass for lack of knowledge, understanding, or decision-making capability that has been defined in previous case precedent addressing this issue.

Legal Analysis

The ADA prohibits discrimination on the basis of disability cited in Title I, Employment; Title II, Local and State Government, Public Transportation; Title III, Public Facilities; and Title IV, Telecommunications.[1] Disability is defined by a physical or mental impairment that substantially limits major life activities, and has been present in the past, or is perceived by others to be present, including unspecified impairment.

This area of caselaw typically focuses on the educational process and achievement. In *Steere* v. *George Washington University School of Medicine*, a medical student challenged his dismissal after 3 years, and requested accommodation.[2] He challenged the dismissal decision based on a learning disability theory alleging violation of the Prohibition of Discrimination

Table 8.1 Learning disability

1. Having a disability
2. Otherwise qualified for benefit
3. Being excluded from benefit
4. Discrimination from disability

Reference: Kaltenberger.[4]

Table 8.2 Substantial limitation

1. Compared to general population
2. Test-taking not a "major life activity"
3. Timeliness less important
4. Not otherwise qualified
5. Procedural not merit-based analysis

Reference: Singh.[5]

Table 8.3 Educational learning disability

1. Consistent, not selective
2. Impact all daily activities
3. Not just academic performance
4. Substantially limited

Reference: Wong.[6]

by Public Accommodations Act.[3] To establish a violation of the provision, the plaintiff must prove that they (1) have a disability, (2) are otherwise qualified for the benefit in question, and (3) were excluded from the benefit due to discrimination because of the disability (Table 8.1).[4] The district court found on appeal that a mere diagnosis alone is not enough to establish the effects of disability. In addition, variable performance, with both success and failure, tends not to support a diagnosis of sustained disability that would require relief. They granted the plaintiff motion for additional time to file, and granted the defendant summary judgment motion in part.

Similarly, in *Singh* v. *George Washington University School of Medicine*, the case involved a medical student with issues related to performance versus disability.[5] Through a complex series of rulings the United States Court of Appeals (USCA), D.C. Circuit found that: (1) the student's "substantial limitation" should be compared to the general population; (2) test-taking was not a "major life activity"; (3) timeliness is less important in the analysis; (4) the complainant was not "otherwise qualified" based on a procedural, rather than merit-based analysis (Table 8.2). They held that the district court did not err in finding the failure to establish the asserted learning disability responsible for the performance.

Lastly, *Wong* v. *Regents of the University of California* came to a similar conclusion with a student who was successful in the basic science years of medical school, but not successful in the latter years of education during clinical rotations.[6] The district court granted the school's motion for summary judgment. The USCA, Ninth Circuit held that this selective failure, suggested to be due to a "learning disability," was not sustainable as rationale for performance, as the disability should be consistent and impact all daily activities, not just academic performance (Table 8.3). The student would have to be "substantially limited" in reading and learning to be "disabled," and this burden was not met by the plaintiff.

Conclusion

As educators, it is therefore necessary and required that we make reasonable accommodations for students, residents, and fellows with disability. Good judgment typically prevails as in cases described in this chapter, in which additional opportunities are offered, as well as providing assistance in the test-taking process. However, we must recognize that accommodation requires a documented disability that significantly impacts the learning process encountered during daily activities.

References

1. US Department of Justice, Civil Rights Section, Disability Rights Section, A Guide to Disability Rights Laws, July 2009.

2. *Steere* v. *George Washington University School of Medicine*, 368 F. Supp, 2d 52 (USDC, DC, 2005).

3. 42 U.S.C. §12182 – Prohibition of Discrimination by Public Accommodations.

4. *Kaltenberger* v. *Ohio College of Podiatric Medicine*, 162 F.3d 432, 425 (6th Cir. 1998).

5. *Singh* v. *George Washington University School of Medicine*, Appellees (No. 09-7032) (USDCA, DC, 2011).

6. *Wong* v. *Regents of the University of California*, 379 F.3d 1097 (US App., 2004).

Americans with Disabilities Act and Access to Facilities

Case

The triage nurse came in to the emergency department (ED) to ask for assistance – a patient needed help to come from her car into the ED. The lift team was activated to come and assist, but even with this extra personnel they had difficulty getting the patient over a curb next to the ED entrance. Finally, they fetched a wheelchair into which the patient was placed and assisted over the curb and taken to the ED for care.

The patient's medical conditions were chronic, mainly related to her congestive heart failure. She was given a diuretic to increase her water output and felt better afterwards. She was offered hospital admission that day, but declined. Her rationale was that she was on her way home, which was approximately 150 miles away. Her physician was there, and the patient wanted to get home tonight. If she had to be admitted to hospital she felt she would rather be closer to home. She seemed stable at this point, with adequate oxygenation, and her vital signs had normalized. After reexamination it was found that her cardiopulmonary status had improved. The patient was ready for discharge, and went home.

About 2 weeks later, hospital administration notified the ED medical director that a claim had been made concerning this patient's lack of physical access to the ED. The patient felt that she was restricted from properly entering the ED, based on some of its design features. With her disability the impact was significant, she said.

The director met with the hospital engineer and administration and went over the design plan for the new ED. The group recognized that one area in the hospital emergency entrance would be inaccessible to some patients. The engineering team and the architect revised the plan and quickly remedied the encumbrance.

The patient was contacted through the patient experience coordinator and replied that she appreciated the response to her claim. However, she had already notified her local state representative about her concerns, as they impacted the Americans with Disabilities Act (ADA).

Medical Approach

It is crucially important for hospital administrators and clinicians to recognize that the ADA has a wide-ranging impact on ED operations. We clearly must address issues of access for people with all manner of disabilities. This has to do with providing the same or similar resources to all patients, including patients who are attempting to access the ED. All reasonable accommodations must be made to allow unencumbered access to the ED, as well as within the ED, to handle patients with all manner of disabilities. Well-established specialty services have been designed for pediatric and geriatric patients as well as for patients who are obese, or are hearing impaired or visually impaired. Patients who have limited mobility may need access requirements for use of a wheelchair or motorized scooter.

Legal Analysis

ADA, specifically Title III, Public Accommodations, requires that architectural standards be followed to prohibit exclusion or unequal treatment of anyone with a disability.[1] This obligation exists even for those with a merely transient interaction with the facility. In *Berthiaume* v. *Yellow Submarine*, a patron who encountered a physical obstruction to entry petitioned for and received an injunction to compel barrier removal and other facility accommodations.[2] The district court heard a plaintiff motion for default judgment, which was awarded. They ordered modification of a public accommodation to make all facilities accessible within

90 days. Interestingly, even though the plaintiff was only a transient visitor and the changes were costly, the defendant was compelled to improve the physical barriers. The court held that even occasional use was significant enough to generate a requirement. In addition, if the net cost of improvements was less than 1% of net revenue, then the cost was not prohibitive as a defense.

Conclusion

Clearly, issues related to disability access are complex and require multidisciplinary input. However, it is often health-care providers who recognize the problem initially, and alert administration to the issues encountered by patients.

References

1. Americans with Disabilities Act (ADA): Title III, Public Accommodations, 28 C.F.R. Part 36 (1991).

2. *Berthiaume* v. *Doremus* DBA Yellow Submarine, No. 6: 2013cv00037 – Document 17 (W.D. Va. 2014).

Assault

Case

The patient was screaming loudly as she was escorted through the emergency department (ED) by security. "I need my medicine, I need my medicine," she seemed to go on shouting forever as they asked the standard medical evaluation questions. It appeared that she was on alprazolam and hydrocodone prescribed by another physician, who would no longer refill the medications for her.

The remainder of the medical history questions were answered without incident. She had no medical concerns and no current localized site of pain. She seemed mainly focused on the refill of her prescription medication. As a last resort, it was decided to medicate her, and she seemed quiet for the time being. The remainder of the medical workup was without abnormality. As the patient was being readied for discharge, she became combative: while the nurse was trying to remove the intravenous access the patient struck her in the face. Security was called, the patient was restrained, and the police were called. They filed an assault report, and took the patient away.

The next day the service excellence coordinator called the ED to say the patient's attorney had filed a complaint concerning the customer service. She wanted to know why the police had been called and suggested that in the future they should call security instead. The staff should be protected but they should not call the police unless there was imminent danger.

Medical Approach

The assault of a hospital ED worker has unfortunately become all too common in the United States today. There are few other professions in which a person's seemingly inappropriate actions would be accepted or tolerated. Typically, most experienced ED workers know the difference between a patient who is "acting out" compared to a patient who truly presents a risk of violence to the staff.

There have been attempts to predict violence to others in advance of the encounter. Lidz et al. selected 357 of 2452 psychiatric patients, judged likely to be violent, compared to matched controls.[1] Violence was reported in 45% of cases overall, with a greater proportion found in those who were predicted to be violent (53% vs. 36%) rather than random acts. Clinical judgment adds to predictive screening accuracy, but overall accuracy is modest at best, with less accuracy in female patients.

Assaultive behavior is pervasive in the general population as well. Houry et al. evaluated a cohort of 971 acutely injured patients, in which 30% (288) suffered intentional assault.[2] There was no documentation of the site in 79%, of the identity in 67%, of police involvement in 46%, of mechanism in 13%, but the perpetrator was an intimate partner in 8%. Even in the ED, the specifics of the assault are often lacking.

Some states have a strict liability standard, so that any assaultive behavior directed toward hospital staff is automatically dealt with by law enforcement. Other states use a case-by-case analysis to decide patient liability for assault.

In 2009, the Commonwealth of Virginia performed a comprehensive analysis of this problem as it relates to emergency medicine.[3] A working group identified a number of factors predisposing to ED violence including lack of reporting, report specificity, variable security, prevalence of mental disorders, drug or alcohol addiction, reluctance to press charges, and variable security training and strategies (Table 10.1). They also performed a state-by-state survey to define the enhanced penalty for simple assault, with penalty enhanced from misdemeanor to mandatory felony. Roughly one-half[26] of states had such statutes, and one-third overall[9] required evidence of physical harm.

Table 10.1 Violence in the ED: predisposing factors

1.	Assaults go unreported
2.	Law-enforcement data not sufficient
3.	Variable security resources
4.	Predisposed by mental illness, alcohol, drug dependence
5.	Reluctance to press charges
6.	Variable security training
7.	Variable prevention strategies

Reference: Hospital Emergency Room Violence.[3]

Legal Analysis

Health-care workers experience the highest rate of non-fatal workplace violence, accounting for 70% of events.[4] There are estimates that as many as 80% of nurses experience at least one violent on-the-job event annually, accounting for one-third of related time off work.

Health-care providers have valid concerns about safety in a number of health-care environments. In *House* v. *SwedishAmerican Hospital*, the plaintiff filed a complaint related to the defendant hospital alleging careless and reckless action that permitted a patient to inflict injury on her in the hospital lounge.[5] The complainant alleged that the hospital "should have known" the patient was dangerous, based on "prior conduct." The trial court awarded a directed verdict to the facility, and the complainant appealed to the Appellate Court of Illinois, Second District. The hospital petitioned to protect all records, patient identification, and documents concerning this incident. The court held the records were "relevant, probative, not unduly prejudicial or inflammatory and that other satisfactory evidence is demonstrably unsatisfactory as evidence of the facts sought to be established." The patient identification was redacted, but then revealed inadvertently in testimony. Information concerning numerous behavioral issues was offered, but previous visit records were protected. The appellate court held that the trial court properly held patient records and nurses' notes confidential. However, they erred in denying the opportunity to depose the patient who allegedly assaulted staff, and remanded to define these activities at the facility. The complexity of these cases is often increased by patient confidentiality obligations.

In *Turnbull* v. *Topeka State Hospital*, the complainant was a psychologist at the hospital who sued the hospital and state as she was allegedly sexually assaulted by a patient.[6] The jury found that a sexually hostile work environment existed, but split over the hospital's responsibility, and awarded a defense summary judgment motion. The United States Court of Appeals, Tenth Circuit held that the decision was not proper, reversed and remanded. They held that although some protective measures were taken by the facility, more were available and should have been implemented.

Conclusion

Across the country, ED staff members work as a team to protect patients and protect each other, and do so successfully on a day-to-day basis. Unfortunately, circumstances sometimes arise in which assaultive behavior is directed toward staff, and this should not be tolerated in health-care facilities.

References

1. Lidz CW, Mulvey EP, Gardiner W. The accuracy of violence toward others. *JAMA*. 1993;269(8):1007–1011. DOI:10.1001/jama.1993.03500080055032.

2. Houry D, Feldhaus KM, Nyquist SR, Abbott J, Pons PT. Emergency department documentation in cases of assault. *Ann Emerg Med*. 1999;34(8):715–719.

3. Hospital Emergency Room Violence (SJR 358, 2009), Report of the Virginia State Crime Commission, Senate Document No. 8, Commonwealth of Virginia, Richmond, VA, 2010.

4. Jacobson R. Epidemic of violence against health care workers plagues hospitals. *Sci Am*. December 31, 2014.

5. *House* v. *SwedishAmerican Hospital*, 564 N.E.2d 922 (1990).

6. *Turnbull* v. *Topeka State Hospital*, 255 F.3d 1238 (2001).

Assisted Suicide

Case

The patient was known in the community as a "self-made man." He had come back from World War II and started his own business funded by The Servicemen's Readjustment Act of 1944 (the "GI bill").[1] He was extremely successful, and well loved in his community. The cancer diagnosis, 3 years earlier, had been difficult for him to bear. The fight was hard, including radiation and chemotherapy, but the cancer progressed to stage IV disease.

He was tired, but wanted to stay home as long as he could. His loving family brought him to the emergency department (ED) for probably the last time. He had stopped eating, couldn't get out of bed, and said he was "too weak." He was promised the standard evaluation and intervention. In this case, doctors would search for things that were easily fixable such as dehydration, low sodium, urinary tract infection, or pneumonia. The patient had talked to his family about this, and told them that his day would come and that he wanted someone to ease his suffering when the time came. He was ready to go and "meet his maker," as he often said to them.

His wife tearfully asked if there was any medicine that might speed his passing. He had seen how fatally wounded soldiers were treated in World War II, and often told her to "just tell that doctor to give me some morphine when the time comes." The physician explained to her that things have certainly become a little more complicated since the war. There are some states in which that type of intervention is allowed. Oregon, for instance, offers an assisted suicide plan for patients and families, but the state that this patient resided in does not.

The patient was, however, offered an alternative to ease his suffering, in the usual fashion. The physician's primary obligation was to provide a supportive situation. The patient should be surrounded by family, they should not feel pain, and they should not be anxious. However, the physician can't provide medicine to actively result in a patient's death. His wife shook her head and said, "I don't understand, doctors are supposed to help people." Again, the physician tried to provide a supportive environment, as far as possible. A benzodiazepine was offered for anxiety and a narcotic analgesic for pain, and the family stayed with their loved one. But, as prescribed by state and federal guidelines, the physician must stop short of active intervention that would result in death. The patient's oncologist was contacted, and she agreed to follow this treatment plan. She considered it unlikely the patient would survive the day.

The facility recognized they did not have a true end-of-life guideline and treatment protocol. They decided to formulate one based on this and other cases encountered at the facility.

Medical Approach

The assisted suicide question has a complex dynamic. Numerous stakeholders are involved – patients, providers, ethics consultants, and people who have a strong opinion based on their experiences watching their loved ones suffer. Some states have moved toward statutory guidelines offering an assisted suicide protocol, while in other states this remains a prohibited action, leaving physicians, providers, and nurses to struggle with the conflicting issues. Most providers attempt to do the right thing by alleviating pain and suffering, which they are obligated to do, but this is often complicated by external rules and regulations.

Oregon enacted the "Death with Dignity Act" initially approved by voters in 1994, and made permanent after numerous appeals.[2] The law allows "physician-assisted suicide," in which a terminally ill patient in Oregon is allowed to self-administer lethal medications prescribed by a physician.

Lee et al. performed an analysis of 3944 physicians based in Oregon, with a 70% (2761) response rate. The study found 60% of the respondents thought physician-assisted suicide should be legal and 46% would be willing to prescribe medication.[3] However, 31% objected on moral grounds, or were concerned about the ability to accurately predict 6-month survival.

Legal Analysis

Similar challenges quickly arose in other states where the question was posed. In *Vacco, Attorney General of New York, et al.* v. *Quill et al.* a group of physicians challenged the constitutionality of physician-assisted suicide.[4] The district court ruled for the state; the United States Court of Appeals, Second Circuit reversed. The Supreme Court of the United States (USSC) held that New York's prohibition on physician-assisted suicide does not violate the Constitution's Fourteenth Amendment Equal Protection Clause.[5] They used a "rationality test" that was related to the state's legitimate interest in preserving life. The rational-basis test suggests that unless a constitutionally based property, class, or liberty interest is being considered, the law will be upheld if it is logically derived from any legitimate governmental purpose.[6]

The Fourteenth Amendment Equal Protection Clause mandates that like cases must be treated in a similar fashion, while dissimilar cases may be dealt with differently, according to *Plyer* v. *Doe*.[7] The USSC held that local school districts were not authorized to selectively deny enrollment to schoolchildren not "legally admitted" into the United States. Here, all within the jurisdiction must be dealt with in a similar fashion, and equality of rights must be maintained.

Likewise, in *Washington* v. *Glucksberg et al.* physicians and terminally ill patients challenged the state's ban on physician-assisted suicide.[8] The USSC held that Washington's prohibition against aiding in a suicide does not violate the Fourteenth Amendment Due Protection Clause.[9] There is no "right" to assistance in committing suicide, asserted as a fundamental liberty interest protected in the Due Process clause. Likewise, the USSC held there to be a legitimate state interest shielding the terminally ill from undue influence.

Table 11.1 End-of-life decision-making

1.	Involve patient and all family members
2.	Ease pain and suffering
3.	Enlist family, friends, and religious organizations for support
4.	Contact primary care and specialty resources for assistance
5.	Utilize hospital ethics committee
6.	Document the rationale for action and plan

Conclusion

It is essential to approach this problem systematically (Table 11.1) First, involve all family members in the discussion to ascertain the patient's wishes. Second, it is paramount to ease pain and suffering. Third, ensure support is offered through family, friends, or religious organizations. Fourth, contact primary care and specialty resources for assistance. Five, utilize the hospital-based ethics committee if one is available. Sixth, document the rationale for one's actions and care plan.

References

1. War Department. (1944) Explanation of the Provisions of "The GI Bill of Rights" (Public Law 346, 78th Congress). Washington, D.C.: US War Department.

2. Oregon State Legislature. The Oregon Death with Dignity Act. Chapter 127. 800–995.

3. Lee MA, Nelson HD, Tilden VP, Ganzini L, Schmidt TA, Tolle SW. Legalizing assisted suicide – views of physicians in Oregon. *N Engl J Med.* 1996;334(5):310–315. DOI:10.1056/NEJM199602013340507.

4. *Vacco, Attorney General of New York, et al.* v. *Quill et al.*, Supreme Court of the United States, No. 95–1858. Decided June 26, 1997.

5. U.S. Const. Amend. XIV, cl. Equal Protection.

6. Wex Legal Dictionary/Encyclopedia/LII/Cornell University. Accessed May 24, 2017.

7. *Plyer* v. *Doe*, 457 U.S. 202, 216.

8. *Washington et al.* v. *Glucksberg et al.*, Supreme Court of the United States, No. 96–110. Decided June 26, 1997.

9. U.S. Const. Amend XIV, cl. Due Process.

Battery

Case

The patient was brought in to the emergency department (ED) by police in conjunction with a motor vehicle accident. He refused to let the ED physician draw his blood, repeatedly saying the hospital "had no right to take his blood." There was a suspicion that he had been driving under the influence (DUI), and law enforcement requested a blood sample to test for alcohol and drugs. The physician tried to talk to the patient again. He was agitated and slightly confused, but insisted there was no way he wanted his blood drawn, he knew his rights, and he had "read the constitution."

The remainder of his medical evaluation was essentially normal. He had no medical complaints and no obvious injuries. The patient said he was ready to go to jail if he had to. Again, the police asked that the blood sample be obtained since there was a fatality at the scene of the accident. The patient was asked again as the staff tried to impress upon him the need to at least get his blood drawn at this point, so he could go on to the next stage of his legal encounter.

One of the law enforcement officers went to obtain a warrant. They were unhappy because this would take time: the patient's alcohol level would decrease during this period, and they didn't want to jeopardize their case. One of the nurses volunteered to talk to the patient: "I think I know him. He'll probably listen to me, I know his family." So the nurse spoke with him for a few minutes. After that the patient allowed blood to be drawn, and was then discharged with law enforcement officers.

The remainder of the hospital shift was uneventful. The next day the physician received a call from the hospital risk management department, suggesting that another nurse at in the department had concerns that the patient was coerced into getting his blood drawn. They had raised an issue with risk management

requesting an opinion. Did the patient truly consent, as he was being incarcerated? This raised concerns of battery.

Medical Approach

The case in which a patient declines a blood draw has come up before, often invoking their constitutional right to determine their testing. They invoke a Fourth Amendment privilege that would prohibit undue search and seizure without a warrant. The Supreme Court of the United States has commented on this issue and stated that a simple blood draw does not rise to the level of undue search and seizure. It is obviously most desirable for the patient to consent, but what happens once we pass that point and the patient denies permission?

Law enforcement personnel should then be instructed to obtain a warrant for this intervention and this is again the next most desirable course. However, in extreme circumstances, or a catastrophic event such as a death at the scene of an incident, a timely blood draw is often required to properly define the patient's capacity. Typically, the defense in a case of operating a motor vehicle under the influence requires excluding the presence of drugs or alcohol as a cause for the altered mental status.

Legal Analysis

These battery cases have a wide variety of outcomes in the health-care setting. In *Duncan* v. *Scottsdale Med Imaging, Ltd.*, the patient consented to the administration of morphine or Demerol, but the nurse administered fentanyl instead for procedural sedation.[1] The trial court dismissed the plaintiff's battery claim, affirmed by the appeal court as there was consent to "an injection."

The Supreme Court of Arizona held that: (1) the injection of a drug against a patient's wishes constitutes battery and (2) Section 12–562 (B) of Arizona's Medical Malpractice Act that prohibits battery in this medical care scenario violates Article 18, Section 6 of the Arizona Constitution as an abrogation of the right to bring action in battery to recover damages.[2,3] However, they did not render a judgment on the medical intervention, remanding to trial court for factual analysis.

In *Cobbs* v. *Grant*, the patient had a series of surgical procedures with complications, some of which were quite uncommon.[4] The Supreme Court of California held that:

> A disclosure need not be made beyond that required within the medical community when a doctor can prove by a preponderance of the evidence he relied upon facts which would demonstrate to a reasonable man the disclosure would have so seriously upset the patient that the patient would not have been able to dispassionately weigh the risks of refusing to undergo the recommended treatment.

They noted the difference between a "lack of informed consent" and "lack of consent." They reserved the battery allegation for the latter, limiting it to surgical procedures performed without consent.

In *Roberson* v. *Provident House*, a nurse inserted an indwelling catheter although the patient objected, and had subsequent complications requiring hospitalization.[5] The trial court dismissed the physician complaint since a medical complaint was not filed with the medical review panel, and they dismissed against the facility with prejudice.[6] The Court of Appeals of Louisiana, Fourth District held since there was no true emergency, absent appropriate informed consent, a battery was committed with damages warranting compensation.

In North Carolina, the Motor Vehicle Driver Protection Act, State Law S.L. 2006–253 amended General Statute 20–139.1 states "when a blood test is specified by a law enforcement officer … a physician, registered nurse, emergency medical technician or other qualified individual … no further authorization is required."[7] This applies to a defendant who has consented, or who is incapacitated and incapable of refusal.

This same directive applies to warrantless search, although the officer will need to provide a written request if solicited, and is held to a probable cause standard. Interestingly, there is debate about whether a warranted body fluid search can be absolutely compelled. There are some who suggest a true forensic analysis requires a contracted health-care provider.

A provider who refuses to perform a sampling procedure may be threatened with a charge of obstructing an officer (G.S. 14–223).[8] Although this provision is theoretically possible it is seldom initiated by law enforcement.

Conclusion

Often the hospital attorney can be consulted for specific information, or the risk management department can help with education to allay fears and help staff to understand the patient's rights and their own responsibilities to both the individual and society. At the end of the day we have obligations to the patient, but to society in general. Indeed, if someone else's health and safety has been jeopardized, then we are required – within proper consent and confidentiality standards – to intervene on behalf of potential patients as well.

References

1. *Duncan* v. *Scottsdale Med Imaging, Ltd.*, 70 P.3d 435, 2003.

2. Arizona Medical Malpractice Act. Arizona Revised Statutes (ARS) §§12–561 (2003).

3. Arizona Constitution: Article 18, Section 6: Recovery of Damages for Injuries.

4. *Cobbs* v. *Grant*, 8 Cal. 3d 229 (1972).

5. *Roberson* v. *Provident House*, 576 So. 2d 992 (1991).

6. Medical Review Panel, Louisiana Revised Statutes (La. R.S.) 40:1299.47. The fact.

7. Motor Vehicle Driver Protection Act of 2006, S.L. 2006–253.

8. North Carolina General Statutes (G.S.). 30 (1) §14–223 (2005).

Chapter 13

Bed Boarding

Case

The emergency department (ED) doctors were there to start their shift, and to take sign out from the departing physician. It was flu season and the hospital was full. There were 12 patients boarding in the ED, some of whom had been there for more than a day. The incoming staff asked if there was any progress in getting beds. The night-time physician was disheartened, as they had had a bad night. He reported the night nursing supervisor said there were no beds anywhere in the hospital.

The morning was busy as well. One of the ED nurses asked for assistance with a patient. She said the patient's temperature was elevated, he was likely septic, and he needed to be started on an antibiotic. The nurse had called the admitting physician, with no response. She said they had been given some holding orders, but no definitive orders for the patient's elevated temperature and low blood pressure. She had asked the counterpart ED physician for help, and was told to call the admitting physician for any additional orders. She said she had tried for the last hour, but there had been no response to the calls.

At this point, the ED physician went ahead to consent to giving orders for antibiotics, cultures, and vasopressors. There was another attempt to contact the admitting physician, still with no response. Finally, there was a response from the admitting physician, who said they had a change of shift as well and that they weren't going to give any orders until the patient got upstairs. The ED physician suggested that admission orders were already provided by the first admitting physician, and that technically this was their patient and they needed to respond to nursing requests for orders. The second hospital physician stated that their practice was not to give any additional orders until the patient got to the admission bed. Until that point, it's an ED patient. Eventually the ED physician ordered

some additional fluid and potassium replacement and eventually the patient went upstairs for admission.

The next morning the ED was notified by the quality improvement committee that a concern had been raised by the admitting physician about the choice of antibiotics, as well as the amount of fluid resuscitation occurring in the ED.

Medical Approach

This is a commonly encountered problem. The bed boarding situation typically occurs in a busy ED, where the accompanying floor service is often overwhelmed as well. The ED is more capable of dealing with an influx of patients – or at least that is the perception of most hospital facilities. Ironically, that assessment is true in a lot of cases, but may not be fair in a work allocation situation.

The admission process requires that once a transfer of service has taken place and the case has been discussed and accepted by the admitting physician, the patient is now technically under their care. The understanding that the accepting physician now takes full responsibility for the patient's care is necessary to provide a clear path for nursing. Unfortunately, in most institutions, the admitting physician often feels that the patient's location actually determines responsibility: as long as the patient is in the ED, they are cared for by the emergency staff. This assessment is in fact incorrect, and it is the responsibility of the accepting physician to provide additional orders until transfer has taken place.

The problem has been pervasive for years, with the impact felt predominantly by the ED. Olshaker et al. in 2006 cited a 91% incidence of overcrowding as noted by ED directors.[1] This overcrowding is attributed to a steady downsizing of hospital capacity, ED closure, increased volume, proportion of uninsured patients, decreased reimbursement, and lack of on-call

Table 13.1 Causes of ED overcrowding

1. Downsizing of hospital capacity
2. ED closure
3. Increased volume
4. Increased proportion of uninsured patients
5. Decreased reimbursement
6. Decreased on-call availability

Reference: DeLia and Cantor.[2]

Table 13.2 Effects of ED overcrowding

1. Longer wait times
2. Increased left without being seen rates
3. Ambulance service disruption
4. Reduced health-care quality
5. Decreased patient safety

Reference: DeLia and Cantor.[2]

capability (Table 13.1). In earlier years, agencies such as the Joint and the General Accounting Office felt the issue was due to inappropriate overuse and was cyclical, not requiring a specific policy response.

The problems associated with ED overcrowding are numerous and significant. The Robert Woods Johnson Foundation Synthesis Project noted overcrowding was associated with decreased care access manifested as longer wait times, increased left without being seen (LWBS) rates, disruptions to ambulance service, as well as reduced health-care quality and decreased patient safety (Table 13.2).[2]

In a meta-analysis of 276 data-based articles, Johnson and Winkleman identified 23 that reported an association between crowding and patient outcome.[3] First, they identified delay interventions, including antibiotic administration, cardiac interventions, and pain management. Second, there was a significant decline in patient satisfaction. Third, there was clear adverse impact on patient outcome with increased mortality. The reasons for adverse impact are complex and may include resource allocation, nursing availability, and uncertainty regarding responsibility for care.

Legal Analysis

The typical question raised is, who is responsible for resource allocation and bed availability decisions? In

Atcherian v. *United States of America*, the patient, who was 38 weeks pregnant, presented for a prenatal visit, was diagnosed with "pregnancy induced hypertension vs. preeclampsia," referred for induction by family medicine and told to report the next day by obstetrics.[4] There was no dispute that the hospital's capacity to perform the induction on the day of presentation was exceeded. The plaintiff alleged it was due to inadequate nursing staffing. The defendant filed a motion in limine, to selectively limit the introduction of evidence from court consideration. They attempted to "exclude any expert opinion that the government had a duty to immediately perform induction as a basis for liability." The district court denied the motion to exclude, and had parties agree that nursing was not the basis for liability and that the proper course of action with limited resources was prompt air evacuation. The parties also agreed the plaintiff cannot recover damages against the government, citing the protection of economic contingencies by the discretionary function exception. However, the Federal Tort Claims Acts (FTCA) of 1946 waives immunity and provides a mechanism for compensating people for negligent or wrongful action of employees of the US government in *Gager* v. *U.S.*, 149 F.3d 918, 920 (9th Circ. 1998).[5,6]

In *Higgins* v. *Salt Lake County*, the complainant sued for her daughter individually and as a guardian ad litem for an assault by a dangerous patient.[7] The patient was taken to an ED with a request for hospitalization, with the request denied allegedly due to a bed shortage. She was referred to a residential treatment facility, and attended sessions there. Subsequently, she was "looking to stab somebody." The trial court held that the defendants owed no third-party duty to protect mother or daughter from a potentially dangerous unrelated mental patient. On appeal, the Supreme Court of Utah affirmed, but on alternative grounds related to governmental immunity.

An additional question is who is responsible for the patient in different geographic areas of the hospital. In *Giles* v. *Anonymous Physician*, the question raised was whether a valid relationship existed between a patient and a hospitalist physician.[8] The patient had had a fall and outpatient surgery was scheduled. Uncomplicated surgery was completed, allegedly followed by postoperative hypotension and hypoxemia. The hospitalist was contacted and presented to the bedside, but found there was no established contracted relationship to care for patients who present to the hospital in this manner. The patient's primary care physician was contacted, and agreed to see her after office hours. She was transferred to the intensive care unit where she succumbed to influenza and pneumonia, according to the pronouncement.

It appeared later that there was a "contract" to provide care to this physician's patients who came through the ED, but apparently not via this outpatient route, and no billing was submitted by the hospitalist.

The trial court awarded a summary judgment verdict to the hospitalist, holding that there was no established duty or physician–patient relationship as affirmed by the Court of Appeals of Indiana.

Conclusion

Most ED physicians will respond to an emergency that occurs with a patient who is still residing in the ED, but the true responsibility moves to the accepting physician. The hospital should establish protocols to improve the bed boarding situation and should define clear care responsibilities. This is important from a customer service perspective, and has a financial impact as well. The medicolegal consideration is that no more than one physician should be involved in any patient care event, in a redundant fashion, unless synergy is thereby gained.

References

1. Olshaker JS, Rathlev N. Emergency department overcrowding and ambulance diversion: the impact and potential solutions of extended boarding of admitted patients in the emergency department. *J Emerg Med.* 2006;30(3):351–356. DOI:10.1016/j.jemergmed.2005.05.023.

2. DeLia D, Cantor J. Emergency department utilization and capacity. *Robert Woods Johnson Foundation, Research Synthesis Report No 17,* July 2009. ISSN 2155–3718. 1–28.

3. Johnson KD, Winkleman C. The effect of emergency department crowding on patient outcomes: a literature review. *Adv Emerg Nurs J.* 2011;33(1):39–54.

4. *Atcherian et al.* v. *United States of America*, Case 3:12-cv-0211-RRB, USDC, D. Alaska, January 23, 2015.

5. Federal Tort Claims Act (FTCA), 28 U.S.C. §§2671–2680 (1994).

6. *Gager* v. *United States*, 149 F.3d 918, 920 (9th Circuit 1998).

7. *Higgins* v. *Salt Lake County*, 855 P.2d 231 (1993).

8. *Giles* v. *Anonymous Physician I et al.*, 13 N.E.3d 594 (2014).

Brain Death

Case

As the paramedics brought the patient in to the emergency department (ED) they were shaking their heads. The patient was a motorcyclist who had been in a catastrophic crash with a car. He was unresponsive and had been intubated at the scene by medics. The providers had done their best for stabilization, placing intravenous access for large-volume fluid resuscitation, monitoring vital signs, and getting the patient quickly to CT scan.

The CT scans of the chest and abdomen were normal, but the head showed a catastrophic hemorrhage, almost engulfing the entire left hemisphere. Neurosurgery was quickly called, and they asked the patient's clinical status. The ED physician stated the patient had no clinical activity whatsoever. There was no overbreathing of the ventilator, no movement at all in the patient, no corneal reflexes. Blood pressure was normal and no other injury was found.

The neurosurgeon stated the patient should have a brain death protocol performed. They felt there was no clinical activity and that a neurosurgical intervention would not be helpful, and went on to their round in the intensive care unit (ICU). Before leaving, they asked for the patient to be admitted to the ICU for additional stabilization and to evaluate the brain function for further decision-making. The staff met with the patient's family, a brother and sister, who asked what the patient's status was and if there was any chance whatsoever for recovery. The brother stated the patient would not have wanted to go on in this condition. The sister said he would have wanted to fight the best he could, and if he did not survive it was his wish to have his organs donated.

The family mentioned that the neurosurgeon had discussed brain death, and they inquired about whether that was indeed the case. The ED physician discussed the brain death criteria, talked to them about the timing of the procedures required, and the

setting in which they would be performed. It was suggested that the ICU was a better place to decide, as well as waiting one additional day to make a decision, to improve accuracy of the prediction. They thanked the ED staff for their care and the patient was transferred to the ICU for additional stabilization and evaluation.

Medical Approach

The most important thing about cases requiring brain death certification is assigning a prognosis as soon as feasible, while still permitting adequate time for recovery. Families typically want to know what will happen, although this is often difficult to determine. It is important to note that the staging of this discussion with the family requires the proper circumstances for brain death certification to be instituted.

First, the decision should be made in the proper timeframe. At least 24 hours of observation is typically recommended, to ensure the patient is in the best possible homeostatic state. Second, the proper geographic location is important; typically this is the ICU, where decisions are made in a controlled setting. Third, the patient's homeostatic needs such as temperature, blood pressure control, oxygenation, and ventilation must be established so that the proper determination can be made. Fourth, the patient will be put through a precise sequence of steps to ensure the evaluation is valid. Fifth, the legal term "brain death" involves a clinical evaluation, as well as evocative testing. Lastly, the lack of ability to breathe on one's own, and the absence of motor activity without the presence of sedatives and muscle relaxants, are required. If all these criteria are met then the patient meets certification requirements for brain death with total loss of cerebral function, which is equivalent to cardiovascular death in most jurisdictions.

The brain death criteria used today are based on the 1995 American Academy of Neurology practice parameters, using a four-step protocol (Table 14.1).[1]

Table 14.1 Brain death certification

1.		Clinical prerequisites
	a	Irreversible and proximate cause of coma
	b	Normal core temperature
	c	Normal systolic blood pressure
	d	Neurological exam consistent with brain death
2.		Clinical evaluation consistent with brain death
	a	Lack of all evidence of responsiveness
	b	Absence of brainstem reflexes
	c	Presence of apnea, absence of urge to breathe
3.		Use of ancillary tests
	a	EEG
	b	CTA
	c	MRI/MRA
	d	TCD
4.		Documentation
	a	Verification of partial pressure of carbon dioxide
	b	Time of death

Reference Wijdicks et al.[1]

Table 14.2 Harvard Ad Hoc Committee of 1968: "brain death" criteria

Clinical criteria	
1.	Unresponsive to normal painful stimuli
2.	Absence of spontaneous movement or breathing
3.	Absence of reflexes
Confirmation	
4.	Absence of EEG activity
Observation	
5.	24 hours of observation

Reference: Harvard Ad Hoc Committee.[4]

First, the clinical evaluation prerequisites include: (1) establishing an irreversible and proximate cause of coma; (2) achieving a normal core temperature; (3) achieving normal systolic blood pressure; and (4) performing a neurological exam sufficient to pronounce brain death. Second, the clinical evaluation consistent with brain death should include: (1) lack of all evidence of responsiveness; (2) absence of brainstem reflexes; and (3) presence of apnea, lack of drive to breathe. Third, ancillary tests used include electroencephalography (EEG), computed tomography angiography (CTA), magnetic resonance imaging and angiography (MRI/MRA), transcranial Doppler (TCD), nuclear scan, or cerebral angiography. Fourth, documentation must include verification of partial pressure of carbon dioxide (P_{CO_2}) and time of death.

The brain death certification criteria are even more meticulous for pediatric patients. In the 2011 update of the 1987 Task Force Recommendations[2] the pediatric exam requires two attending examiners with an interposed observation period of 12 hours for infants (>30 days) and children and 24 hours for term newborns (37 weeks to 30 days).

Legal Analysis

The discussion has long passed "cardiac standstill" to the concept of "brain death," in which criteria have matured following innovations in diagnostic testing. In *Commonwealth* v. *Siegfried Golston*, a criminal act was committed leaving a man "brain dead."[3] The defendant appealed the murder conviction, claiming that death was not properly established. The Harvard Ad Hoc Committee on Brain Death in 1968 promoted three clinical criteria including: (1) unresponsive to normal painful stimuli; (2) absence of spontaneous movement or breathing; and (3) absence of reflexes, accompanied by EEG confirmation followed by 24 hours of observation to identify irreversible coma (Table 14.2).[4] The trial court held that the "brain death" criteria were correctly applied and the decision was affirmed by the Supreme Judicial Court of Massachusetts, Suffolk.

In *Janus* v. *Tarasewicz*, the time of death became significant for consideration of an insurance policy and time of death of husband and wife, where the patient had no blood pressure or pulse, but persistent cardiac electrical activity.[5] They again cited the Harvard Ad Hoc Committee confirming the widely accepted criteria that have matured over time.[4,5] These criteria include: (1) unreceptivity and unresponsivity to intensely painful stimuli; (2) no spontaneous movement or breathing for 1 hour; (3) no blinking, no swallowing, and fixed and dilated pupils; (4) two flat EEGs with a 24-hour intervening period; (5) absence of drug intoxication or hyperthermia (Table 14.3).

However, in *In re Haymer* the circuit court and affirmed by the Illinois Appellate Court, refused to establish criteria for determining brain death, because they noted that the advent of new research and technologies would continue to change the tests used for determining cessation of brain function.[6] They merely required the diagnosis of death be made in accordance

Table 14.3 Harvard Ad Hoc Committee: examination of brain death

1.	Unreceptivity and unresponsivity to intensely painful stimuli
2.	No spontaneous movement or breathing for at least 1 hour
3.	No blinking, no swallowing, and fixed, dilated pupils
4.	Flat EEGs taken twice with at least a 24-hour intervening period
5.	Absence of drug intoxication or hyperthermia

Reference: Harvard Ad Hoc Committee.[4]

with "the usual and customary standards of medical practice."

In *Brophy* v. *New England Sinai Hospital*, an extremely active man suffered an intracranial hemorrhage, and was left with a devastating neurological injury.[7] He was technically not brain dead, but his family advocated for withdrawal of support, while providers did not. The probate judge held that the hospital and its medical staff should not be compelled to withhold food and water from a patient, contrary to its moral and ethical principles, when such principles are recognized and accepted within a significant segment of the medical profession and the hospital community.

The Supreme Judicial Court of Massachusetts, Norfolk held that:

> when there is substantial disagreement in the medical community over the appropriate medical action, it would be particularly inappropriate to force the hospital, which is willing to assist in and transfer the patient to take affirmative steps and the provision of nutrition and hydration. A patient's right to refuse medical treatment does not warrant such an unnecessary intrusion upon the hospital's integrity.

However, a recent case, *Winkfield* v. *Children's Hospital Oakland*, found that although the patient had been certified as brain dead, an injunction was filed continuing life support until transfer could be made to a long-term care facility.[8] The patient's mother filed suit for her minor daughter with the district court to file a temporary restraining order to prevent discontinuation of her artificial airway, maintain ventilatory support, and place a tracheostomy and feeding gastrostomy to facilitate transfer to another facility.

The superior court granted the injunction to maintain ventilation, but denied the other requests including the invasive procedures. This court held an evidentiary hearing, where an independent, court-appointed physician from a prominent medical school ultimately concluded the patient met brain death criteria and was legally "deceased." The court ultimately felt that it did not have subject-matter jurisdiction, and asked plaintiff to show cause that it should not. The patient was released to the coroner who issued a death certificate. She was released into the custody of her mother who assumed responsibility for her during transfer to another location where the invasive procedures where performed, and she continued to be cared for. Her legal representatives have presented evidence that she may have some level of responsiveness, so is not "brain dead," and have filed a medical malpractice action.

Conclusion

It is clear that this field is constantly undergoing rapid evolution, as both technological capabilities and patient and family expectations grow. Health-care providers need to continually update their knowledge and their capability to assist in the determination of patient survival and functional outcome.

References

1. Wijdicks EFM, Varelas PN, Gronseth GS, Greer DM. Evidence-based guideline update: determining brain death in adults. Report of the Quality Standards Subcommittee of the American Academy of Neurology. *Neurology* 2010;74:1911–1918. DOI:10.1212/WNL.0b013e3181e242a8.

2. Nakagawa TA, Ashwal S, Mathur M, Mysore M, Society of Critical Care Medicine Section on Critical Care, American Society of Pediatrics Section on Neurology, and the Child Neurology Society. Guidelines for the determination of brain death in infants and children: an update of the 1987 Task Force recommendation. *Pediatrics*. 2011;128(3):e720–e740. DOI:10.1542/Peds.2011–1511.

3. *Commonwealth* v. *Siegfried Golston*, 373 Mass. 249 (1977).

4. A definition of irreversible coma. Report of the Ad Hoc Committee of the Harvard Medical School to examine the definition of brain death. *JAMA*. 1968;205(6):337–340.

5. *Janus* v. *Tarasewicz*, 135 Ill. App.3d 936 (1985).

6. In re Haymer, 450 N.E.2d 940 (1983), 349, 354–355.

7. *Brophy* v. *New England Sinai Hospital*, 497 N.E.2d 626 (1986).

8. *Winkfield* v. *Children's Hospital of Oakland*, Temporary Restraining Order, No. RG13-707598, Super Ct Cal., December 23, 2013.

Chapter 15

Care of Children

Case

It appeared that she was normally a happy child, playing with her brother and doing the usual things children her age do. When she came into the emergency department (ED), she managed a weak smile. Her mother stated that she had been sick all week. She had a cough, felt nauseous, and couldn't keep anything down. She had no fever, urinary complaints, or recent trauma.

The physical exam was essentially normal, but her lips were dry and parched. The blood work, urinalysis, and chest radiograph were normal. However, her white blood cell count was significantly elevated at 25.5 cells/mm^3.

She felt a little better with rehydration, but still looked ill. The nurses reported the mother wanted to leave and take her child home. The physicians spoke with the mother again and recommended further evaluation. The mother declined and said, "Give me the form to sign, I need to go."

Once again, she was offered further evaluation, discussion with the pediatrician or social service assistance to help with any family needs, which she again declined. The mother's sister arrived and told her, "You can't take her home, they will call the police." The mother screamed, "They can't do that, she's my daughter." She consented to stay for the remainder of her daughter's evaluation, and the child was eventually discharged with a diagnosis of gastroenteritis with dehydration resolved.

Medical Approach

The epidemiology of medical malpractice in pediatric emergency care patients was reported in 1995 by Selbst et al. who found that 96% of cases occur in the ED and 4% in the urgent care center (UCC) based on a 2283 closed claim cohort from a 16-year period

(1985–2000).[1] The cases involved boys (59%) and those less than 2 years of age (47%), who were ultimately diagnosed with missed meningitis, appendicitis, fracture, and testicular torsion, with the first two diagnoses associated with the greatest mortality.

The study of pediatric discharge against medical advice (DAMA) establishes some trends and patterns. Paul performed a study of 39 pediatric patients from 2007 to 2009 evaluated in a United Kingdom ED for acute illness.[2] The majority (82%) of patients were seen within 2 hours of presentation, 56% (22) had parents who signed the form. The admission rate was 15% (6) with all children less than 5 years of age. Lastly, the predominant reason for leaving the hospital was the parent's perception that the child was healthy and not in need of further health care, according to 21% (8) of families.

Little has been written about the factors that persuade a pediatric physician to allow a parent to discharge their child against medical advice. The factors that influence include first, their ability to do something about the parent's rationale for the DAMA request, their impressions of the care provided by the parents and their own legal liability.[3] This group of pediatric residents generally felt positive about their interaction with the parents, and would care for the child again if readmitted.

These cases are often problematic: no one knows a child better than the parents. However, parents can sometimes exhibit suboptimal judgment concerning their child's health and well-being. We should always try the least invasive, least restrictive approach, making every attempt to convince patients, or families of patients, that we have instituted the proper medical decision-making. It is often helpful to enlist other family members, both parents, the child's pediatrician, and hospital-based resources, such as social services, to assist parents in their decision-making.

If at that point the physician still cannot make headway, external regulatory or judicial influence may be required. The first step is to contact Children, Youth, and Family Services, which can often do a fitness assessment of parents to ensure the interests of the child are being followed. If it is felt that the parent's deviations from normal medical standards are so severe as to require removal of the child from the home, then judicially imposed guardianship may be imposed. The least invasive method possible should be implemented, avoiding a more permanent controversy, which is always the most desirable course.

Legal Analysis

The health-care system has always had special focus on the care of children. In *Smith* v. *Richmond Memorial Hospital*, the patient presented at 33 weeks of pregnancy with premature rupture of membranes.[4] The patient was transferred to a larger facility by physician verbal order, with some delay as a result of emergency medical services (EMS) requiring payment for the transfer. After evaluation at the receiving facility, an emergency cesarean section was performed and the child was delivered with severe brain damage, according to the records. The trial court sustained a demurrer without leave to amend, on the ground that the motion for summary judgment failed to state a valid Emergency Medical Treatment and Labor Act (EMTALA) claim.[5] The hospital defended by claiming the patient had to arrive at the ED, and secondarily a child with an emergency medical condition (EMC) born at the facility did not "come through the ED" to activate a valid EMTALA claim.[6] The Supreme Court of Virginia held that the statute in a literal interpretation applied to an EMC or active labor, as was clearly the case here. They affirmed in part, reversed in part, and remanded for further consideration as the burden to file a valid EMTALA claim was met.

In *Thing* v. *La Chusa*, a minor was struck by an automobile. The mother proceeded to the scene, saw her unconscious child, and after care filed a lawsuit.[7] The trial court granted the defendant's motion for summary judgment, ruling that a claim for intentional infliction of emotional distress (NEID) could not be established as she did not "contemporaneously and sensorily perceive the event." Bystander claims from intentional infliction of emotional distress are recoverable only if the plaintiff: (1) is closely related to the

Table 15.1 Bystander recovery for intentional infliction of emotional distress

1. Closely related to victim
2. Present at scene of injury
3. Aware of it causing injury to victim
4. Suffers emotional distress
5. Beyond that of normal witness

Reference: Dillon.[8]

victim; (2) is present at the scene of the injury-producing event and aware that it is causing injury to the victim; (3) suffers emotional distress beyond that which would be experienced by a disinterested witness.

In *Dillon* v. *Legg* the Supreme Court of California affirmed, holding the plaintiff could not recover as she was not present at the scene nor necessarily aware of the tragedy (Table 15.1).[8]

Conclusion

The least desirable outcome is intervention by security or law enforcement if the patient's family tries to physically remove the child from the facility in an unsafe medical situation. In that case the family's behavior will need to be controlled until an objective analysis can be performed by an objective agency or group that may require judicial intervention to best protect the welfare of the child.

References

1. Selbst S, Freidman MJ, Singh S. Epidemiology and etiology of malpractice lawsuits involving children in US emergency departments and urgent care centers. *Pediatr Emerg Care*. 2005;21(3):165–169.

2. Paul SP, Remorin R. Discharge against medical advice (DAMA) – a study. *West London Med J*. 2010;2(3):17–27.

3. Macrohon BC. Pediatrician's perspectives on discharge against medical advice (DAMA) among pediatric patients. *BMC Pediatr*. 2012;12:75. DOI:10.1186/1471-2431-12-75.

4. *Smith* v. *Richmond Memorial Hospital*, 416 S.E.2d 689 (1992).

5. EMTALA, 42 U.S.C. §1395dd (1988).

6. *Loss* v. *Song*, 1990 WL 159612 (N.D. Ill. 1990).

7. *Thing* v. *Chusa*, 771 P.2d 814 (1989).

8. *Dillon* v. *Legg*, 68 Cal.2d 728 (1968).

Code Response

Case

About an hour before the end of the night shift, a Code Blue response was called on the hospital medical ward. This was a small hospital facility, and it was the emergency department (ED) physician's responsibility to respond to codes. Other members of the ED physician practice group were worried about this and had previously voiced their concerns regarding their medicolegal liability. The physicians had to respond to floor codes while still managing their responsibilities in the ED. They agreed with this concept as they had always felt that since the facility was small and there were no other physicians in the hospital at night, it was obviously their duty to respond. There was a hospitalist, but they were typically not trained in critical care procedures, which was the hospital's rationale for not having them respond to house code events.

An elderly patient with cancer had just had an asystolic cardiac arrest. The patient was intubated and the usual round of pharmaceutical interventions, including epinephrine and one dose of atropine, was performed. At one point, after there was no response to 15 minutes of cardiopulmonary resuscitation (CPR), the physician talked to the family members, most of whom seem resigned to the patient's fate. There was one daughter who seemed distant from the rest. She complained about her siblings' opinion and said their mom really didn't know. The patient was bad one day, and great the next. The rest of the family looked away when she spoke. The physician returned to the ED and finished her shift. Approximately a year later, while leaving the ED, the physician was met by a constable who presented a summons for appearance. It was a notice of intent to file suit concerning the care provided in that patient care encounter.

The provider had an appointment with the hospital attorney a week later and expressed her dismay.

How could she be sued when her only involvement was that she provided care to a code patient during an emergency, where nothing was done incorrectly? The hospital attorney acknowledged the concern, but this was a comprehensive lawsuit that involved everybody in the care chain including the patient's primary care physician, the surgical consultant, the oncologist, and the ED physician based on the response to the code. He said that it happened "all the time," and advised the physician not to worry because he expected there would be a dismissal from the case.

The following year the physician received a deposition request to appear concerning this case, again listing her as a defendant. The hospital attorney stated he was unable to get the plaintiff attorney to dismiss any physicians from the lawsuit and it would continue as intended. Again, the ED physician stated she had responded in an emergency situation and that the appropriate level of care was provided.

Medical Approach

This is an all-too-common scenario in emergency medicine. Typically, a smaller hospital has minimal night staff coverage and the ED physician is often called to respond to floor code events, as the only physician in the hospital. However, sometimes it is difficult to undertake responsibilities in the ED as well as ongoing care on the floor.

Emergency physicians are often concerned about the medicolegal responsibility of responding to a code in a different area of the hospital in a hurried fashion, while still maintaining their ED responsibilities as their priority.

Legal Analysis

Physicians assume that responding to resuscitation events outside of their normal area of responsibility is accompanied by "Good Samaritan" legal protection. There is a patchwork of statutory authority and caselaw regarding the Good Samaritan defense that differs from state to state.[1] The idea behind this is that societal good is enhanced when individuals act to benefit others without a defined contractual obligation or liability to do so.

In *HIRPA* v. *IHC Hospitals*, a physician responded to a cardiopulmonary arrest emergency on an obstetric patient who was not under his care.[2] He assumed responsibility for the code event in light of his qualifications as an internal medicine and emergency medicine physician, and suit was filed after an adverse outcome. The United States Court of Appeals, Tenth Circuit held that statutory immunity was offered in Utah to the physician providing emergency care to a hospitalized patient, where there was no pre-existing duty to do so.[3]

In *Harris* v. *Soha*, the emergency physician requested the assistance of the on-call anesthesiologist for assistance in an acute airway emergency.[4] After an untoward outcome it was alleged that the anesthesiologist had an obligation to respond and provide this care, as was customary. The Florida First District Court of Appeals upheld the trial court's directed verdict in favor of the physician, based on the state's Good Samaritan Act.[5]

Conclusion

It is important as an emergency physician always to provide the appropriate service to patients, families, and other hospital staff members. But it is also the physician's duty to recommend that fair and equitable coverage be arranged for emergency responses. In a significant number of hospitals there is now a transition from the physician's primary service to the hospitalist medicine physicians. This requires each facility to look at its own individual case mix, resources, and capabilities and to come up with a safety plan that benefits the patients within their community by establishing an effective response system.

References

1. Sutton V. Is there a doctor (and a lawyer) in the house? Why our Good Samaritan laws are doing more harm than good for a national public health security strategy: a fifty-state survey. *J Health Biomed Law.* 2010;VI:261–300.

2. *HIRPA v. IHC Hospitals Inc.*, Supreme Court of Utah, No. 960180. Decided: November 14, 1997.

3. Utah Code Ann. §58-12-23 (1996), Good Samaritan Statute.

4. *Harris* v. *Soha*, 2009 WL 2049173, *1 (Fla.App.1st Dist.).

5. Fla. Stat. & 768.13 (2)(c)(1) (2009).

Commitment

Case

The patient's chief complaint was, "I want to hurt myself." Unfortunately, this is a complaint we hear far too often in the emergency department (ED). She had tears streaming down her face, as she sobbed quietly. There were job issues, and some boyfriend issues as well. She said she wanted to take pills, had saved some up, and had made two previous suicide attempts. Her mother came in and said she had concerns about her daughter's behavior as well. There had been on-and-off issues with her boyfriend, which was "not a new problem."

The patient's boyfriend arrived, and briefly argued with the mother. The patient said she wanted to go home with her boyfriend. The physician informed her that in the circumstances, it would be wiser for her to remain in the hospital. She screamed that she wasn't staying. The physician discussed her suicide risk with the on-call psychiatrist, who recommended admission. She again screamed, "No one can keep me here against my will." Her mother was happy with the admission decision.

Although the patient was being monitored, she made it to a phone and activated a "Condition Help" alert, stating she was being "held against her will." The team responded and quickly discontinued the alert. This was discussed with the patient advocate, who then had a better understanding of the situation.

Medical Approach

These cases are often a complex matrix of psychiatric, psychosocial, and societal stress issues. Some patients may overstate their desire to harm themselves, then become reticent later. Others may initially understate their risk, and then go home and attempt to harm themselves.

It is crucially important to have an objective understanding of the suicide risk based on known parameters. These include patient's gender, the presence of alcohol or drug abuse, the support systems they have, whether they are married or divorced, whether they have had a previous suicide attempt, and the potential lethality of that attempt. We can then move through the process from the least restrictive to the most restrictive intervention. This means trying to protect the patient's rights of self-determination, while still protecting their health and well-being.

Legal Analysis

The concept of *parens patriae* dictates that the state or governmental agency has the obligation to care for someone who is in dire need of treatment or care.[1] Mental health advocates have cited *Rogers* v. *Okin*, a Massachusetts case citing constitutional protections (Ad. I, IV, V, VIII, XIV) concerning medication and restraint, even for those involuntarily committed.[2-7] Seven types of acute psychiatric emergencies were defined, providing a helpful construct that was ultimately rejected by the district judge. First, suicidal behavior either with serious intent or gesture. Second, assaultive behavior toward self or others. Third, the destruction of property. Fourth, the presence of extreme anxiety or panic. Fifth, bizarre behavior. Sixth, acute or chronic emotional disturbance with the potential to interfere with daily function. Seventh, the necessity of an immediate medical response to prevent or decrease severe suffering or worsening of the patient's clinical state (Table 17.1).

In *Zinermon* v. *Burch*, the respondent alleged that the petitioner deprived him of liberty without due process, by admitting him as a "voluntary" mental health patient, when he was incompetent to give informed consent.[8] He alleged that he was deprived of the constitutional rights afforded by the safeguards instituted in conjunction with the involuntary commitment of a mentally ill patient. The district court dismissed the

Table 17.1 Acute psychiatric emergencies

1. Suicidal behavior or gesture
2. Assaultive behavior
3. Property destruction
4. Extreme anxiety or panic
5. Bizarre behavior
6. Emotional disturbance interfering with daily living
7. Necessity of immediate response to prevent worsening

References: Swartz[1]; Rogers.[2]

plaintiff's case on a procedural basis as the state statutory protections were adequate, just not followed in this case. The United States Court of Appeals, Eleventh Circuit upheld the decision since the deprivation was not anticipated, and post-deprivation remedies were still available to him.

In *In re James E.*, the district court held that a patient voluntarily committed to a psychiatric facility could have their stay extended, if their behavior decompensated and the state filed a petition for voluntary/judicial admission.[9] The appellate court affirmed the right to protect society, while still attempting to preserve the patient's rights in doing so.

Conclusion

There is a judicial predisposition to ensure societal safety in a decompensated patient scenario, while still ensuring protection of constitutionally mandated safeguards. We should always involve family, when appropriate, and appeal to their sense of self-worth and reliance, as well as trusting in the system to preserve the best outcome possible for the patient if mandatory hospitalization is required.

References

1. Swartz MS. What constitutes a psychiatric emergency: clinical and legal dimensions. *Bull Am Acad Psychiatr Law*. 1987;15(1):57–68.

2. *Rogers* v. *Okin*, 478 F Supp 1342 (D. Mass. 1979).

3. U.S. Const. Amend. I.

4. U.S. Const. Amend IV.

5. U.S. Const. Amend V.

6. U.S. Const. Amend VIII.

7. U.S. Const. Amend XIV.

8. *Zinermon et al.* v. *Burch*, 494 U.S. 113 (1990).

9. In re James E (*The People of the State of Illinois, Appellee* v. *James E., Appellant*), Docket No. 93608 – Agenda 8, November 2002.

Communication

Case

The patient was in her late fifties, but looked older. She had a previous cardiac history, as well as a prior pulmonary embolism (PE). She had had breast cancer earlier in life, but was cured after radiation and chemotherapy. The cardiac workup had been done, and was essentially negative. Then a CT angiogram (CTA) was ordered to rule out PE, but the patient remembered she might have had a contrast dye reaction in the past so this test was placed on hold for evaluation. If the clinical scenario indicated a need to order the test, it was felt that a ventilation–perfusion (VQ) scan, which could be done safely, was warranted. The clinical likelihood was considered significant enough that she was prepped for a CT scan the next day and received an empiric dose of a low molecular weight heparin. These issues were discussed with the admitting physician and the patient was transferred to the floor for the night. During the handover discussion the admitting physician was reminded the patient had a previous history of breast cancer and that she had a clinical condition that could be consistent with PE as indicated by either tachycardia or hypoxemia.

The treating emergency department (ED) physician was off the next day, but returned the day after. He found out that the patient had been admitted and had an untoward outcome due to PE. The ED staff stated the patient was admitted with a diagnosis of PE and they treated her with enoxaparin (an anticoagulant). It was suggested during the admission that the medication had been stopped, as the admitting medicine team thought the presentation was more consistent with congestive heart failure.

One week later there was a call from the quality committee, who wanted an explanation. The ED physician again explained the patient had been admitted with a diagnosis of PE and had been treated with an anticoagulant. At some point, the care plan had been changed even after the patient's risk factors were discussed. The committee agreed, and they were evaluating other parts of the health-care chain.

Medical Approach

The transition of care process is often complicated and requires optimal communication to avoid issues. There are obviously individual preferences and variance in practice. For that reason, it is desirable to use tools to assist the transfer of care process that address the admission, consultation, specialty consultation, transfer of care to higher acuity unit, or discharge.

The ED is a high-risk, rapid-turnover area especially prone to difficulty in care transition. Maughan et al. evaluated 110 ED handover sessions of 992 patients, noting errors in 13.1% (130) and omissions in 45.1% (447),[1] while laboratory errors and omissions were noted in 3.7% (37) and 29.2% (290), respectively. The errors were increased with longer handover times and prolonged length of stay, and decreased with the use of written or electronic support materials to assist with the transition.

Even objective data, such as vital signs, can be miscommunicated. Venkatesh et al. reported on 1163 patients during 130 ED shift rounds, in which 74% (116 of 154) patients with hypoxia and 42% (66 of 117) with hypotension did not have this finding communicated on shift changeovers.[2] Overall, 14% (166) of the handovers included a vital sign error of omission or miscommunication. Interestingly, multivariate analysis examining factors such as ED occupancy found no correlation with miscommunication.

Clearly, the more objective criteria that are available for this transfer procedure and protocol, the better the patient's quality of care. The protocol for transfer of care and service may involve specific information transfer, call and check-back reports, dual redundant care resources, and electronic tracking.

Table 18.1 Strategy to improve ED handover process

1.	Reduce the number of unnecessary handovers
2.	Limit interruptions and distractions
3.	Provide a succinct overview
4.	Communicate tasks, anticipate change, have a clear plan
5.	Make information available for direct review
6.	Encourage questioning and discussion of assessments
7.	Account for all patients
8.	Signal a clear moment in the transition of care

Reference: Cheung and Kelly.[3]

The American College of Emergency Medicine (ACEP) Section of Quality Improvement and Patient Safety has generated a practical strategy for this high-risk shift-change period.[3] First, reduce the number of unnecessary handovers in the department. Second, limit interruptions and distractions as much as practicable. Third, provide a succinct overview to encourage efficiency. Fourth, communicate outstanding tasks, anticipate changes, and have a clear plan for transition. Fifth, make information readily available for direct review. Sixth, encourage questioning and discussion of patient assessments. Seventh, account for all patients in the department in the transition process. Eighth, signal a clear moment in the transition of care so that accountability is defined (Table 18.1).

The handover between emergency physician and hospitalist was evaluated by Apker et al.[4] The emergency physicians talked more during handover (67.4% vs. 32.3%) than hospitalists. The content of discussions focused on patient presentation (43.6%), professional environment (36%), and assessment (20.3%), with questions accounting for less than 10% of the dialogue.

Another high-risk area is the transition to hospital admission, typically involving a hospitalist service. Arora et al., in an expert consensus statement, recommend the use of a verbal handover, supplemented with written documentation in a structured format; or a technological solution.[5]

Pham et al. described the concern that the growth of hospitalist programs increases the burdens on coordination of care, and blurs accountability for post-discharge care.[6] These programs are more likely to employ standardized routines to ensure coordinated transitions between hospital admission and discharge.

Legal Analysis

Communication is an essential part of the transition of care process. In *Thomas* v. *Corso*, the patient presented to the ED after a pedestrian–motor vehicle accident and was admitted to a facility with on-call physicians and no resident physician assistance.[7] The nurse contacted the surgeon and discussed hypotension and tachycardia, but then the patient died. The surgeon acknowledged responsibility for the patient, but suggested that nursing communication implied he did not need to come in. The trial court awarded financial damages to the family; the physician and hospital defendants appealed. The Court of Appeals of Maryland affirmed the trial court judgment was not in error.

In *Kelley* v. *Middle Tennessee Emergency Physicians*, the patient presented with chest pain, was diagnosed with a myocardial infarction, and underwent a cardiac catheterization procedure 2 months before presenting to the ED with similar complaints.[8] The ED physician stated it was his normal practice to communicate with the patient's primary care physician (PCP), which was done in this case. He also attempted to contact her cardiologist, and spoke with the covering cardiologist discussing a normal-appearing EKG and troponin, and a discharge plan was generated. She followed up with her PCP and was told to follow up with cardiology. She subsequently attempted to notify the cardiology group of her chest pain, prior to her visit. However, she returned to the ED before the on-call cardiologist called back, and suffered an acute cardiopulmonary arrest. The trial court granted the defense summary judgment motion, holding that no valid patient–physician relationship existed with the cardiology group. This decision was reversed by the Court of Appeals and affirmed by the Supreme Court of Tennessee, Nashville remanding for reconsideration. They held that the consult by the ED physician with the on-call cardiologist for her cardiologist, in which there was a verbatim reading of the catheterization report by the ED physician, likely established the patient–physician relationship, and a subsequent duty. However, the final determination will rest again with the trial court jury.

Conclusion

The more this process becomes standardized, using electronic, reproducible, and recordable means, leaving less individual variation, providing more redundant services and controls, the more it will make for a better patient care transfer process.

References

1. Maughan BC, Lei L, Cydulka R. ED handoffs: observed practices and communication errors. *Am J Emerg Med.* 2011:29:502–511. DOI:10.1016/j.ajem.2008.12.004.

2. Venkatesh AK, Curley D, Chang Y, Liu SW. Communication of vital signs at emergency department handoff: opportunities for improvement. *Ann Emerg Med.* 2015;66:125–130. DOI:10.1016/j.annemergmed.2015.02.025.

3. Cheung DS, Kelly JJ, American College of Emergency Physicians Section of Quality Improvement and Patient Safety. Improving handoffs in the emergency department. *Ann Emerg Med.* 2010;55(2):171–180. DOI:10.1016/j.annemergmed.2009.07.016.

4. Apker J, Mallak LA, Applegate EB, Gibson SC, Ham JJ, Johnson NA, Street RL. Exploring emergency physician-hospitalist handoff interactions: development of the handoff communication assessment. *Ann Emerg Med.* 2010;55(2):161–170. DOI:10.106/j.annemergmed.2009.09.021.

5. Arora VM, Manjarrez E, Dressler DD, Basaviah P, Halasyamami L, Kripalani S. Hospitalist handoffs: a systematic review and task force recommendations. *J Hosp Med.* 2009;4(7):433–440.

6. Pham HH, Grossman JM, Cohen G, Bodenheimer T. Hospitalists and care transitions: the divorce of inpatient and outpatient care. *Health Aff.* 2008;27(5):1315–1327. DOI:10.1377/hlthaff.27.5.1315.

7. *Thomas v. Miller*, 288 A.2d 379 (1972).

8. *Kelley v. Middle Tennessee Emergency Physicians*, 133 S.W.3d 587 (2004).

Competence and Capacity

Case

This was the elderly woman's second visit to the emergency department (ED) in the last 2 weeks. She had fallen late last week and had a laceration and a slight concussion. She was back again today, as the family stated she had fallen again and this time had injured her wrist. This visit also revealed a forearm radial head fracture.

The family was concerned she was getting to the point where living by herself was not appropriate. They offered to try to get someone to stay and care for her, but she declined this option, saying she had always taken care of herself. She and her husband had always been self-sufficient, and had always done well together.

The ED physician again suggested that perhaps someone should stay with her, and she should be evaluated for a different living arrangement. She became angry and stated she had always managed her own affairs and finances. When this was explored further it appeared one of her utilities had been shut off because she had forgotten to pay a few bills recently. The provider conducted a Mini-Mental State Exam (MMSE) and found she indeed had some definite deficits. They suggested she should perhaps be admitted to the hospital to be further evaluated.

"You can't keep me here," she exclaimed. Social service intervention was offered, as well as an attempt to call her primary care physician (PCP), which she refused. Her family said she became irascible and angry with them as well. The staff went to make another call to her PCP, but the nurse summoned the physician because the patient was dressed and heading out the door. She was intercepted and redirected back to her room. She said she was going home, and if no one was taking her she was walking. The physician pointed out that since it was 20°F (−7°C) outside, walking home was probably not appropriate. She countered that she would walk 5 miles a day when she was younger. The family stated again that she was unsafe to go home and there were concerns about her decision-making, so she was admitted to the geriatric unit. Although she said she would go, she wasn't happy about it. As social service came to chat with her she attempted to throw them out of the room as well.

Medical Approach

Having one elderly parent survive the other is a more frequent occurrence as our population ages. The survivor has a diminished ability to go on alone without their spouse. Typically, when an elderly husband and wife function as a unit they often mask each other's potential deficiencies. Once one is gone, more problems seem to surface than when they were working as a team. Often the survivor is unwilling to be admitted to the hospital, because they don't want to lose their independence. But it is clear they are not capable of living independently.

The most important thing is to make sure of the elderly patient's safety. It is clear that as long as the elderly patient is capable of making their own decisions, caring for themselves, and meeting their financial needs they should live independently as long as they can. But, once they are deficient in any or all of these respects, then it is incumbent upon us to evaluate their situation and provide the best possible care. This may take the form of a more supervised living arrangement, or other assistance.

Formal analysis suggests that *competence* refers to the ability to make the proper legal judgment, while *capacity* refers to the ability to make clinical decisions.[1] The current standard of care is to have the physician determine the patient's capacity to consent, and to decide whether to seek substituted judgment or judicial review. We strive for an optimal balance of patient autonomy and safety.

Perhaps, the most difficult area in which to intervene is assessing capacity in the setting of alleged self-neglect.[2] At times, patients may retain their decision-making capacity, while still existing in marginal living conditions. The key then is if they have the capacity not only to recognize a tenuous living arrangement, but to extricate themselves from that situation.

Legal Analysis

The competence issue comes to the forefront in questions related to controversies of care. In *The Matter of William Schiller*, the patient who presented to the ED required a lower extremity amputation to prevent gangrene and was judged to be not capable of consent for the procedure by an examining psychiatrist.[3] The court granted the order to show cause, relying on *Barnert Memorial Hosp. Ass'n* v. *Young* (1972), in which the court appointed a family member as a special guardian to consent to an amputation in an adult patient incapable of consent.[4] The Superior Court of New Jersey, Chancery Division, observed that the patient usually selects their surgeon, but this is often not the case in the ED. The court appointed a special guardian with the capacity to consent to this procedure as the patient did not have the mental capacity to knowingly consent or refuse.

In *Miller* v. *Rhode Island Hospital*, the patient presented to the ED because of a motor vehicle accident after significant alcohol intake.[5] When asked about his injuries, he said they were multiple and he couldn't see because of the blood in his eyes. His fiancée, who was brought to the bedside and asked to consent for a diagnostic peritoneal lavage, referred to his sister for consent. The plaintiff declined to have the procedure, but was told he was not capable of deciding the state of his own injuries because of his drinking. He attempted to sit up but was physically restrained. A local anesthetic was administered and the procedure was performed. He signed out against medical advice (AMA) the next day. The trial court found the physician and facility liable for performing a procedure the patient declined, awarding compensatory and punitive damages. The defense expert testified that a life-threatening emergency existed, the state of intoxication rendered the physical exam unreliable, and the patient was not competent to consent. The trial court excluded this testimony, holding it commented on medical not legal competence:

> Legal competency is the assumption that an individual has a presumptive right to informed consent, compared to medical competence that is the result of the fact based subjective evaluation of whether an individual has the ability to consent to treatment, and what treatment is an individual's best interest.

The Supreme Court of Rhode Island heard the appeal from the physician and the hospital. They alleged that the patient was not competent to consent to surgery, based on his very high alcohol level. They held that his consent capacity may have been impaired, but the jury was required to consider evidence that would add to or detract from this premise. The defendants' appeal was sustained, judgment of the Superior Court was vacated and remanded for a new trial.

Conclusion

A crucial part of a proper mental status evaluation is the MMSE, which allows one to determine competence and decide on subsequent decision-making capability. If the patient is indeed competent, it is important to work with them to maintain their home situation. If the patient is not competent to make decisions, then health-care professionals should strive to make the best decision possible for their health, welfare, and safety.

References

1. Applebaum PS. Assessment of patient's competence to consent to treatment. *N Engl J Med.* 2007;357:1834–1840. DOI:10.1056/NEJMcp074045.

2. Naik AD, Lai JM, Kunik ME, Dyer CB. Assessing capacity in suspected cases of self-neglect. *Geriatrics.* 2008;63(2):24–31.

3. In the Matter of William Schiller, 372 A.2d 360 (1977).

4. *Barnert Memorial Hosp. Ass'n* v. *Young*, 63 N.J. 578 (1972).

5. *Miller* v. *Rhode Island Hospital*, 625 A.2d 788 (1993).

Confidentiality

Case

The emergency department (ED) was even more busy than usual. There were patients in the hallways as there was difficulty admitting patients to the hospital that day. For reasons of efficiency, patients were being evaluated in the hallway. The staff did what they could to maintain as much privacy as possible in the evaluation. However, history taking and some parts of physical exams were done in an open hallway.

Things seem to go reasonably well, in that all patients were seen and evaluated. Some patients were amused and one joked that it was "just like on TV here." Patients were discharged later that afternoon and evening, and some patients were sent to the floor. The last patients were moved into rooms for the remainder of their ED stay.

Some two weeks later there was contact from the patient experience coordinator, stating that one of the patients who had been in the hallway on that particular day had filed a complaint. There were concerns about confidentiality violation during the ED visit, relating to the lack of privacy created by the hallway bed boarding.

Medical Approach

We all recognize the need for patient confidentiality and most emergency medicine systems have ongoing training, education, and protocols to that effect. However, there are days when normal geographic boundaries and protections are unfortunately violated because of the need to care for many acute patients.

Perceptions of privacy and confidentiality in ED patients were reported by Olsen and Sabin.[1] They found 36% of patients overheard other patient conversations, while inappropriate staff comments were overheard by 1.6% of patients. Patients felt more comfortable relating their history in a walled room. Interestingly, the walled room allowed patients to hear more hall noise, while a curtained room allowed

conversation in the adjacent room space to be overheard. It is especially important to consider patient confidentiality in a busy ED setting.

Interestingly, physicians have a broad range of expectations regarding patient confidentiality. Elger reported the evaluation of patient vignettes by 378 primary care physicians and 130 hospital physicians compared to the evaluation by law school professors, medical students, and law school students.[2] They found that between 4% and 57% of physicians did not feel there were violations of confidentiality. Community physicians, students, and law professors reported a higher proportion of violations than the hospital physicians.

Legal Analysis

The typical concern is compromised patient confidentiality. In *Moses* v. *McWilliams*, the patient presented to the ED and was diagnosed with a pelvic infection, had surgery, and filed suit alleging malpractice.[3] The hospital retained an underwriting adjusting company to manage the claim. The company retained a medical expert witness, who contacted the patient's physician, without notifying her attorney or the patient herself. The trial court dismissed the appellant trespass action against the physicians, hospital, and underwriter. They then appealed this violation of patient confidentiality; and ex-parte discussion, in which the contact with an interested party or judge without attorney notification is improper. The Supreme Court of Pennsylvania reversed the trial court order and summary judgment for the defense for breach of confidentiality and inducement. They held there is a reasonable expectation of patient privacy and confidentiality that would have required the patient's consent to release.

In *Grand Jury Investigation* v. *Morgenthau*, an unidentified assailant allegedly stabbed a victim. Two years later a police investigation sought hospital ED records, specifically triage logs, for any individual fitting this description with a potential consistent injury.[4] The hospital asserted a patient–physician confidentiality privilege to maintain privacy of patient records under Civil Practice Laws and Rules (CPLR) 4504 (a).[5] The hospital felt the subpoenas would breach the statute, the district attorney held them in contempt, and the hospital moved to quash the subpoenas. The Court of Appeals of New York granted the district attorney leave to appeal, but affirmed the appellate decision to quash the subpoenas. The Supreme Court of New York denied both motions, but ordered the hospital to produce records for camera inspection. The Appellate Division unanimously reversed and granted the motion to quash the subpoenas, holding that, "The assessment of the nature and cause of the injury triggering production of the relevant documents involves an inherently medical evaluation."

In *Alsip* v. *Johnson City Medical Center*, the patient presented to the ED with a sore throat and was discharged with antibiotics. He returned the next day, a CT scan was performed and a specialist was consulted.[6] The specialist performed a procedure in the ED, encountered a bleeding complication, was informed of other medical history, and took the patient to the operating room after a delay in room availability. The patient died after a prolonged illness. The family filed suit for alleged malpractice. The trial court granted the defendant physician's motion for ex-parte communication with the patient's other physicians without consent. The sole legal authority appears to have been *Kilian* v. *Med. Educ. Assistance Corp., No. 22477* (2003), which permits ex-parte communication between defendant's counsel and plaintiff's physicians in a medical malpractice action if the following conditions are met (Table 20.1):

1. Court of pending action must authorize contact pursuant to defendant motion with plaintiff notice.
2. Information must only relate to condition for which treatment was sought and any time-relevant treatment for injury from the alleged malpractice where the defendant physician was still involved.
3. No defendant physician will be present.
4. No general discussion of malpractice cases and their practice impact.[7]

The trial court granted the plaintiff motion for interlocutory appeal, but stayed the order for appellate review. The Tennessee Court of Appeals struck down

Table 20.1 Medical malpractice ex-parte defense communication

1.	Court must authorize defense motion
2.	Specific to treated condition or consequences
3.	No defendant physician presence
4.	No general malpractice discussion

Reference: Kilian.[7]

the trial court order. The Supreme Court of Tennessee affirmed the Court of Appeals judgment and remanded for further proceedings. The issue balances society's legitimate desire for medical confidentiality against the medical malpractice defendant's need for full disclosure of all the patient's relevant health information. Although they recognize the need to obtain all relevant information, there are other approaches than the ex-parte communication pathway offered.

However, occasionally there are concerns related to the health-care provider's confidentiality in the setting of a medical panel review or malpractice litigation. For example, the Indiana Medical Malpractice Act requires that actions for medical negligence must be submitted to the medical review panel as a prerequisite to further legal action if a claim of more than $15,000 is sought in damages.[8] The act does provide the capacity for a contemporaneous court filing, provided there is no identifying information for the provider defendants (Table 20.2).

In *Kho* v. *Pennington*, the representative of the deceased patient filed a medical negligence claim with the Indiana State Medical Panel and there was a concurrent legal filing with identification of the defendants.[9] One of the defendant providers filed a motion for summary judgment alleging he did not care for the patient, and her lawyers dismissed him with stipulation. He subsequently commenced an action against the malpractice claimant, her attorney, and the law firm alleging emotional suffering, embarrassment, undue negative publicity, injury to reputation, and mental distress. The Court of Appeals affirmed the trial court's grant of summary judgment against the physician. However, the Supreme Court of Indiana held that this violation of physician defendant identity confidentiality provision is actionable as a violation of a statutory-based obligation. They held that the summary judgment was erroneously granted, prohibiting the statutory negligence claim for the undisputed violation of the physician confidentiality provision.

Table 20.2 Indiana Medical Malpractice Act: conditional exception

Section 4: Claim >$15,000 must be presented to the review panel
1. Court filing cannot contain any defendant identifier
2. Claimant prohibited from pursuing action
3. Court prohibited from taking action except setting trial date
4. Complaint amended once panel presentation met

Reference: Indiana Medical Malpractice Act.[8]

Table 20.3 Maintaining confidentiality in high census conditions

1. Take limited history out of hearing range of others
2. Establish geographic boundaries as feasible
3. Adequate spacing to ensure privacy
4. Activate hospital efficiency program to facilitate turnover

Conclusion

It is crucial to recognize that even in times of undue ED stress it is necessary to maximize available resources to maintain patient confidentiality. First, limited history should be obtained out of the hearing range of other patients and families. Second, geographic boundaries should be established as much as possible. Third, patients should be geographically isolated by spacing, when appropriate, while still ensuring patient safety. Fourth, hospital efficiency maneuvers should be activated to allow patients from the ED to be either admitted or discharged rapidly to increase the hospital's available bed space (Table 20.3).

References

1. Olsen JC, Sabin PR. Emergency department patient perceptions of privacy and confidentiality. *J Emerg Med.* 2003; 25(3):329–333. DOI:10.1016/S0736-4679(03)00216-6.

2. Elger BS. Violations of medical confidentiality: opinions of primary care physicians. *Br J Med Pract.* 2009;October:e344–e352. DOI:10.3399/bigp09X472647.

3. *Moses* v. *McWilliams*, 549 A.2d 950 (1988).

4. *Grand Jury Investigation* v. *Morgenthau*, 779 N.E.2d 173 (2002).

5. 2012 New York Consolidated Laws CVP – Civil Practice Law & Rules Article 45-CPLR 4504 (a): Evidence Physician, Dentist, Podiatrist, Chiropractor and Nurse.

6. *Alsip* v. *Johnson City Medical Center*, 197 S.W.3d 722 (2006).

7. *Kilian* v. *Med. Educ. Assistance Corp.*, No. 22477 (Washington County Law Court May 19, 2003).

8. Indiana Medical Malpractice Act: §34-18-8-4: Prerequisites to Commencement of Action; Presentation of Claim to Medical Review Panel, §34-18-8-7:Commencement of Action While Claim Being Considered by Medical Review Panel.

9. *Kho* v. *Pennington*, 875 N.E.2d 208 (2007).

Consultation

Case

As he was looking at the digitized image of the head CT scan on his computer monitor, the emergency department (ED) physician heard a voice from behind. It was the radiologist who said he was heading home, and he wanted to give someone the findings of the previous scan. He discussed an acute finding and then a more chronic abnormality that required additional referral. The physician asked the radiologist about the scan of the current patient, which was a pediatric head scan. He suggested that on closer inspection the CT "looked okay," but that was "unofficial" because technically he was off shift, and someone else would be reading the scan. The physician said his input was appreciated, because the lumbar puncture had to be performed here acutely. The radiologist said he would be back the next day, and an official read on the scan should be sent to the ED shortly. The ED staff waited for approximately another hour, without receiving a CT scan report. The child's fever was getting higher, and he was becoming a little more somnolent.

A lumbar puncture was performed, and he seemed to be a little worse clinically. He required admission, as the antibiotics ceftriaxone and vancomycin were started. The physician again reviewed the CT scan that had not yet been read by a radiologist. He called the incoming radiologist, who said that by and large, it looked okay, but that there was a little worsening and perhaps compromise of the interventricular space. The radiologist suggested this could be associated with worsening of the intracranial pressure. Radiology suggested that as the lumbar puncture had already been performed, the child would be okay. However, the patient was in fact more somnolent or sleepy and was admitted to the intensive care unit (ICU). The physician spoke with the attending pediatrician the next day and heard that the child had improved somewhat. But the radiology final report noted an increase in intracranial pressure as noted on the subsequent scan with loss of gray–white matter differentiation and effacement of sulci.

Subsequently, a call was received from risk management, who was concerned the lumbar puncture had been performed in the setting of an intracranial pressure alteration. The "curbside consult" with radiology was discussed. Although the attending radiologist who was going off shift said the CT looked normal, the neuroradiologist who subsequently read it officially thought it might be associated with an increased intracranial pressure. The clinical outcome was fine, but a concern was raised by the pediatric intensive care physician.

They concluded the procedure was appropriate, but that better coordination was needed on the reading and processing of critical findings between the radiologists and the ED staff.

Medical Approach

Often in the hospital setting we rely on consultation with our colleagues to improve patient care both on a primary care and specialty level. Most often there is an official consult with the medical evaluation, assessment, and treatment plan, but sometimes a curbside consult, or an unofficial opinion, may be offered. If one asks a colleague for an opinion and they give a helpful recommendation, without noting on the record the consult has been made, there is no official consultation. It is crucial to recognize that this type of consultation may not offer medicolegal protection, and should be avoided if possible. Such an informal consultation is appropriate, if at all, only for a brief, single event, low-complexity question.[1] Even then, there are numerous caveats, and this is not a recommended practice unless it is crucial for patient care at that point in time.

The primary care community has had exposure to the informal consultation process. Olick performed an analysis of the risk of legal liability in the informal consultation setting.[2] Courts have consistently ruled that there is no physician–patient relationship if an informal consultation is requested. Therefore, from the primary care perspective, if a consultant is asked for a curbside consult, no medicolegal protection is offered to the requesting physician, whatever the method of communication.

From the consultant perspective, Fox et al. suggested that the informal consultation is an obligation to the wider community of patients and physicians.[3] They also cite the risks associated with superficial involvement in the care of a specific patient without any formal recognition. They recommend that a proper consultation ensures accountability for the patient, the referring physician, the specialist, and the facility.

Legal Analysis

The caselaw in this area centers around the theme of a consultant suggesting uncertainty about the formal consultation. In *Cogswell* v. *Chapman and Eichner*, an infant suffered an eye injury, presented to the ED, and was seen by the physician's assistant (PA).[4] The PA was advised by the ED physician to contact the ophthalmologist who had a consulting/courtesy status at the facility. The ophthalmologist questioned and advised the PA, but did not want to personally examine the patient. The family testified the patient was examined by the ED physician, given a prescription for eye drops, and told to take acetaminophen (Tylenol or Advil) for pain. The ED physician stated he had no direct contact with the ophthalmologist, was surprised he did not want to evaluate, but did not call himself. The ophthalmologist stated he did not see patients in the ED, did not receive payment for these courtesy consults, did indeed ask questions concerning the patient, and did not feel he needed to evaluate based on those responses. The Supreme Court denied the defendant's summary judgment motion requesting dismissal due to the absence of a physician–patient relationship. The Appellate Division of the Supreme Court of the State of New York affirmed, holding that the totality of circumstances, including the telephone questioning and the discharge plan, established a relationship with the ophthalmologist.

In *Oja* v. *Kin*, the patient was brought to the ED with a facial gunshot wound. The specialty consultant was on call that evening.[5] This on-call physician was allegedly contacted three times that evening, but the ED resident was informed the physician was not feeling well and could not appear, and was told to find another physician. The patient was eventually transferred to another facility, where he died during an operative procedure. The trial court granted a summary judgment motion for the defendants, and plaintiff appealed. The Court of Appeals affirmed holding that the phone call dialogue did not establish a patient–physician relationship as every call to the consultant stated they could not appear and another physician should be found.

In *Diggs* v. *Arizona Cardiologists*, after conferring with the cardiologist, the ED physician diagnosed the patient with chest pain and discharged her home, where she died three hours later.[6] The ED evaluation consisted of an EKG with an electronic interpretation of myocardial infarction, but the ED physician thought her physical presentation was more consistent with pericarditis. He felt this conflict required discussion with a cardiologist. Coincidentally, a cardiologist was in the ED seeing another patient, although he was not on call. He offered to hear about the patient's presentation, reviewed the EKG, and agreed with the discharge plan, to follow up in their office in 10 days. The official EKG interpretation was that an acute myocardial infarction was present.

The trial court exonerated the cardiologist, holding that the interaction amounted to an informal consultation that did not give rise to the duty of care. The Court of Appeals of Arizona, Division 1, reversed the grant of summary judgment to the cardiology defendant and remanded the case for further consideration. They held that as soon as the cardiologist rendered an opinion, the ED physician subordinated to his decision-making, and the consultant effectively became a care provider to this patient.

In *Schroeder* v. *Albaghdadi*, the patient was transported to the ED with shortness of breath two weeks after three-vessel cardiac bypass.[7] The evaluation revealed evidence of a heart attack of uncertain age and a high potassium level. The cardiologist was contacted for admission and requested the EKG should be faxed to his home. Although the conversation was in dispute retrospectively, the cardiologist called back, suggesting the patient could be sent home with office follow-up in a day or two. This conversation was documented by the ED physician on the physical exam form. The cardiologist alleged the ED physician told him the EKG looked abnormal, but not that the patient had recent bypass surgery, and did not relate the laboratory information. The patient returned the next morning and suffered a cardiopulmonary arrest. The family filed suit, and the trial court presented an alternative jury instruction assuming two considerations in the finding of negligence in which the cardiologist, (1) was not told about the high potassium level and did not interpret the EKG correctly, or (2) had a more comprehensive responsibility for proper EKG interpretation, evaluation, diagnosis, and admission. The trial court jury found for a defense verdict, and the appeal followed. The Court of Appeals of Iowa found error in that the jury warranted an instruction that would have allowed the capacity to find fault beyond mere EKG misinterpretation. The judgment was reversed, and remanded for consideration. They held that the trial court usurped the jury's ability to determine liability by presenting the either/or instruction.

In *Mead* v. *Legacy Health System*, the patient presented to the ED with severe low back pain and leg weakness, so the ED attending physician and resident were concerned about cauda equina syndrome.[8] They ordered an MRI which demonstrated an L3–4 disk herniation, and contacted the on-call neurosurgeon. The ED physician presented the case, requested admission, and documented the discussion. The neurosurgeon allegedly recommended discharge and bed rest, which the ED physician recommended against, and settled on primary care admission at the surgeon's request. The neurosurgeon felt that if the patient worsened, he would be contacted. He was apparently contacted after a number of attempts by various providers and performed surgery with residual deficit. The trial court jury concluded that no valid patient–physician relationship existed. The Court of Appeals of Oregon reversed and remanded for new trial with preemptory instruction to the jury on the patient–physician relationship.

The consensus of jurisdictions that have considered the question is that a physician–patient relationship can arise:

> by the implied consent of the physician based on indirect contact between the physician and the patient thorough telephone communication between a hospital emergency room physician and an on-call physician concerning the care of the emergency room patient. The pivotal inquiry is whether the on-call physician affirmatively participates in care of the patient. That affirmative participation exists if the on-call physician undertakes to diagnose or treat the patient.

The Court of Appeals of Oregon concluded that the on-call physician who affirmatively undertakes to diagnose or treat an ED patient over the telephone implies consent to a physician–patient relationship for the purposes of negligence liability.

Conclusion

Often the consultant asks, "Do I have to put a note in the record"? The answer should be yes, for the protection of the patient, the consulting physician, and the physician requesting the consult. In addition, to be fair to the consultant, a written order request for consultation is required so that proper procedure is followed, and the consultant is protected too.

References

1. Manian FA, Janssen DA. Curbside consultations: a closer look at a common practice. *JAMA*. 1996;275(2): 145–147.

2. Olick RS, Bergus GR. Malpractice liability for informal consultation. *Family Med*. 2003;35(7):476–481.

3. Fox BC, Siegel ML, Weinstein RA. "Curbside" consultation and informal communication in medical practice: a medicolegal perspective. *Clin Infect Dis*. 1996;23:616–622.

4. *Cogswell* v. *Chapman and Eichner*, 672 N.Y.S.2d 460 (1998).

5. *OJA* v. *Kin*, 581 N.W.2d 739 (1998).

6. *Diggs* v. *Arizona Cardiologists*, 8 P.3d 386 (2000).

7. *Schroeder* v. *Albaghdadi*, No. 6-1024/06-0243 (2007).

8. *Mead* v. *Legacy Health System*, 220 P.3d 118 (2009).

Controlled Substances

Case

The patient was well known to the system. He had made multiple visits to the emergency department (ED) for various pain complaints. There was usually an accompanying administrative complaint if his preferred medications were not prescribed. These requests were accommodated by some providers, but others would not provide additional prescriptions for controlled substances. One particular practice is based on the presence or absence of objective findings rather than subjective report of pain. In this instance, the patient had fallen and injured his right ankle. It was quite badly swollen, a grade III sprain. He was prescribed hydrocodone and acetaminophen, and was discharged home.

Later that evening a police officer who had come by the ED for another purpose stated the patient had been in a motor vehicle accident. It was a minor accident and he was suspected of driving under the influence. During his arrest, he stated he had just left the hospital, after he was prescribed pain medications. "They prescribe them to me all the time, they know I have a problem."

Two weeks later, the physician was subpoenaed as a witness concerning the accident and allegedly prescribing controlled substances while the patient was operating a motor vehicle.

Medical Approach

The prescribing of controlled substances is perhaps one of the most controversial issues in the practice of acute care medicine today. Numerous external regulatory agencies are intimately involved in prescribing practice. There are recommendations to prescribe more analgesics, to monitor under-prescribing and to ensure pain control; while other agencies hope to monitor and restrict overprescribing practice.

Physicians have a clear moral, ethical, and legal obligation to relieve suffering. Reasons offered for the potential under-treatment of pain, described as barriers to effective pain relief, are summarized in Table 22.1.[1] First, insufficient knowledge concerning the assessment and treatment of pain. Second, the failure of health-care professionals and institutions to make pain relief a priority. Third, lack of accountability for providing effective pain relief. Fourth, physician concerns about regulatory scrutiny of their prescribing practice. Fifth, persistence of myths and misinformation about addiction, tolerance, and adverse side effects.

Brennan et al. discussed the premise that pain management is a fundamental human right as described by the World Health Organization.[2] They suggest an etiology related to the biomedical model of disease focusing on pathophysiology, rather than quality of life. They suggest we are at an inflection point, where an unreasonable failure to treat pain is viewed worldwide as poor medicine, unethical practice, and abrogation of a fundamental human right.

However, Denisco and others have questioned the problem of opiate misuse and chronic pain treatment.[3] They point out the increasing trend for opioid prescription availability for chronic non-cancer pain and a potential association with opioid misuse. The intersection of these two public health problems remain a concern, and is an ongoing matter of significant controversy.

Medical professional organizations have weighed in on this difficult issue. The Emergency Nurse Association (ENA) approach is to accept the patient's subjective pain assessment, provide education, use evidence-based assessment tools, collaborate, use thorough documentation, and emphasize dignity and respect.[4] The Washington Emergency Department Opioid Prescribing Guidelines were promulgated by a multidisciplinary group, specifying defined treatment

Table 22.1 Barriers to effective pain relief

1. Insufficient knowledge concerning pain management
2. Failure to make pain management a priority
3. Lack of accountability to provide effective pain relief
4. Regulatory scrutiny concerns
5. Persistence of addiction myths

Reference: Rich.[1]

protocols and goals to treat chronic pain in the ED setting.[5]

Legal Analysis

The caselaw can be problematic as well. In *Bergman v. Wing Chin, MD and Eden Medical Center*, the plaintiffs prevailed in a suit alleging pain under-treatment and involving both the physician and the facility.[6] The patient had a five-day stay in a nursing facility, where his pain was rated between 7 and 10 on a 10-point pain scale. On the day of discharge, however, the pain was rated 10. The patient had a presumptive diagnosis of lung cancer, declined further treatment, requested discharge to hospice, and succumbed within a week. The family felt pain treatment standards were not met and could be enforced by the legal process. In conjunction with a pain treatment advocacy group, they filed a medical board complaint against the treating physician. The medical board declined to take any action. The family, with assistance, filed an action based on the California Elder Abuse and Dependent Adult Civil Protection Act §§15600–15675, and prevailed with a significant financial award.[7] Patients also have rights related to pain control interventions as mandated by the Joint Commission dictating the assessment, monitoring, and treatment achieving pain control goals.[8]

In addition, physicians can be blamed after injury or death in the setting of prescribed medications. In *Posner* v. *Walker*, the Florida District Court of Appeals reversed the trial court ruling awarding damages to the patient's family for an inadvertent prescription drug overdose.[9] The physician, a board-certified orthopedic surgeon, managed the patient's long-standing back pain with 30-day narcotic analgesics prescriptions and physical therapy. The patient was referred to the pain service, refused the recommendation, and was discharged from the physician's care.

She then allegedly obtained multiple prescriptions for various narcotic analgesics and benzodiazepines from different providers, as well as from the ED. After an ED visit for a traumatic injury, she died at home. The family representatives alleged negligence in that the physician should have weaned her from the narcotic analgesics to prevent her death. The trial court originally awarded a $1.9 million verdict, which the appeal court overturned, stating the physician's treatment strategy was appropriate, and the plaintiff's representative failed to establish a causal link to this untoward outcome.

In *Iodice* v. *United States of America*, after a car crash an action was filed against the United States pursuant to the Federal Tort Claims Act.[10] The plaintiff alleged that employees of the Veterans' Administration (VA) hospital negligently dispensed narcotics, and failed to institute, enforce, and monitor adequate policies that proximately and foreseeably caused his injuries. The patient had been treated for 15 years after an accident, was allegedly prescribed excessive pain medication, was listed in a monitoring registry, and his family requested prescription limitation. The district court dismissed their complaints, which was affirmed by the United States Court of Appeals, Fourth Circuit. The question raised was whether a third-party victim could bring a properly pled negligence action against the patient's medical care providers. Even if such a claim exists under state law, the plaintiffs had not alleged the facts to support such a claim. However, the VA had more responsibility than the typical social host in an intoxication action.

Conclusion

It is a constant struggle to balance patients' pain control needs, service expectations, dependence or tolerance, and evidence-based medical standards. As always, our goal is to ensure the best care possible for patients, which sometimes requires multidisciplinary care pathways.

References

1. Rich BA. Physician's legal duty to relieve suffering. *West J Med.* 2001;175(3):151–152. PMCID: PMC 1071521.
2. Brennan F, Carr DB, Cousins M. Pain management: a fundamental right. *Anesth Analg.* 2007;105(1):205–221. PMID 17578977.

3. Denisco RA, Chandler RK, Compton WM. Addressing the intersecting problems of opioid misuse and chronic pain treatment. *Exp Clin Psychopharmacol.* 2008;16(5):417–428. DOI:10.1037/a0013636.

4. Emergency Nurses Association. *Care of patients with chronic/ persistent pain in the emergency setting.* (Des Plaines, IL: ENA, 2014).

5. Washington Emergency Department Opioid Prescribing Guidelines. July 2011, www.washingtonacep.org/painmedication.htm.

6. *Bergman* v. *Wing Chin*, and Eden Medical Center, No. H205732-1 (Cal. App. Dept Super Ct 1999).

7. California Elder Abuse and Dependent Adult Civil Protection Act §§15600–15675.

8. Patient Rights. Accreditation Manual (Oakbrook Terrace, IL: Joint Commission for the Accreditation of Healthcare, 2000), RI 1.1.

9. *Posner* v. *Walker*, 930 So. 2d 659 (2006).

10. *Iodice* v. *USA*, 289 F.3d 270 (2002).

Criminal Charges

Case

The staff physician was nominated to serve on the hospital credentialing committee. During the first meeting, there was discussion concerning a potential addition to the medical staff. This new member of the medical staff came highly recommended with excellent evaluations, a good training background, and fellowship training as well. It appeared there were a couple of items still missing from the file, so the application was tabled until the next month's meeting, according to the staff credentialing guidelines.

At that next credentialing committee meeting, it was time for a final approval vote. Those present then noted the criminal background check returned a felony charge in a different state. This had apparently not been noted by the state medical licensing board. Discussion with the physician stated he had indeed committed that infraction, however, he stated it was not a felony but a misdemeanor and his lawyer would be in touch. On further checking, it appeared there was a valid felony charge in a different state. In addition, one of the committee members found the information on an Internet search. The state licensing board for that state had a moral turpitude clause and the facility declined the credentialing application and appointment to medical staff.

Approximately one month later the medical staff office received a summons of suit, alleging wrongful denial of privileges based on improper motives. The physician stated that refusing to appoint him was anticompetitive, economically inclined, and discriminatory. The case was referred to the hospital attorney for assistance.

Medical Approach

The judicial standard for most credentialing committees is that hospitals historically have been given fairly wide scope to make their own decisions concerning credentialing and staff privileges. However, physicians have challenged the credentialing process about issues that appear on their record. Clearly, in this case, there was a criminal infraction that was listed as a felony. Many state licensing boards have a moral turpitude clause that rules out appointing anyone with a felony on their record to the clinical staff.

Legal Analysis

In similar cases the facility alleges quality issues, while the physician alleges anticompetitive activity. The first cluster centers on alleged behavioral issues affecting staff privileges. In *Westlake Community Hospital* v. *Superior Court*, a physician sued two private hospitals, staff, board, and committee members over revocation of staff privileges after committee credential review and recommendation.[1] There was extensive due process involving the hospital chief of staff, ad hoc evaluation, and executive committee, all of which arrived at a decision to revoke staff privileges. The Supreme Court of California felt that a physician who is denied staff privileges must exhaust all available internal remedies before instituting any judicial action, including seeking damages. However, the court rejected the defense premise of absolute immunity when a quasi-judicial proceeding denies or revokes staff privileges. If denial of privileges action is found to be improper in a mandate action, an excluded physician may proceed in tort against the hospital, board, or committee members. The Supreme Court of California held that a preemptory writ of mandamus should issue, directing the trial court to vacate the challenged order insofar as such orders deny defendant motion for summary judgment with respect to the revocation of staff privileges (Code Civ. Proc. §437c, 6th para).[2] However, the plaintiff must set aside the quasi-judicial revocation before she may maintain the tort action for damages.

In *Bryan* v. *James A. Holmes Regional Medical Center*, a staff physician had his clinical privileges terminated after a lengthy internal disciplinary process, and additional disciplinary incidents after the review started.[3] The staff at the facility thought he was an excellent surgeon, tackling difficult cases, but he was allegedly difficult to work with. He alleged that he offered constructive criticism, and that due process was not followed in this action. The trial court concluded that facility had revoked his staff privileges in violation of bylaws, awarding $4.2 million in damages for breach of contract. The trial court decision was reversed by the United States Court of Appeals (USCA), Eleventh Circuit, finding that the hospital was immune from liability in monetary damages under the Health Care Quality Improvement Act of 1986, and under Florida state law.[4,5] They held that since the physician was not entitled to recover financial damages, the hospital post-trial motion for judgment as a matter of law denial was reversed.

Other facilities have encountered and addressed issues that may rise to the level of criminal activity. In *Landefield* v. *Marion General Hospital, Inc.*, a staff physician had his clinical privileges revoked after allegedly removing, disrupting, or discarding mailbox contents belonging to other physician recipients, activity which was captured on a hidden camera in the physician lounge.[6] The hospital's medical executive committee voted to suspend and the physician then requested a post-suspension hearing. The hearing board issued a non-binding recommendation that he be reinstated with an extensive list of probationary conditions. The board declined, as there was allegedly evidence that patient health information records were corrupted as well. The physician alleged that his aberrant behavior was due to an undiagnosed mental illness, and that with treatment he could return to effective practice. The board established a treatment and recovery plan with requirements for rehabilitation. The physician reapplied within two weeks, was declined, and obtained privileges at another facility 4 months later. The physician filed suit alleging he was "otherwise qualified" except for his illness, if "reasonable accommodation" was made for his "handicap." He contended his discharge was violative of Section 504 of the Rehabilitation Act of 1973, guaranteeing certain rights to people with disabilities.[7] The district court ruled for the defendant, ruling that the plaintiff had not proven a prima facie case that this handicap was the sole cause of this behavior. The USCA, Sixth Circuit affirmed the trial court decision, as there was ample evidence, and hospital consensus in decision-making, to support the denial of the physician's clinical privileges.

Conclusion

For most credentialing decisions, it is best to start with a wide-ranging evaluation followed by a state medical licensing board inquiry. Often the hospital must wait for the licensing board to make an official decision, which delays the hospital credentialing committee decision.

References

1. *Westlake Community Hospital* v. *Superior Court*, 551 P.2d 410 (1976).

2. California Code of Civil Procedure §437c: Summary Judgment.

3. *Bryan* v. *James E. Holmes Regional Medical Center*, 33 F.3d. 1318 (1994).

4. Florida Statute Annotated §395.0193 (51993): Licensed Facilities; Peer Review; Disciplinary Powers; Agency or Partnership with Physicians.

5. Health Care Quality Improvement Act of 1986 (HCQIA), 42 U.S.C. §§11101–11152 (1988) & Supp IV (1992).

6. *Landefield* v. *Marion General Hospital, Inc.*, 994 F.2d. 1178 (1993).

7. §504 Federal Rehabilitation Act of 1973, 29 U.S.C. §701 et seq.

Chapter 24

Criminal Acts

Case

The chief complaint for the patient's visit to the emergency department (ED) was multiple skin lacerations. The nurse told the ED physician she had some concerns about the presentation, which seemed a little unusual. When the patient was examined he was found to have a wound on his back which looked more like a stab wound than a laceration. In addition, he had some abrasions on his hands. The physician asked what had happened. The patient said he had slipped and hit some broken glass, and that was how he got the cut on his back. The physician ordered some radiologic imaging, and found no pneumothorax or evidence of vascular injury. The surgeon was then consulted for additional help with management. The patient became a little irate and said that he had to leave: "Could you just sew this thing up so we can go?" His girlfriend also said they had to go, because they had children at home.

At this point security began to check if local law enforcement had any concerns. They said they were obliged to contact law enforcement, either due to the alleged criminal concern or due to the potential for an alleged assault, which also would require mandatory reporting to law enforcement. The local police responded quickly and said there had been a burglary, and the alleged perpetrator had been confronted and possibly injured by the homeowner. Security asked the ED physician if they were to keep the patient here until the police arrived. She replied that she wasn't sure if they were allowed to do this, but security should follow their appropriate protocol. The physician would try talk to the patient to help him understand the circumstances.

Medical Approach

Cases such as this are often problematic, being at the intersection of patient confidentiality and the mandatory law-enforcement reporting obligations. These obligations tend to be based on state statutory regulations that list alleged criminal acts and the obligation to report. Some are in the patient's best interest and are meant to be protective. Anyone who has undergone an assault that involved infliction of bodily force, or use of a weapon in that assault, is truly a victim. There is also a requirement to protect the public, when there is an allegation that a crime has been committed or someone else in society is at risk from ongoing violent acts.

These cases often present with complex interactions resulting in a moral, ethical, and legal quandary. The treatment pathway is inherently obvious, but the interface with the legal system presents a challenge.

There is a distinction in reporting requirements, in which the incident in question "comes to the attention," or the patient "comes under treatment" of the reporting physician before the obligation is triggered.[1] As an example, the Arizona Law Mandatory Reporting Statute states the physician is obligated to report any gunshot wound likely to have been inflicted by an unlawful act and to notify the "chief of police" immediately.[2]

The problematic choices are these: first, in a healthcare setting should one, from an ethical perspective, report suspected criminal activity occurring outside the facility? Our primary job is to deliver health care, and the reporting could prevent those predisposed from seeking health care in the future. Second, are we obligated from a legal perspective, and can we be held liable for failing to report? The answer is clearly yes, based on the severity of the infraction, occurrence in a vulnerable population, or where reporting is compulsory under the law. Third, can a patient be prevented from leaving to await law enforcement? The answer is typically no, unless law enforcement has an active warrant and require the patient to remain on the premises until their arrival. Patients who present a significant danger to themselves or others can be restrained under an involuntary commitment premise.

Ideally, the patient will be convinced to have the appropriate medical treatment, as well as having the appropriate officials notified and involved. Referring to this as a public safety issue, rather than a law enforcement intervention, can often help the patient and family to understand the situation.

Legal Analysis

The interface between law enforcement and patients in the ED can often be complicated. In *People v. Cage*, the sheriff service was summoned twice to a residence for a family altercation.[3] A patient was transported to the ED with a deep facial laceration. The ENT consultant asked him what happened. The patient (a minor son) related the history of an alleged deliberate act by his mother and grandmother. The defendant was convicted of aggravated assault with the injured party's statement to law enforcement awarded evidentiary value. It survived a hearsay exception challenge since the utterance was made in the context of medical decision-making by a physician providing care, rather than in the setting of law enforcement intervention. The trial court convicted the defendant, affirmed by the court of appeal as well as the Supreme Court of California. They relied on the Supreme Court of the United States (USSC) decision in *Crawford v. Washington* (2004) for determining when the Confrontation Clause of the Sixth Amendment prohibits the use of hearsay evidence, an out-of-court statement offered for its truth against a criminal defendant.[4,5] *Crawford* protects the accused against hearsay uttered by one who spoke at a witness if the declarant neither takes the stand at trial nor was otherwise available for cross-examination by the accused. It allows "testimonial statements" that may occur in the setting of law enforcement, or by extension a medical inquiry.

In *Chavez* v. *Martinez*, a suspect who was allegedly armed with a knife struggled for an officer's gun, achieved control, and was shot by another officer.[6] The suspect was taken to the ED and was questioned by police while receiving treatment for a sustained period. The questioning was intermittent and lasted 10 minutes over a 45-minute period. The suspect objected to the questioning, and allegedly did not receive a Miranda warning.[7] He was never charged with a crime, and his answers were not used in any criminal prosecution. He filed suit under 42 U.S. Code §1983, establishing a civil action for deprivation of rights, claiming his Fifth Amendment not to be compelled to testify against himself, or his Fourteenth Amendment, substantive due-process right to be free from coercive questioning.[8,9] The district court granted summary judgment to the patient as to the officer's qualified immunity claim. The patrol supervisor took an interlocutory appeal to the United States Court of Appeals (USCA), Ninth Circuit, which affirmed the district court's denial of immunity. They held that a reasonable officer, "would have known that persistent interrogation of the suspect despite repeated requests to stop violated the suspect's rights." The USSC granted certiorari and issued a judgment stating no constitutional rights were violated through a complex series of decisions. However, the only opinion to gain a majority vote was the concurrence that remanded the case to reconsider the substantive due-process case.

In *Johnson* v. *Deep East Regional Narcotics Trafficking Task Force*, a series of warrants were executed and a home was entered but the suspect was not found. The occupant of the home was asked if she had any medical needs, although there was no contact with any of the officers.[10] However, later in the day she presented to the ED with chest pain and was hospitalized for 3 days. She filed suit under 42 U.S.C. §1983 alleging violation of her Fourth Amendment right to be free of unreasonable search and seizure.[8,10,11] The court granted summary judgment motions for the officers, holding they were entitled to qualified immunity and no actionable police policy deviation was pled. The USCA, Fifth Circuit affirmed the dismissal.

Conclusion

Patients with trauma or exacerbation of chronic medical conditions often present to the ED in the setting of law enforcement intervention, for diagnosis, treatment, and medical clearance. Because these are often unusual or unique cases, clear security protocols are required regarding the rules health-care providers should follow. The goal of physicians, nurses, security, and law enforcement personnel is to care for the patient's health and well-being, as well as for society in general.

References

1. Smith HM. Legal requirements for notification, in *Ethics in Emergency Medicine*, eds. K. Iverson, A. Sanders, D. Mathieu and A. Buchanan, 2nd edition (Baltimore, MD: Williams and Wilkins, 1995), pp. 92–97.

2. Arizona Revised Statutes, Article 1: Prevention of Offenses, Title 13–3806.

3. *People* v. *Cage*, 155 P.3d 205, 56 Cal. Rptr. 3D 789 (2007).

4. *Crawford* v. *Washington*, 541 U.S. 36, 124 S. Ct. 1354 (2004).

5. U.S. Const. Amend VI.

6. *Chavez* v. *Martinez*, 538 U.S. 760 (2003).

7. *Miranda* v. *Arizona*, 384 U.S. 436 (1966).

8. 42 U.S. Code §1983, Civil Action for Deprivation of Rights.

9. U.S. Const. Amend V.

10. *Johnson* v. *Deep East Texas Regional Narcotics Trafficking Task Force*, 379 F.3d 293 (2004).

11. U.S. Const. Amend IV.

Death Certification

Case

The patient was still relatively young, in his late forties. He had some heart disease and hypertension and was cared for by a local primary care physician (PCP). He had chest pain that began at home and was in full cardiac arrest when the medics brought him into the emergency department (ED). The ED staff continued the usual resuscitative efforts without avail. After 20 minutes of additional resuscitation he was still in asystole and the code was called, discontinuing resuscitative efforts.

The nurses asked for a physician to fill out the death certificate. It was explained to the patient's family that the ED doctor would be the certifying physician, discussing the events that happened today. But the actual cause of death would need to be filled out by the patient's PCP. The PCP was called, the circumstances of his patient's presentation were discussed, and he was asked if he would be the certifying physician for cause of death. He was a little hesitant, and said that although the patient did have heart disease, his death was unexpected and he would prefer to have the coroner called.

The coroner was called and the circumstances surrounding the patient's presentation were discussed. The coroner concluded that at least on his initial evaluation based on the patient's age, presentation, and past health history, this was not an unexpected death. He then suggested that since the ED physician had spoken with both the PCP and the coroner's office, all parties should discuss and arrive at the certification confirmation. That certification and authorization process was then done with the PCP certifying a cause of death, and the patient was taken to the morgue.

Medical Approach

The certification process can sometimes be complicated in the emergency setting. There is a pronouncing physician, typically an ED staff member who evaluates, treats, and cares for the patient, and establishes time of death. The certification process typically involves the PCP, who performs a hierarchical analysis of the patient's actual health conditions and then decides the ultimate cause of death.

Lastly, the coroner is involved in particular types and circumstances of cases that may center on the unexpected nature or unusual circumstances of a death. Unexpected deaths are those in which an individual who seemed otherwise healthy then suffered a catastrophic sudden death. The unusual circumstances of concern are deaths of young people, elderly patients who are in the health-care setting with low-risk conditions, or people who are incarcerated.

The physician's responsibility for proper death certification can be taxing in a busy ED. The importance of proper documentation cannot be underestimated. There are repercussions for the deceased patient, families, and public health initiatives. The pronouncing physician is responsible for filling out the certificate, compliant with established guidelines, usually within 72 hours.[1] The certifying physician is complemented by the physician who was in charge of the patient's condition that resulted in death, or in attendance at time of death. The certifying physician should definitively specify the primary condition causing death, followed by the secondary or contributing cause, lastly the underlying disease cause with duration of onset. Proper documentation is especially important since these matters are often disclosed as part of a public record.

Legal Analysis

In *People* v. *Holder*, an issue arose concerning a completed and certified death certificate.[2] The trial court found the defendant guilty of vehicular manslaughter and he appealed his guilty verdict. He alleged that guilt had not been proven beyond a reasonable doubt, citing the death certificate as part of the rationale. They cited the fact that the certificate did not have an "underlying cause" specified and was blank, as well as an "accident" description in the "injury information" space. The California Court of Appeals affirmed the trial court judgment, stating that in totum there was clear sufficiency of evidence to convict. Health and Safety Code 10252 provides that the coroner shall state on the death certificate, that "the disease or condition directly relating to death, antecedent causes, other significant conditions contributing to death and such other medical and health section data as may be required of the certificate, and the hour and day in which the death occurred."[3] Section 10577 of the same code declares that a properly certified copy of the certificate is prima facie evidence of the facts stated therein.

In *The Home News* v. *State of New Jersey, Department of Health*, the cause of death was sought from the release of the death certificate from a pediatric murder victim.[4] The local newspaper cited the Right-To-Know Law, formalizing the common-law right to inspect public documents as their rationale.[5] However, the New Jersey Annotated Code (NJAC) 8:2A-1.2 provides an exclusion exception allowing the cause of death to be omitted from the released certificate unless the executor, surviving spouse, or parent consents, or previous consent was provided.[6] The Supreme Court of New Jersey held that the public good benefits outweighs the individual benefit of the confidentiality of the death certificate. They reversed the appellate court judgment, dismissing the plaintiff complaint and requiring disclosure of the complete death certificate.

In *Esgro* v. *Trezza*, the petitioner filed for an order of exhumation of her deceased husband, since no autopsy was ever performed, and the physician accused of negligence was the certifying physician for cause of death.[7] The patient presented in cardiac arrest shortly after an office visit. This trial court order issued an exhumation order and then stayed that order allowing the superior court a chance to rule. The writ of certiorari was denied as there was no compelling reason to review, or order an exhumation. The benefits of exhumation over the signed death certificate were not substantiated by the petitioner so it was declined by the District Court of Appeal of Florida, Fourth District.

Conclusion

The coroner's involvement often includes forensic analysis and a legal determination of cause of death, either natural or unnatural. The coroner is required to investigate all unnatural deaths, deaths in which the primary physician is unable to state the cause of death, or when the deceased did not have a physician. However, families typically want to know the medical cause of death. This is usually obtained in the routine process of health-care delivery, but is sometimes still distinct and different from what is normally expected. In that case, additional autopsy intervention may be required to define the actual cause of death.

References

1. Physician's Responsibility in Death Registration. Chapter 4 – Registration of Deaths. Vital Signs Registration Handbook, Death Edition, 2006 Revision A; 13–17.

2. *People* v. *Holder*, 230 Cal. App. 2d 50.

3. New Jersey Health and Safety Code §10252, 10577.

4. *The Home News* v. *State of New Jersey, Department of Health, et al.*, 224 N.J. Super. 7, 539 A.2d. 736.

5. New Jersey Statutes Annotated. §47:1A-1.4.

6. New Jersey Death Regulations. §8:2A-2.1.

7. *Esgro* v. *Trezza*, 492 So. 2d 422 (1986).

Decision-Making

Case

The patient was born with cerebral palsy, and had quite limited physical capability. Her cognitive ability was not impaired, and her parents were able to maintain her at home for most of her childhood and adolescence. But once she became an adult, her parents' resources were limited, and they were unable to care for her in a proper way. She was living in a group residential home, so that she could be better assisted in her daily activities. She had been healthy and happy there in the month since her transition, but had recently become ill with fever due to recurrent urinary tract infections.

A recent episode required that she be hospitalized with what appeared to be urosepsis. As the paramedics were driving in, she began to have agonal respirations. As they transported her to the emergency department (ED) the staff quickly started broad-spectrum antibiotics, including aminoglycosides. They were able to resuscitate her sufficiently to be admitted to the intensive care unit (ICU).

When the admission was discussed with the intensivist, she asked if the patient had an advance directive. The ED physician said that this was complicated. There was an advance directive from the residential home stating she was to be a full code, with no limitations on resuscitative effort applied. However, her parents who were with her stated she had suffered enough and they wanted to let her go. At this point, the intensivist asked what she should do. The ED physician pointed out that the institutionalization process often involves a transfer of guardianship so that the facility and/or guardian has the responsibility for medical decision-making. Obviously, the parents would be acting in the patient's stead since she was not competent to make a decision in her current condition, and their wishes were in disagreement with the advance directive completed by the legal guardian.

It was suggested that social service and case management input might be helpful and the patient was then transferred to the ICU. Certainly, an ethics consult or legal counsel review may be warranted, if decisions are at odds.

Medical Approach

The patient's right of self-determination is well established and continues as long as they are competent. Once they lose their competence, their treatment can be directed by a pre-stated advance directive stating their wishes, which cannot be overturned by another party. If there is no such advance directive, then there is a "substituted judgment" argument, in which the nearest relative – in this case the parents – must make a decision based on the patient's likely wishes in that clinical situation.

Legal Analysis

In *The Matter of Claire C. Conroy*, the question raised was whether life-sustaining treatment may be withheld or withdrawn from an incompetent, institutionalized elderly patient with severe, permanent mental and physical impairments and limited life expectancy.[1] The nephew and guardian of an incompetent patient in a nursing facility sought discontinuation of a nasogastric tube being used for nutrition. No question was raised concerning the relative's intention, and her submission supported removal. The trial court agreed that removal of the tube should be permitted as the patient's life had become "impossibly and permanently burdensome." The guardian ad litem appealed, and the patient died with the feeding tube in place. However, the Appellate Division reversed the trial court's decision. The Supreme Court of New Jersey reversed the appellate decision, holding that these considerations should be "conducive to the humane, dignified and decent ending of life." Subjective requests are used for support limitation when requests are clearly stated, while objective tests are used when the wishes of the patient are not clearly known. The Supreme Court of New Jersey held that life-sustaining treatment may be withheld or withdrawn if either of the "best interests" tests – limited objective or pure objective test – is satisfied.

- The "limited objective" test requires that, (1) trustworthy evidence exists that the patient would have refused the treatment, and (2) the decision-maker is satisfied that the burden of continuing life with treatment outweighs the benefits of life. This test is used when there is some, but not definitive, evidence of a pre-stated wish to withdraw.
- The "pure objective" test criteria are met when the burdens "clearly and markedly" outweigh the benefits of life; support can then be withdrawn. This test is used when the patient does not have a clearly documented support limitation request.

In *Cruzan* v. *Director, Missouri Department of Health*, the patient was left in a "persistent vegetative state" and rendered incompetent after a motor vehicle accident.[2] Her parents and co-guardians petitioned for a court order to withdraw support (feeding and hydration) after it was clear there was no possibility of cognitive recovery. The Supreme Court of Missouri held there was no clear and convincing evidence that the patient had any desire to have medical treatment withdrawn under any circumstance, and parents lacked the ability to make that request. The Supreme Court of the United States granted certiorari and affirmed the lower court's decision. They held that state's policy right to prolong life prevailed over the patient's right to refuse treatment. There was no "clear and convincing" evidence that the patient desired treatment to be withdrawn. Likewise, they held there was no guarantee that family members would always act in the best interests of incompetent patients, and because an erroneous decision to withdraw is irreversible, the higher evidentiary standard is required.

Significant time has passed since this seminal case, and opinions have changed. The critically ill patient

Table 26.1 Emergency consent issues

1. Decide patient's decision-making capacity
2. Emergency exception if no capacity
3. Override treatment or non-treatment decisions

Reference: Palmer and Iserson.[3]

who refuses treatment poses an ethical dilemma and a significant challenge to the emergency physician (Table 26.1).[3] First, the ED physician is often left to decide the patient's capacity, which can be complicated. Second, when the patient lacks decision-making capacity, there is an emergency exception to the informed consent process. Third, what is the ethical or legal premise of overriding the patient's desire for treatment or no treatment?

Conclusion

If a patient is institutionalized and there is an application by the patient and family members to be the guardian, the objective appraisal of that institution is to analyze the question of resuscitation as if the individual or the guardian then has the right to decide the ultimate care course. Typically, that process is required if a memorialized advance directive document does not exist. However, if guardianship rights have been transferred to a governmental or regulatory agency, then that patient decision-making capacity may have been transferred as well. If there is conflicting decision-making between family and institution, then legal and judicial support are often required to decide the best course for the patient.

References

1. In the Matter of Claire C. Conroy, 486 A.2d 1209.
2. *Cruzan* v. *Director, Missouri Department of Health*, 492 U.S. 917 (1989).
3. Palmer RB, Iserson KV. The critical patient who refuses treatment: an ethical dilemma. *J. Emerg Med.* 1997;15(5):729–733.

Difficult Patient Encounter

Case

The patient had missed dialysis again. This was not a first-time event: he missed his dialysis treatment appointments two or three times a month, on average. Each time the patient returned for emergency dialysis, giving various reasons for having missed his appointment. The emergency department (ED) performed standard laboratory screening including an EKG, chest radiograph, and laboratory tests to evaluate for a dangerously high potassium to justify the emergency dialysis. The patient was slightly hypovolemic, but the potassium was not at an emergency level for a dialysis patient. The ED physician contacted nephrology, who asked that the patient be admitted and they would once again do emergency dialysis. Once again, the nephrologist or renal physician would discuss the need for some potential counseling for this patient who missed dialysis appointments so often, resulting in significant harm to their health and state of well-being.

A call to the medical admitting team caused some consternation, as this patient made multiple visits requiring admission. They agreed to come down to see the patient. When the ED physician went to review the findings the patient asked her what was going on, saying he wanted a room upstairs "immediately." The ED physician told the patient she would see what could be done. She called the admitting team again, and let them know the patient's concerns. They replied they were busy, and would come down as soon as they could. They had already admitted this patient three times in the past month under similar circumstances, but the ED physician reminded them that each event was different and the patient still required admission.

When the ED physician went back to discuss the findings with the patient, she found him eating a fast food lunch – hamburger, French fries, and orange juice – that had been brought in by a family member. He had earlier been offered a hospital lunch tray with diabetic and potassium restrictions, but had refused it. The patient and family were told the admitting team would come down. He would receive dialysis now and be admitted some time that day. Both the family and patient insisted they wanted him admitted to the hospital immediately. The ED physician told them that this process was already in the works, but she would voice their concerns. She suggested to the charge nurse that getting a bed sooner would be a good idea. The charge nurse said she already knew about this issue as the family had called the patient advocate. They had just called a Condition Help, summoning the code response alert team that can be activated by family or friends. Here, the family had the ability to notify another group of health-care providers that they were in need of care in the current health-care setting. The admitting team then responded to the Condition Help response and told the patient they would be down to admit him once his dialysis was completed. He would be admitted after that because there were no telemetry beds available at that point in time.

The patient was subsequently admitted to hospital later in the day and filed various concerns and complaints about his hospital visit.

Medical Approach

Encounters with difficult patients are becoming far too common in the emergency hospital setting. These events are stressful both for the patient and for the health-care system. The patient involved is usually someone who has a chronic illness, with multiple recurrent hospital visits. Difficult patient–physician relationships are found more commonly in those with multiple chronic medical conditions, complicated by psychiatric or chronic pain issues, exacerbated by socioeconomic stressors.

Table 27.1 Difficult patient encounters: incidence 15%

Physician factors
1. Age < 40 years
2. Work hours > 55 hours per week
3. Subspecialty practice
Patient factors
4. Psychosocial problems
5. Substance abuse

Reference: Krebs et al.[1]

Table 27.2 Problematic patient encounters

Patient characteristics
1. Violent
2. Demanding
3. Aggressive
4. Rude
5. Secondary gain
6. Multiple non-specific complaints
7. Psychosomatic issues

Reference: Steinmetz and Tabenkin.[2]

Table 27.3 Difficult patient encounters

	Comparison OR, 95% CI, P < 0.05
Patient factors	
1. Mental disorder	2.4, 1.1–1.8
2. More severe symptoms	1.6, 1.04–2.3
3. >5 somatic symptoms	1.4, 1.1–1.8
4. Poorer functional status	0.005
5. More unmet expectations	0.005
6. Less satisfaction with care	0.03
7. Higher utilization of care	<0.001
Physician factors	<0.001
8. Poorer psychosocial attitudes	23 vs. 8%

Reference: Jackson and Kroenke.[3]

Table 27.4 Difficult patient encounters: incidence 10.3–20.6%

Patient factors
1. Psychosomatic symptoms
2. Mild personality disorder
3. Axis I major disorder

Reference: Hahn et al.[4]

Krebs et al. have described an incidence of 15% of adult patient encounters from a sample of 1391 family, internal medicine, and specialty physicians.[1] However, they focused on the physician interface and reported associated factors to include age less than 40 years, work hours more than 55 hours per week, subspecialty practice, and a greater number of patients with psychosocial problems or substance abuse (Table 27.1).

However, Steinmetz and Tabenkin reported in a family medicine survey that the more problematic patients are not those with difficult medical problems, but those who are violent, demanding, aggressive, rude, and seeking secondary gain.[2] They characteristically present with multiple non-specific complaints and other psychosomatic issues (Table 27.2).

Furthermore, Jackson and Kroenke found that one of every six patient encounters are perceived as difficult by physicians.[3] They evaluated 500 adult primary care patients, where 15% were found to be difficult. Difficult encounter patients were more likely to have a mental disorder (OR 2.4; 95% CI 1.1–1.8), more than 5 somatic symptoms (OR 1.4; 95% CI 1.1–1.8) and presented with more severe symptoms (OR 1.6; CI, 1.04–2.3). They also tended to have poorer functional status, more unmet expectations ($P = 0.005$), less satisfaction with care ($P = 0.03$), and higher utilization of health services ($P < 0.001$) However, they also noted that clinicians with poorer psychosocial attitudes experienced more difficult encounters (23% v. 8%; $P < 0.001$ (Table 27.3).

Hahn et al. developed the Difficult Doctor–Patient Relationship Questionnaire (DDPRQ) completed by the treating physician utilizing a 30-question Likert scale assessment.[4] This survey classified 10.3–20.6% of patient encounters as difficult. They did not find any major demographic, provider, or medical diagnosis correlates. The strongest association was found with patient psychosomatic symptoms, mild personality disorder, and axis I major disorder, often occurring in combination. The study is limited to its status as a derivation set analysis (Table 27.4).

The problem is deeply entrenched, so what is the solution? Elder et al. focused on a group of "respected" family medicine physicians to attempt to arrive at a potential solution.[5] They interviewed 102 physicians rated as excellent and recommended in a nationwide survey of medical school faculty. The proposed model confronts the problem of opposition, misuse of power,

Table 27.5 Approach to the difficult patient–physician interface

	Problem
	Problem
1.	Opposition
2.	Misuse of power
3.	Compassion fatigue
	Solution
4.	Collaboration
5.	Appropriate use of power
6.	Empathy

Reference: Elder et al.[5]

Table 27.6 Judicial intervention for intrusive treatment for non-consenting patients

	Factors in decision
1.	Incompetent or refuses consent
2.	Medical director petitions probate court in county
3.	Guardian ad litem appointed to guard patient interests
4.	Necessity of reasonableness of prescribed treatment
5.	Court ordered intervention

Reference: *Price* v. *Sheppard.*[7]

and compassion fatigue by utilizing collaboration, accompanied by the appropriate use of power and empathy (Table 27.5).

Legal Analysis

The difficult patient can be involved in administrative complaints, but is less commonly involved in the legal process. The key is to prevent the "difficult patient" from interfering with one's medical judgment.

In *Jarvis* v. *Levine*, a patient was committed to a mental institution after a lethal violent crime.[6] He was described as a "quite difficult" patient, who could fail to cooperate with treatment programming, group therapy, individual counseling, or psychological interviews. As well, he was described as caustic, derogatory, and sarcastic in staff interactions. Most recently, he refused treatment, although records reveal improvement in the past. These difficult behaviors adversely impacted the treatment plan. The state questioned whether state medical personnel could forcibly administer medication to a non-consenting patient. The Supreme Court of Minnesota cited *Price* v. *Sheppard* (1976), which established a pretreatment judicial review before imposition of "intrusive forms of treatment on non-consenting patients:

1. If the patient is incompetent to give consent or refuses consent or his guardian other than the persons responsible for his commitment also refuse consent, before more intrusive forms of treatment may be utilized, the medical director of the state hospital must petition the probate division of the County Court in the county in which the hospitals located for an order authorizing the prescribed treatment;

2. The court shall appoint a guardian ad litem to represent the interests of the patients;

3. In an adversary proceeding, pursuant to the petition, the court shall determine the necessity of reasonableness of the prescribed treatment." (Table 27.6).[7]

They held that patients are protected from intrusive medical treatment, although the pretreatment judicial review was required and not completed. Damages were not recoverable, as they followed statutory procedures. The case was remanded to the originating court for reconsideration.

In *Kassen* v. *Hatley*, the patient had been listed in the "difficult patient file" due to experience by the provider and at other institutions.[8] The file recommended she be referred to her home agency rather than admitted to the hospital, unless she had significantly different symptoms than on previous presentations. During this presentation to the psychiatric ED she was not admitted, because her conduct was consistent with past behavior, and there was a dispute over returning her medication. The Supreme Court of Texas felt that the ED nurse and physician did not admit because of the difficult patient file that indicated hospitalization was not therapeutic. Only on appeal did the defendants argue that the need to allocate scarce state hospital resources among potential patients also influenced the decision. If there was no basis for the decision not to admit except for therapeutic considerations, then their exercise was medical only and they are not entitled to official immunity. The court held that the defendants failed to prove conclusively that they exercised governmental discretion. They affirmed the appeal court decision that reversed the summary judgment for the physician and directed verdict for the nurse defendant, remanding for further consideration on the immunity issue.

Conclusion

These issues with an ED population are often not remediable in this environment. There are often associated psychosocial stressors, economic disadvantage, issues with drug and alcohol dependence, or premorbid psychiatric illness. These patients are best served by a multidisciplinary team approach focusing on frequent unplanned ED or hospital visits, significant patient non-compliance with the medical regimen, and a disproportionate frequency of administrative complaints.

References

1. Krebbs EE, Garrett JM, Konrad TR. The Difficult doctor? Characteristics of physicians who report frustration with patients: an analysis of survey data. *BMC Health Serv Res*. 2006;6(6):128.

2. Steinmetz D, Tabenkin H. The "difficult patient" as perceived by family physicians. *Fam Pract*. 2001;18(5):495–500. DOI:10.1093/fampra/18.5 495.

3. Jackson JL, Kroenke K. Difficult physician encounters in the ambulatory clinic: clinical predictors and outcomes. *Arch Int Med*. 1999;159(10):1069–1075. DOI:10.1001/archinte.159.10.10690.

4. Hahn SR, Thompson KS, Wills TA, Stern V, Budner NS. The difficult doctor-patient relationship: somatization, personality and psychopathology. *J Clin Epidemiol*. 1994;47(6):647–657. DOI:10.1016/0895-4356(94)90212-7.

5. Elder N, Ricer R, Tobias B. How respected family physicians manage difficult patient encounters. *J Am Board Fam Med*. 2006;19(6):533–541.

6. *Jarvis* v. *Levine*, 418 N.W.2d 139 (1988).

7. *Price* v. *Sheppard*, 239 N.W.2d 905 (1976).

8. *Kassen* v. *Hatley*, 887 S.W.2d 4 (1994).

Discharge Instructions

Case

"That's a pretty bad cellulitis," the nurse said. She asked if the patient had been seen yet. The emergency department (ED) physician said she was going to go and talk to him. As she looked at his leg, she was concerned as well. It was beefy red from the knee to the ankle. The patient stated he had cut his leg on a chain-link fence a few days back.

The ED physician ordered the standard blood work, radiographs, and ultrasound and administered a first dose of intravenous clindamycin. The patient started to improve and felt better. He had fluids administered and something for pain, and said he wanted to go home. He had work responsibilities at home that he could complete without going into the office. The ED physician thought this was a reasonable plan and they would continue the clindamycin and pain control medication. The patient was instructed to visit his primary care physician (PCP), or return to the ED if symptoms got worse. The physician repeated the discharge instructions and suggested again that if there was any worsening he would need to come back to the ED for reevaluation. The patient was discharged with his prescriptions and was appreciative of the care provided.

The next week the medical director asked the physician if she remembered the patient who had been evaluated the previous week with cellulitis. The patient had reported he went to another hospital in a much worse condition. The medical director was concerned the patient had been discharged inappropriately. The treatment plan and its rationale was discussed. The medical director pointed out that although the patient had been given clear instructions to return if his clinical condition worsened, he had not specifically been told what to do if he failed to improve. He subsequently stayed home for the next week and continued to be symptomatic, but felt he was not able to work,

due to an overly literal interpretation of the discharge instruction recommendations.

Medical Approach

The provision of discharge instructions is one of the most important parts of the ED evaluation. It should be done by both the physician and the nurse. The physician takes the operative role of asking for any additional questions concerning the patient's visit. Often if nursing staff go back and ask again, the patient will then offer a different set of questions that could be reevaluated by the physician.

It is important to note that the patient's understanding of what they are told can be limited by social circumstances, psychosocial stressors, and educational understanding. Again, it is crucially important they understand when they should seek additional care, which is typically the greatest uncertainty for patients. They should be told to return if they worsen, but also if they fail to improve over time. It is also helpful to give patients specific targets for their recovery, or vital sign abnormalities that they should return specifically for. The more specific the goals and guidelines are, the easier it is for patients to understand the discharge instructions. In addition, it is important to have them follow up with their PCP as soon as convenient or necessary, rather than some arbitrary delay of 2–3 days after their ED visit.

A combination of factors may result in a significant adverse impact on compliance with ED advice. The compliance with ED follow-up physician evaluation recommendations may be as low as 27.8%.[1] This may be improved by providing individualized directed instructions with follow-up resource identified, specifying time, location, and contact for the resource.[2] The easier the process is made for the patient, the more likely they are to comply, although non-compliance can occur even in the best of circumstances.

Table 28.1 Proper discharge instructions: important factors

1. ED care does not substitute for comprehensive medical care
2. Post-ED discharge follow-up is important
3. Follow-up with your personal physician
4. Establish specific referral time interval
5. Post-discharge referral physician will be provided
6. Contact referral physician if condition worsens or fails to improve
7. Return to ED if referral resource is not available

Reference: Castillo.[3]

Table 28.2 Continuous Treatment Doctrine Elements

1. Original Disease Condition
2. Specific Course Of Treatment
3. Physician Who Instituted Care

Reference: *Ganess* v. *City of New York*

Legal Analysis

In *Castillo* v. *Emergency Medicine Associates MD*, the patient presented to the ED with abdominal pain and nausea for several months.[3] She was diagnosed with a urinary tract infection and discharged with antibiotics and specific written follow-up instructions. She was to follow up with her own doctor within 3–4 days, and contact the on-call specialist or return to the ED if she worsened or failed to improve. The instructions were all-encompassing and directed, specifying a number of critical factors. First, the ED services were rendered on an emergency basis and are not a substitute for comprehensive medical attention. Second, it is important that you follow-up for said medical condition. Third, follow-up with your specific pre-established physician. Fourth, follow-up should be mandatory within a specified timeframe for a recheck. Fifth, the facility will provide an on-call primary or specialty follow-up physician, if there is no pre-established physician relationship. Sixth, should your condition worsen, any new symptoms develop, or you do not recover as expected, please contact the doctor you were given for follow-up care. Lastly, if you cannot reach the doctor, you should return to the emergency department (Table 28.1).

The patient's condition was alleged to have worsened. She recontacted the ED to speak with the physician she saw previously. The on-shift ED physician prescribed a different medication over the telephone. The patient returned 5 days later with a bowel perforation requiring operative intervention. Initially, she filed suit alleging negligent treatment, which was dismissed voluntarily to file an amended complaint alleging the physician group was liable for the acts and omissions of their agents.

The Continuous Treatment Doctrine (Table 28.2) prevents the statute of limitations for medical malpractice litigation from being applied as long as the course of treatment, for the original disease condition is provided by the physician, who instituted the treatment are all present.[4] This doctrine addresses the undesirability of having to discontinue treatment to engage in litigation, when the original treating physician would have the best chance of intervening to avoid a negative outcome.

However, the court found the continuing treatment doctrine did not apply as the ED provided episodic care with a patient–physician relationship that ended upon her discharge, and dismissed the claim as being time barred. The United States Court of Appeals, Fourth Circuit concurred with the trial court dismissing the claim as well.

In *Johnson* v. *Jamaica Hospital Medical Center*, the patient arrived at the ED with a gunshot wound of the lower extremity and was ultimately cared for by the chief of orthopedic surgery.[5] He was discharged with an external fixator in place. His discharge instructions stated he should "stay off the leg, keep it dry and not touch the pins." Approximately 2 months later, he developed a severe infection requiring multiple surgical procedures and a prolonged recovery. The plaintiff filed suit alleging malpractice based on the provision of negligent discharge instructions, failing to provide proper instructions on pin maintenance. The Supreme Court granted the defendant hospital motion to dismiss, but the Appellate Division reversed, holding that a prima facie case for standard of care violation was met. The plaintiff expert testified that the pins required daily cleaning, and the instruction not to touch them was in violation of that standard. They held that it was more probable than not that the increased incidence of infection was related to inadequate discharge instructions.

Conclusion

A successful medicolegal approach to the ED discharge instruction process requires careful attention to detail. Some authorities recommend providing maximum detail and specificity, while others feel that for the advice to be most effective it is more important for the patient to be aware of broader thematic follow-up trends, such as failure to improve.

References

1. Vukmir RB, Kremen R, DeHart DA, Menegazzi J. Compliance with emergency department patient referral. *Am J Emerg Med*. 1992;10(5): 413–417.

2. Vukmir RB, Kremen R, Ellis G, DeHart DA, Plewa MC, Menegazzi J. Compliance with emergency department patient referral: effect of computerized discharge instructions. *Ann Emerg Med*. 1993;22(5):819–823.

3. *Castillo* v. *Emergency Medicine Associates MD*, 372 F.3d 643 (2004).

4. Ganess v. City of New York, 85 N.Y.2d 733 (N.Y. 1995).

5. *Johnson* v. *Jamaica Hospital Medical Center*, 800 N.Y.S.2d 609 (2005).

Disruptive Provider Behavior

Case

The word quickly spread through the hospital that the surgeon was having a really bad day. First, they had to change his operating suite because of a problem with the room. Then there was an anesthesia delay, due to decreased staff availability. The final straw came when the robotic arm broke for his scheduled surgical procedure at 9 a.m. When the surgeon heard about the robotic arm, he began to scream and curse in the anesthesia preoperative staging area. This diatribe was overheard by staff, patients, and families. One of the anesthesiologists, a friend of the surgeon's, was summoned to de-escalate the situation.

Although the substance of his complaints was usually founded in fact, it was felt that the way he expressed himself was not helpful to his fellow workers. There was no debate about the inappropriateness of the setting in which the comments were made, or of the public discussion of the work circumstances. The staff felt the surgeon's complaints should be directed at administration, not at them. They were trying their best to move the patients through the operating room in difficult circumstances. Interestingly, the staff agreed with the surgeon's sentiments: there had been recent staffing cuts and equipment unavailability.

He cooled down and started his next case. The remainder of the day went on uneventfully. The next day the patient advocate received a family complaint concerning the surgeon's behavior.

Medical Approach

Problems occur every day in medicine, and the key is to navigate through these issues efficiently and effectively. Discussing difficult issues such as this in public is not an appropriate or effective way to resolve such matters. The public should not be exposed to work-related discussions. Likewise, matters are not likely to be improved in this open-air discussion forum.

Hospital facilities are given wide scope in privileging decision-making by medical staff, including professional medical competence and other non-medical considerations. Discriminatory, anticompetitive, or financial motivation for these actions may be alleged.

Legal Analysis

In *Miller* v. *Eisenhower Medical Center*, a family physician appealed a judgment denying his petition for a writ of mandate compelling the facility to grant him staff privileges.[1] His petition for a hearing according to medical staff bylaws was denied as "untimely." Physician witnesses to the judicial proceeding described good professional competence. However, a compilation of comments included, "little impetuous about things he wanted done," "in the long run most were very constructive ideas," "had heard rumors of interpersonal conflicts, but none witnessed or experienced," and "expressed himself forcefully and vigorously." The Supreme Court of California reversed the trial court judgment, directing a peremptory writ of mandate directing the defendant to set aside their privilege declination. They were compelled either to grant privileges, or to undertake further proceedings. This case may have turned on the lack of conclusive evidence and the declination of the due-process right awarded in the medical staff bylaws.

In *Oksanen* v. *Page Memorial Hospital*, the appellant alleged the facility's medical staff and board of trustees conspired to exclude him from the medical staff, violating the Sherman Antitrust Act.[2,3] The importance of this challenge was far-reaching as the peer review process is the cornerstone of the privileging and credentialing system. There were allegations of abrasive behavior, including verbal outbursts, the use of profanity and a "volatile personality." He responded that he was concerned over patient safety issues, and referred patients to other facilities. The relationship continued to deteriorate until staff privileges were revoked. The trial court held that the medical staff and board of trustees were indeed one entity that could not conspire with itself, and dismissed the claim overall, distancing an alleged workplace dispute from federal antitrust law. However, the United States Court of Appeals, Fourth Circuit reversed the granting of summary judgment and reheard the case en banc. However, they ultimately arrived at the same decision as the trial court on the theories presented.

In *Kibler* v. *Northern Inyo County Local Hospital District*, a physician was granted staff privileges and the facility brought action due to alleged threatening verbal assaults and threats of physical violence, including assault with a firearm.[4] The physician was suspended, and then staff privileges were reinstated by written agreement. As part of that agreement, he was compelled to attend anger management classes and forbidden to bring a firearm onto the hospital premises. He subsequently filed suit alleging defamation, abuse of process, and interference with the practice of medicine. The hospital quickly responded, moving under a section 425.16 theory, the Anti-SLAPP statute, to strike this complaint as a Strategic Lawsuits Against Public Participation (SLAPP), a suit brought solely to harass the defendants.[5] The trial court agreed and the court of appeal affirmed that the peer review process was an "official proceeding authorized by law" subject to a special motion to strike. The Supreme Court of California agreed to hear the appeal, focusing on the question of whether the hospital peer review process qualifies as an "official proceeding." They affirmed the judgment of the court of appeal.

Conclusion

The judiciary typically allows the hospital wide latitude in decision-making, unless an egregious due-process error has occurred. The perspective is that, historically, the hospital or medical system is more likely to make a correct decision than the individual physician, although it is clear there are individual cases in which that assumption has turned out not to be true.

References

1. *Miller* v. *Eisenhower Medical Center*, 27 Cal 3d. 614 (1980).

2. *Oksanen* v. *Page Memorial Hospital*, 945 F.2d. 696 (1991).

3. Sherman Act, 15 U.S.C. §§1–7 (1890).

4. *Kibler* v. *Northern Inyo County Local Hospital District*, 46 Cal. Rptr. 3d. 41 (2006).

5. California Code of Civil Procedure CCP S 425.16, subd (a). The Anti-SLAPP Statute.

Chapter 30

Do Not Resuscitate

Case

The chief complaint listed on the registration sheet was "worsening pneumonia." The patient had come from a nursing home and been treated with antibiotics at that facility for 7 days with pneumonia. He seemed to be doing poorly and he had a Physician Orders for Life-Sustaining Treatment (POLST) resuscitation form that stated he wanted "everything done." The intensive care unit (ICU) team was called down in anticipation of the admission.

With some additional interventions, he certainly improved. He received steroids and a beta-agonist. As it turned out, his disease was not pneumonia but bronchitis with reactive airway disease, as he had severe chronic obstructive pulmonary disease (COPD).

The resident physician returned from a discussion with family and reported that the patient's family had reversed the resuscitation order and now wanted him to have a Do Not Resuscitate (DNR) order. The ED physician pointed out that the resuscitation order itself was fairly explicit. The patient wanted everything done, including dialysis. The resident was reminded that the patient's ultimate location for medical care did not truly depend on resuscitation status so much as on the patient's physician and nursing needs for additional care. The patient's son had power of attorney (POA) and had signed the new form on the resident's recommendation. The ED physician pointed out that the family were required to present a valid Health Care Power of Attorney (HCPOA) document, which is not the same as a POA. As an alternative, they could contact at least one other family member to corroborate the information. That would be a good start to address the conflict with the advance directive or POLST form. The patient was then taken to the ICU.

Later that week, the chair of the ethics committee contacted the ICU and suggested that the patient's

resuscitation status was indeed still intact. In addition, contact with a second family member confirmed that the son who claimed to have POA was mistaken. The patient did well in the ICU and returned to the nursing home within a few days.

Medical Approach

End-of-life therapy can be a complicated, stressful time for all involved. The key to success is an advance directive, typically written from a legal perspective, offering conceptual care guidelines. The POLST form typically focuses on medical operational questions, providing clear directional orders to guide care. In the past, this directive took the form of a DNR instruction, specifically citing interventions to be excluded from the medical care regimen.

These documents should be contemplated and completed by the patient at some calmer point in time. The family may assist in the formulation process, but may not alter or influence the patient's wishes once complete. This document needs to be followed and adhered to by health-care providers. The family cannot change the course or alter the document if the patient is competent.

If the patient becomes incapacitated, the document will specify whether to follow it as written, or to refer to another for interpretative assistance. The "follow as written" version does not allow change by an outside interested party. The "outside interpretative assistance" version typically is offered by the individual who holds the HCPOA, who has the capacity to direct subsequent care once the patient becomes incapacitated. A POA document typically focuses on legal and financial matters rather than health-care decision-making issues.

Any time there is a conflict in end-of-life decision-making, one must seek written confirmation. In lieu of written evidence of intent, agreement among family members allows at least a preliminary direction for the care to proceed.

The caselaw has progressed over time in the approach to resuscitation, the right to life, and the right of self-determination.

Legal Analysis

For historical perspective, we offer several cases to illustrate the change in end-of-life care expectations. They often involve a court-appointed guardian in the decision-making mix of family and physician. Early on, these cases involved the question of withholding cardiopulmonary resuscitation (CPR).

In *Superintendent of Belchertown State Sch.* v. *Saikewicz*, the patient suffered from severe congenital mental disability and was legally incompetent.[1] The probate court ruled that radical chemotherapy should not be administered in this case. The Massachusetts Supreme Judicial Court left some uncertainty in the care and course of an end-of-life patient. Some felt that it created the premise that unless a judicial determination of support limitation has been made, the physician has the duty to provide all resuscitative interventions possible even with physician and family agreement on support limitation. A more balanced reading of the decision, including the explanatory notes and dissent, suggests this to not be the result or intent. If the person was incompetent from birth, they were not required to receive lifesaving treatment. The Massachusetts Supreme Judicial Court held that the decision was consistent with attending physician opinion, generally accepted medical views, no State interest proven sufficient to counterbalance the patient's right to privacy and self-determination, affirming the probate judge's decision to withhold treatment.

Any uncertainty was quickly put to rest. In *The Matter of Shirley Dinnerstein*, an elderly woman suffering from advanced dementia was bed-bound in a nursing home, in a vegetative state.[2] Here, the family and the physician were in agreement that she was to be a "no code," in which no invasive resuscitative procedures should be performed. The guardian ad litem appointed by the probate court opposed this, and the case was referred to the appellate court. The Massachusetts Appeals Court ruled that in the case of unremitting, incurable mortal illness, the court does not prohibit any course of medical treatment. The lawfulness of the physician order to institute, or not provide, resuscitative intervention in the setting of cardiorespiratory arrest does not require judicial order or decision. The case was remanded to the probate court to enter a judgment in accordance with the request for declaratory relief.

In *Matter of Warren*, the public administrator appealed the trial court order denying him authority to withhold CPR, in a patient with bilateral amputations who suffered severe episodes of sepsis, and was left in a persistent vegetative state.[3] The trial court ruled that the treating physician confused the concepts of low likelihood of survivability and futility, and there was no indication of the patient's wishes. They felt there was evidence to support resuscitation in the setting of sepsis. The Missouri Court of Appeals reversed the trial court, concluding that the treating physician was in the best position to determine the necessity of life-prolonging interventions. They held that the appointed guardian had the statutory authority to make medical decisions and consent to or withhold treatment in the best interest of the patient without judicial authorization.

The latter cases involved withholding of specific life-prolonging interventions in patients with disease states beyond recovery. In *The Matter of Earle N. Spring*, an incompetent person was receiving life-prolonging hemodialysis.[4] The patient's wife and his son, who was appointed temporary guardian, petitioned the probate court to limit support. The judge found that the patient, if competent, would choose not to receive the life-prolonging treatment. The trial court ordered and was affirmed by the appeal court that the son and wife should make the decision regarding the continuation or limitation of the dialysis treatment. This was followed by appointment of a guardian ad litem, after the son petitioned to be conservator of the property, who requested additional appellate review. The Supreme Court of Massachusetts ruled that decision-making should remain with the family rather than a court-appointed guardian.

In *William Francis Bartling* v. *The Superior Court of Los Angeles County, Glendale Adventist Medical Center*, the court was asked to decide if life support in the form of mechanical ventilation could be withdrawn from a competent, but likely incurable, patient after complications of a lung biopsy procedure.[5] The patient and wife requested removal of mechanical ventilation and challenged the denial injunction by the trial court. There was complete patient and family consensus with an offer to relieve the facility of any potential legal liability. The California Court of Appeals, Second

Table 30.1 DNR: stepwise approach

1. Patient wishes followed if competent
2. Patient unable to understand, or desire to limit, enter decision tree
3. If reversible condition or unclear, no DNR
4. If irreversible, DNR is appropriate
5. Discuss with those with expertise
6. Discuss with family; if consensus, DNR is appropriate
7. If disagreement exists, ethics committee or hospital counsel involved
8. External judicial review may be required, if differences persist
9. Monitor for change in course

Reference: Lee and Cassell.[6]

Appellate Division clearly felt the trial court erred, and the patient was competent to choose his own course. As the final irony, although the patient petitioned with the utmost urgency he died prior to this ruling.

The ethical and legal framework for the decision not to resuscitate was described by Lee and Cassell, suggesting a stepwise approach.[6] First, the patient's wishes should be honored if competent. Second, if the patient is unable to understand or expresses wishes to limit resuscitative efforts, one should enter the decision tree. Third, if the condition is reversible or prognosis is unclear, then no DNR is indicated. Fourth, if the condition is irreversible, the DNR order is appropriate. Fifth, this decision needs to be discussed with those who have expertise in predicting prognosis. Sixth, discuss the decision-making with family; if consensus exists the DNR order should be written. Seventh, if disagreement exists, the ethics committee or hospital counsel should be involved. Eighth, external judicial review may be required if differences persist. Ninth, always be aware of change in patient status, either improving or worsening; be prepared to change course (Table 30.1).

Conclusion

The terminology has recently changed again, with attempts to combine the attributes of the advance directive, DNR, and "do not intubate" documents. Although the POLST form, initially developed in 1993 in Oregon, was designed to be as clear as possible, unexpected challenges in its interpretation and implementation do exist in the ED.[7]

References

1. *Superintendent of Belchertown State Sch.* v. *Saikewicz*, 373 Mass. 728 (1977).

2. In the Matter of Shirley Dinnerstein, 6 Mass. App. Ct. 466 (1978).

3. Matter of Warren, 858 S.W. 2d 263 (1993).

4. In the Matter of Earle N. Spring, 380 Mass. 620 (1980).

5. *William Francis Bartling et al.* v. *The Superior Court of Los Angeles County, Glendale Adventist Medical Center et al.*, 163 Cal. App.3d, 186 (1984).

6. Lee MA, Cassel CK. The ethical and legal framework for the decision to not resuscitate. *West J Med.* 1984;140(1):117–122.

7. Jesus JE, Giederman JE, Venkat A, Limehouse Jr. WE, Derse AR, Larkin GL, Heinrichs CW; On behalf of the ACEP Ethics Committee. Physician orders for life-sustaining treatment and emergency medicine: ethical consideration, legal considerations, legal issues and emerging trends. *Ann Emerg Med.* 2014;64:140–144. DOI:10.1016/j.annemergmed.2014.03.014.

Documentation

Case

When the patient presented to the emergency department (ED) her chief complaint was chest pain. The nursing triage note said she had upper abdominal pain and lower chest pain for a day. There were no other cardiac-type symptoms such as shortness of breath or vomiting, although there had been some nausea. By the time the physician went to see her, the patient denied any chest pain whatsoever. However, she reported earlier abdominal pain, which came on after she had eaten some questionable food the previous evening. No one else in the house was sick, but she had previously had some food intolerance before. She was certain that was what this episode of discomfort had been. It had alleviated with antacids she had taken at home.

The standard testing for abdominal pain was complete, including liver function tests and lipase which were completely normal. She was discharged home with a prescription for a proton pump inhibitor (PPI), a drug that reduces acid production in the stomach, and instructed to follow up with her primary care physician. The ED physician had finished the dictation, the discharge instructions, and final documentation as the patient was discharged home.

The patient returned 2 days later, and was admitted with a non-ST elevation myocardial infarction (STEMI) cardiac event. She received a percutaneous cardiac stent and did well. The provider received a call from the quality committee who asked about the documentation of the first visit. They stated there was inconsistency in the documentation, in that both registration and nursing had documented chest pain as the chief complaint, but the physician had documented abdominal pain. The ED physician replied that the patient had only had abdominal pain in their interview, and that chest pain was not present when she was asked.

The quality committee asked if the ED physician had documented and reconciled the difference in history in the charting in the electronic record. She stated that she was not certain, but would check. The quality committee also cautioned her to not have any casual public discussion about the case with nursing staff.

Medical Approach

It is crucially important in any medical record to have internal consistency in data and information. If something is found to be conflicting in the record, it should be reconciled by re-interviewing the healthcare providers involved. If the inconsistency in documentation cannot be resolved, this should be stated and acknowledged to demonstrate attention to detail and interest in producing the most accurate medical record possible.

An interesting phenomenon encountered in medicolegal analysis is that the public may have different perceptions of provider history believability. They believe the providers who perform the initial screening, such as registration and nursing, are more objective and provide a purer history, as it occurs earlier in the process. Advanced practice providers (APP) and physicians subsequently refine the accuracy of the report, which may change over time. This often leaves a medicolegal quandary that needs to be resolved.

One of the areas of concern in a busy ED is attention to detail in documentation to address patient care, medicolegal issues, and billing considerations. Emergency medicine documentation is risk-prone because of the unpredictable and often chaotic environment, high-risk conditions, multiple transitions of care, decreased patient care continuity, and extensive charting requirements (Table 31.1).[1]

It has always been assumed that the busier the department, the higher the risk of error. Dawdy et al. evaluated 833 patient charts, examining high-risk

Table 31.1 Difficulties in emergency department documentation

1.	Chaotic, unpredictable environment
2.	High-risk medical conditions
3.	Multiple transitions of care
4.	Decreased patient care continuity
5.	Extensive charting requirements

Reference: Yu and Green.[1]

conditions (chest pain, abdominal pain, and chronic obstructive pulmonary disease [COPD]) and comparing 11 predetermined criteria.[2] They reported a linear increase in documentation errors in written but not dictated charts with an increase in patient entry rates.

Fordyce et al. evaluated 1935 ED patients, identifying a 17.8% (346) overall error rate with 13% categorized as documentation errors.[3] Patients involved in errors were more likely to be older and have a higher visit intensity, but 98% did not have an adverse outcome ($P < 0.0001$).

Legal Analysis

Health record documentation often comes under scrutiny for a host of evidentiary issues. In *Housley* v. *Cerise*, the patient, who was pregnant at the time, slipped in a rental property, and presented to ED. She was then referred to another ED, and was admitted with premature rupture of membranes.[4] A suit was filed for the fall, plaintiff was awarded damages by the trial court, then reversed by the appeal court. The fall history was corroborated by family, but was not in the ED records. Allegedly, neither ED medical record, mainly focused on the nursing documentation, related a history of a fall or physical evidence of bruising. The nurses testified that normally this information would be documented. However, the Supreme Court of Louisiana reversed the appeal court decision, reinstating the trial court judgment for plaintiff. They held that there was factual evidence of a fall, and a temporal association indicating causation with a medical event even though not documented.

Conclusion

Often in a litigation setting, the jury finds the history from the "pure of heart," typically nursing staff, to be the most credible in the legal decision-making. Another important issue in high-risk litigation scenarios is to avoid casual conversation about patient care events, participation, and outcome that might be discoverable.

References

1. Yu KT, Green RA. Critical aspects of emergency department documentation and communication. *Emerg Med Clin North Am*. 2009;27(4):641–654. DOI:10.1016/j.emc.2009.97.008.

2. Dawdy MR, Munter DW, Gilmore RA. Correlation of patient entry rates and physician documentation errors in dictated and handwritten emergency treatment records. *Am J Emerg Med*. 1997;15(2):115–117. DOI:10.1016/S0735-6757(97)90078-4.

3. Fordyce J, Blank FSJ, Pekow P, Smithline HA, Ritter G, Gehlbach S, et al. Errors in a busy emergency department. *Ann Emerg Med*. 2003;42(3):324–333. DOI:10.1016/S0196-0644(03)00398-6.

4. *Housley* v. *Cerise*, 579 So. 2d 973 (1991).

Domestic Violence

Case

The patient had been to the emergency department (ED) a few times previously with a discharge diagnosis of non-specific abdominal pain. She had been seen by the physician at least once for this complaint. She was back in this time with a blackened eye and an arm injury. When she was asked what happened, she said that she fell down the steps. After some time in the evaluation process, the ED physician suggested she seemed to have an unusual injury complex to be associated with that sort of event. The physician asked her what really happened. After some encouragement, she looked away and said, "he hit me." The ED staff addressed her medical concerns, and luckily she had no serious injury. Her CT scan was normal, and eye exam did not reveal any corneal injury. Thankfully, the wrist radiograph revealed no broken bones or fractures, just a significant sprain.

As the physician was getting ready to complete the evaluation, as part of the discharge plan, the patient was asked if she had a safe place to go. She said yes, that she would stay with her sister. Social work had already spoken to the patient. The physician asked her if she wanted to speak with the domestic violence advocate, but she said she did not. Again, she was reminded that, although we did not walk in her shoes, health-care staff would always be vigilant about domestic violence, and intervention or staff assistance would always be available if she ever needed it. She was asked again if she wanted to file a police report, and again she declined.

The patient's sister then came in, and after an emotional exchange the patient had a change of heart. The sister said this hadn't been the first time the partner had been violent, and his behavior wasn't going to get any better. Initially, the patient agreed to talk with police, and the staff offered that they often dispatch a domestic violence unit to assist. After another emotional discussion with her sister, the patient declined once again to speak with anyone. The sister asked the ED physician, "How come you don't just call the police?" The physician explained that in their state there is a statute giving the domestic violence victim the ultimate right to decide in the setting of non-lethal assault.

The patient would stay with her sister. Social services came back to provide outpatient advocacy contact information, and she was advised to return to the ED if she had a change of heart on the reporting, or any other needs.

Medical Approach

Domestic violence is one of the most pervasive problems encountered in the ED. All individuals and relationship types can be affected. It is often the bellwether symptom where there are significant psychosocial and environmental stressors in the community. Patients often present with a nondescript symptom complex such as abdominal pain, trauma, dizziness, headache, and multiple somatic complaints, subconsciously hoping that someone will discover the real issue.

The prevalence of domestic violence in the ED as reported in Abbot's evaluation of 418 women and their current male partner was 11.7% (217) (95% CI, 8.7–15.2%).[1] Of the 230 patients without male partners, 5.6% (13) presented with an episode of domestic violence within the last month, and the lifetime event presence was 54.2% (95% CI, 50.2–58.1%).

Often the existence of male victims of domestic violence is not appreciated in the ED. Mechem et al. evaluated 866 patients in the ED setting and found a 12.6% (109) incidence of violence inflicted by their female partner within the last year.[2] Only 19% of patients contacted the police, 14% required medical attention, 11% filed charges or filed for a restraining order, and 6% received follow-up counseling.

Wadman's study clarified our greatest concern and fear, that patients had visited the ED before their final victimization.[3] They identified 139 female homicide victims, in which 24.5% (34) cases were found to be related to domestic violence. The medical records of 53.3% (8) of the 15 victims yielded suggestive evidence of battery.

Most states recognize these issues are complex, with economic dependence of the victim, recidivism by the perpetrator, and increased potential for additional violence. State statutes have made the unfortunate calculated decision that the victim is truly the only one who knows all the risks involved. This means that if their domestic partner commits an assault that is not of high lethality, the victim can decline to file a law enforcement report. There is a strict liability modifier, mandating reporting as assault of high potential lethality, typically involving use of a weapon.

Legal Analysis

In *Nash* v. *State of Indiana*, the trial court jury convicted the defendant of rape and he appealed the conviction.[4] The grounds for appeal focused on the ED evaluation. First, the nurse was allowed to testify that the patient stated she was attacked by her estranged husband pursuant to Indiana Evidence Rule 803,[4] over his hearsay objection.[5] Second, the medical records were admitted as evidence where the attack was described, as records of a regularly conducted business activity. The appeal court affirmed, holding that the evidence was properly admitted as a hearsay exception as it was performed routinely in the practice of emergency medicine.

Hearsay is a statement, other than the one made by the declarant while testifying at trial, offered to prove the truth of the matter asserted, and is inadmissible unless admired pursuant to a recognized exception (Indiana Evidence Rule 801 (c), 802).[5] There are 24 accepted exceptions to the rule against hearsay, and these are not excluded, regardless of whether the declarant is available as a witness (Table 32.1).

For a hearsay statement to be admissible as a statement for the purposes of medical diagnosis or treatment, the following elements are required: (1) it must be made for the purpose of medical diagnosis or treatment; (2) it must describe medical history, symptoms, pain sensations, "or the inception or general character of the cause or external source"; and (3) it must be "reasonably pertinent to diagnosis and treatment" (Table 32.2).

Table 32.1 Rule 803: Exceptions to the rule against hearsay

1.	Present sense impression
2.	Excited utterance
3.	Then existing mental, emotional, or physical condition
4.	Statement made for medical diagnosis or treatment
5.	Recorded recollection
6.	Records of regularly conducted activity
7.	Absence of a record of a regularly conducted activity
8.	Public Records
9.	Public records of vital statistics
10.	Absence of a public record
11.	Records of religious organizations concerning personal or family history
12.	Certificates of marriage, baptism, and similar ceremonies
13.	Family records
14.	Records of documents that affect an interest in property
15.	Statements in documents that affect an interest in property
16.	Statements in ancient documents
17.	Market reports and similar commercial publications
18.	Statements in learned treatises, periodicals or pamphlets
19.	Reputation concerning personal or family history
20.	Reputation concerning boundaries or general history
21.	Reputation concerning character
22.	Judgment of a previous conviction
23.	Judgments involving personal, family or general history or a boundary
24.	Other exceptions

Reference: Indiana Rules of Evidence, Rule 803.[5]

Table 32.2 Hearsay exception for purpose of medical diagnosis or treatment

1.	Made for the purpose of medical diagnosis or treatment
2.	Describing medical history, symptoms, pain, sensations
3.	Reasonably pertinent to diagnosis and treatment

Reference: Indiana Rules of Evidence, Rule 803.[5]

In *State of Washington* v. *Moses*, the jury convicted the defendant of murder and appeal was filed again alleging improper admission of ED medical records and testimony.[6] The police arrived at the scene of an alleged domestic violence assault and transported the patient to the ED for evaluation. The trial court admitted the testimony under the "excited utterance" hearsay exception for the declarant; and from the ED physician and social worker, where the patient victim identified her assailant, as statements made for medical diagnosis or treatment.[7] The ED physician interviewed both patient and children, referred to social services, and testified to the event and assailant identified.

The defendant challenged the admission, arguing these out-of-court statements concerning a prior incident violated the Sixth Amendment Confrontation Clause, "where in all criminal prosecutions, the accused shall have the right to confront witnesses who might testify against them."[8] The Supreme Court of Washington held that an out-of-court testimonial statement cannot be admitted unless the declarant is unavailable and the defendant had a prior opportunity to cross-examine.[9,10] The Court of Appeals of Washington affirmed the trial court decision, but remanded for consideration of exceptional sentencing. They held that at the time the patient had no way of knowing that the statements to the ED physician might be used at a subsequent trial. Therefore, they were not testimonial under a Crawford analysis.

Other states feel the requirement is too high a standard for the victim and adopt a mandatory reporting strategy, transferring the burden to law enforcement so the victim is not blamed for "turning someone in." This approach tries to minimize the risk to the victim from repeated assaults. The concern is that the patient will be dissuaded from seeking medical care for this reason.

Conclusion

Either approach has the goal of empowering and protecting the patient as much as possible. Our responsibility is to ensure a proper safety plan for the patient, which may include admission in some cases. It is incumbent upon us to be aware of our local environment and be familiar with the obligatory reporting statutes as well as other resources available to the population at risk from domestic violence.

References

1. Abbott J, Johnson R, Koziol-McLain J, Lowenstein SR. Domestic violence against women: incidence and prevalence in an emergency department population. *JAMA*. 1995;273(22):1763–1767. DOI:10.1001/jama.1995.03520460045033.

2. Mechem CC, Shofer FS, Reinhard SS, Hornig S, Datner E. History of domestic violence among male patients presenting to an urban emergency department. *Acad Emerg Med*. 1999;6(8):786–791. DOI:10.1111/acem.1999.6.issue-8/issuetoc.

3. Wadman MC, Muelleman RL. Domestic violence homicides: ED use before victimization. *Am J Emerg Med*. 1999;17(7):689–691. DOI:10.1016/S0735-6757(99)90161-4.

4. *Nash* v. *State of Indiana*, 754 N.E.2d 1021 (2001).

5. Indiana Rules of Evidence §§801–803(4): Definitions, Rule Against Hearsay, Exceptions To Rule Against Hearsay: Statements Made for Medical Diagnosis.

6. *State of Washington* v. *Moses*, 119 P.3d 906 (2005).

7. Washington Rules of Evidence ER 803 (a)(4):Hearsay Exceptions; Availability of Declarant Immaterial.

8. U.S. Const. Amend VI.

9. *Crawford* v. *Washington*, 541 U.S. 36 (2004).

10. Washington State Courts, Rule ER 803 Hearsay Exceptions; Availability of Declarant Immaterial.

Driving Impairment

Case

The paramedics brought the patient in to the emergency department (ED) after a minor motor vehicle accident (MVA). The patient's car had veered off the road and struck a concrete barrier, but no one appeared to be hurt. He had a passenger with him, who stated the driver, who was her husband, had a seizure, which appeared to cause the accident. The patient had a known seizure disorder from a previous head injury, but he had not had a seizure for years. He had been taking his medicine and was obviously distraught. He drove a truck as a delivery man. He told his wife, "No, I didn't have a seizure, I just must've fallen asleep a little, I was daydreaming." She said, "No, you had a seizure."

The workup was essentially normal. He had some laboratory work, EKG, and head CT scan all of which were normal, and his anti-seizure medication was at a therapeutic level. The patient was given the good news that everything was okay and that he could go home. However, the seizure issue in relation to his driving would have to be addressed. He was told the state bureau of motor vehicles would be contacting him regarding the seizure, and was cautioned not to drive until the reevaluation. He responded angrily, pointing out that driving was what he did for a living, and cautioned his wife not to say any more.

The ED staff had further discussion with the patient, pointing out he was lucky this accident hadn't injured him or anyone else. How would it be the next time, if someone was injured because he had a seizure? He seemed to understand the rationale and was resigned to his fate. The physician filled out the state licensure paperwork, his driver's license was revoked until a later reevaluation; and he was referred to neurology for a safe seizure-free interval to reinstitute his license.

Medical Approach

It is crucial to investigate drivers involved in MVAs for causes of infirmity, such as chest pain, a syncopal episode, or a small stroke that made them pass out. Bystanders and family can often help to corroborate an event and in this case a seizure event is almost certain. The use of intoxicants poses the possibility of additional liability of reporting.

Runge et al. evaluated the incidence of driving under the influence (DUI) and its association with MVAs and injury.[1] They evaluated 187 patients, where 28% (53) were charged and 17% (32) convicted of a DUI offense. The likelihood of being charged with a DUI decreased as injury severity increased. Repeat offenders are charged more often, but this does not result in a greater number of convictions.

Most states have obligatory reporting requirements, in which health-care professionals are obliged to refer the patient immediately for evaluation by the state's bureau of motor vehicles for driving safety. Some states have no obligatory reporting or referral requirement, but either way, there is a moral obligation for the health-care provider to ensure no one else is harmed. If there is a substantial likelihood of a repeat event, or if there is any likelihood of a repeat event, then the patient should be referred to the bureau of motor vehicles for driving assessment. The patient should be cautioned not to drive and this should be documented in the discharge instructions.

The Pennsylvania statutory code states it is a physician's duty to advise the department of transportation of a patient's potential lack of fitness to operate a motor vehicle.[2] However, courts seem reluctant to impose strict liability for failure to report allegations.

The obligation to report a potentially unsafe driver can cause considerable consternation. The impact of a mandatory physician reporting system for cardiac patients potentially unfit to drive has been studied by Simpson et al.[3] They evaluated 1.3% (994) cases in which a driver's license was suspended for cardiac reasons, compared with an estimated 72,407 that would have been suspended if the Canadian Cardiovascular Society's Consensus Conference guidelines on driving fitness were followed.[4] If all drivers with significant cardiac illness were suspended from driving, as many as 29.2 serious events could have been avoided. However, only 1.4% (13 of 929) of road fatalities were attributed to medical illness in the driver.

Legal Analysis

In *Hospodar* v. *Schick*, a patient prone to "blackout" episodes, previously diagnosed with a seizure disorder, was under specialty medical care when his car struck another vehicle, resulting in multiple fatalities.[5] This event was due to a "blackout" episode, and there had been previous such events. There were two subsequent specialty evaluations, with discussion of seizure in the differential, but no ongoing treatment was ordered. The treating physician's response to the "physically/mentally competent to drive" question on the department of transportation form was, "I don't know." The fatal accident occurred 5 months later. The trial court held there was liability for alleged failure to report. In Pennsylvania there is an affirmative physician duty to advise of a potential lack of fitness to operate a motor vehicle.[6] The Pennsylvania Department of Transport Medical Advisory Board sets out specified disorders or disabilities in any patient 16 years of age or older that must be reported within 10 days of discovery by the examining physician, including epilepsy and periodic loss of consciousness, attention, or awareness from whatever cause (Table 33.1).[7]

The Superior Court of Pennsylvania felt there was no third-party duty owed to the parties affected, and reversed the trial court's judgment. They held that the Pennsylvania Supreme Court established in *Estate of Witthoeft* v. *Kiskaddon* (1999) that the motor vehicle code did not create, explicitly or implicitly, a private cause of action against a physician when a patient causes an accident and the physician fails to comply with the notification requirements of the rule.[8]

In *Norvell License*, the driver had a coughing paroxysm resulting in a fatal car crash and an involuntary manslaughter charge. His driver's license was

Table 33.1 Pennsylvania driver's license impairment notification: Pennsylvania Code §83

1.	Any patient 15 years of age
2.	Notify within 10 days
3.	Epilepsy (§83.4)
	Seizure free
	Personal physician
	One year
	Treated or not
4.	Physical and medical standards (§83.5)
	Examining physician
	Condition likely to impair
5.	Periodic loss of consciousness, attention, or awareness

Reference: Pennsylvania Code §83.[7]

suspended for 3 months.[9] The court held that "a driver, stricken with illness, not reasonably to be anticipated, is not chargeable with negligence if the illness is the sole cause of the accident in the absence of any other testimony which could show a lack of due care." The common pleas court held that since there was no evidence of lack of due care, the defendant should not have had his driving privileges revoked. If the illness was unpredictable, the driver is not responsible. The order was vacated and his operating privileges were restored.

Likewise in *Sikorski* v. *Johnson*, the patient was alleged to have poor control of his diabetes, resulting in a fatal MVA, and his medical clinic should have foreseen this outcome.[10] They filed suit alleging the patient's negligent failure to control his diabetes, while the clinic should have been aware as well. The trial court held and the Supreme Court of Montana affirmed that there was no third-party duty to report, as the state had no statutory duty to suspend the driver's license,[11] and the clinic was immune from liability for good-faith reporting of an issue or event.[12]

Conclusion

Inability to drive can often be an undue burden for the patient, but it is important to balance the risks and benefits of individual versus societal harm. Unfortunately, we are often obliged to report a seizure, or any other medical condition that impairs driving ability, either by statute or by moral obligation.

References

1. Runge JW, Pulliam CL, Carter JM, Thomason MH. Enforcement of drunken driving laws in cases involving injured intoxicated drivers. *Ann Emerg Med.* 1996;27(1):66–72. DOI:10.1016/S0196-0644(96)70299-8.

2. Pennsylvania Motor Vehicle Code, Chapter 15, 75 Pa. C.S.A. §1518 (b).

3. Simpson CS, Klein GJ, Brennan FJ, Krahn AD, Yee R, Skanes AC. Impact of a mandatory physician reporting system for cardiac patients potentially unfit to drive. *Can J Cardiol.* 2000;16(10):1257–1263.

4. Simpson C, Ross D, Dorian P, Essebag V, Gupta A, Hamilton R et al. CCS Consensus Conference 2003: Assessment of the cardiac patient for fitness to drive and fly – executive summary. *Can J Cardiol.* 2004;20(13):1313–1323.

5. *Hospodar* v. *Schick*, 588 Pa. 765 (Pa. 2006).

6. Title 75 Pa.C.S.A. §1501 et seq.: Licensing of Drivers.

7. Title 67 Pa.Code §83: Physical and Mental Criteria Licensing of Drivers.

8. *Estate of Witthoeft* v. *Kiskaddon*, 557 Pa. 340, 733 A.2d 623 (1999).

9. Norvell License, 85 Pa. D. & C. 385 (1952).

10. *Sikorski* v. *Johnson*, 143 P 3d 161 (Mont 2006).

11. Montana Code Annotated §61-5-206, MCA (1999): Authority of Department to Suspend License or Driving Privileges.

12. Montana Code Annotated §37-2-312, MCA: Physician's Immunity from Liability.

Drug and Alcohol Abuse

Case

The patient came in to the emergency department (ED) with a laceration to the dorsal surface of his hand that had occurred while he was using a power saw at work. He had cut through the back of his hand, dividing his extensor tendons with an associated fracture and loss of sensation as well. The bleeding was controlled and the physician began intravenous antibiotics, administered a tetanus shot and morphine for pain, and contacted the hand surgeon for further evaluation.

At that point, the patient's employer arrived and asked about his employee's situation. He was already in the patient's room by the time the physician appeared. The situation seemed friendly enough. The physician asked the patient if it was appropriate that his employer was there to discuss his circumstances, and he said it was. It was a small family-owned business, and they were cousins.

The employer ushered the physician outside and asked if she could do a drug test. There had been some concerns over time that the patient was taking prescription pain medicine. The physician pointed out to him that it was the patient's right to consent or not consent. Unless there is an obligatory testing requirement, the patient has the right to decide whether they will be tested or not.

When his boss had left the room, the patient asked what he had to say. The discussion concerning a drug test was mentioned. The patient said he would prefer not to be tested, although he thought that his contract said he had to if the employer asked. The employer insisted that it had to be done and was again told the patient would not consent unless there was written evidence he had to. Otherwise there was no legal obligation to do so. The boss said he was going back to the office to look it up, then left and did not return. The patient had his injured hand repaired by plastic surgery, had a good outcome, and regained the use of the hand.

Medical Approach

These cases can often be difficult, since the prevalence of substance use is increasing. Rockett et al. studied the self-reported vs. actual incidence of 1502 ED patients with intact cognition and not in custody.[1] The highest self-reported incidence was found for alcohol (47% of males, 26% of females), marijuana (11% of males, 6% of females), and benzodiazepines (7% of males, 10% of females). The overall rate for eight targeted substances, after correction for underreporting, is 61–69% for men and 44–56% for women (Table 34.1). So, in this ED population approximately half the patients were found on screening to be using targeted substances.

London and Battistella evaluated the trauma population as reported in the National Trauma Data Bank with 996,225 patients evaluated at 258 facilities from 1998 to 2003.[2] They found only half of the patients admitted for injury were screened for alcohol, with 50% testing positive for alcohol. Likewise, only 36.3% of patients were tested for drug use, and 46.5% yielded positive results (Table 34.2).

Legal Analysis

In *Schmerber* v. *California*, the petitioner was arrested for driving under the influence (DUI) while receiving medical care at the hospital.[3] The police directed the physician to draw a blood sample to test the alcohol level, even after the patient's alleged refusal of blood draw. He contended that the blood withdrawal and use of this evidence violated his constitutional rights by denying his Fourth Amendment right to not be subjected to unreasonable search and seizure, Fifth Amendment right against self-incrimination, due-process rights of the Fourteenth Amendment, Sixth

Table 34.1 Self-reported vs. actual substance use for ED patients not in custody

	Substance	Incidence (%)	
		Male	**Female**
1.	Alcohol	47	26
2.	Marijuana	11	6
3.	Benzodiazepines	7	10
4.	Overall	61–69	44–56

Reference: Rockett et al.[1]

Table 34.2 Substance use in trauma patients (National Trauma Data Bank, 996 225 patients)

	Substance	Incidence (%)	
		Screened	**Positive**
1.	Alcohol	50	50
2.	Drug use	36.3	46.5

Reference: London and Battistella.[2]

Amendment right to counsel, and the due-process rights afforded in the Fourteenth Amendment.[4–6] The California Supreme Court upheld the conviction, and that decision was also affirmed by the Supreme Court of the United States (USSC).

In *Ferguson* v. *City of Charleston*, the court addressed the question of whether diagnostic testing to obtain evidence of criminal conduct can be done without the patient's consent.[7] The case was complicated by the circumstances where pregnant women were being screened for illicit substances at the time of delivery, and subsequently prosecuted because the newborn was positive for drugs of abuse as well. In these uniquely emotive circumstances the USSC agreed to "take the case as it comes to us" and concluded that the punitive nature of the intervention made the Fourth Amendment "unreasonable search and seizure" argument compelling. The appeal court decision was reversed and case remanded for proceedings consistent with this opinion.

Interestingly, Boldt evaluated substance use and the complex interaction of patient confidentiality, brief screening, and comprehensive intervention for this issue,[8] concluding that providers' uncertainty over confidentiality of screening and legal jeopardy may possibly have inhibited their ability to engage in these activities.

The patient typically has the right to consent, but by the time the issue arises they have often been medicated already. Often the patient will decline to have drug sampling done. Employers are usually insistent that testing should be done, but they cannot compel it unless there is a written contractual requirement for the employee to consent. Typically, when testing is mandated it is done in another setting where forensic analysis is possible. However, if the hospital is the designated mandatory testing location and there is a contract stipulation to do so, then the patient must submit a specimen. In this case the patient should be told that the testing was required on the basis of factors external to the ED staff, such as their employment contract.

Conclusion

If there is no such stipulation for testing, patients are certainly free to decline. The only caveat would be if the patient had a reason to have a urine drug screen based on their medical concerns. Then it would be mandated as part of their medical care, but not part of a forensic analysis. A particular case in point might be concern about a sympathomimetic agent, such as cocaine or methamphetamine, being used surreptitiously by a patient who is heading to the operating room, because this could have an adverse impact on the patient and the anesthetic plan might have to be changed depending on the result.

References

1. Rockett IRH, Putnam SL, Jia H, Smith GS. Declared and undeclared substance use among emergency department patients: a population-based study. *Addiction*. 2006;101(5):706–712. DOI:10.1111/j.1360-0443.2006.01397.x.

2. London JA, Battistella FD. Testing for substance use in trauma patients. *Arch Surg*. 2007;142(7):633–638. DOI:10.1001/archsurg.142.7.633.

3. *Schmerber* v. *California*, 384 U.S. 757 (1966).

4. U.S. Const. Amend IV.

5. U.S. Const. Amend V.

6. U.S. Const. Amend VI.

7. *Ferguson* v. *City of Charleston*, 532 U.S. 67 (2001)

8. Boldt RC. Confidentiality of alcohol and other drug abuse treatment information for emergency department and trauma center patients. *Health Matrix Clevel*. 2010;20(2):325–362.

Duty to Warn

Case

The emergency department (ED) staff had been down this road numerous times before with this patient. He often complained of suicidal or homicidal ideation. He was usually angry and wanted either to harm himself or to harm someone else. Typically, the scenario was complicated by drugs or alcohol and often some family stressors were involved. Sometimes he was admitted to the hospital, while other times he went home with a safety plan in place. He was well known for this behavior. His family was friendly and often came in to help him through his distress.

The latest event seemed to emanate from a squabble with his wife. He threatened to harm her, but had no formulated plan. He seemed intoxicated and had a standard screening laboratory profile and a head CT scan, all of which were normal. His family came in and so did his wife, and there appeared to be some reconciliation between them. After an extensive discussion with his intensive case manager, it seemed like there was consensus that the safety plan was in place and the patient was discharged home with his wife.

Later that evening, there was a police call that a man was at home brandishing a firearm. His family was out of the house, but he was intoxicated and belligerent. About an hour later, law enforcement personnel came to the ED with the patient in custody; it was the man who had been there earlier in the day. He had brandished a firearm but allowed his family to leave the house, which was fortunate for all involved. He was then reevaluated and admitted to the psychiatric ward.

The next day a call was received from the risk management department, questioning why the patient was sent home. Was there indeed a duty to warn the public or specifically his family concerning his behavior? The provider stated the patient had made no threats against the public in general, only a vague threat

toward his wife. He had done this before and had left the ED with both extended families, with everyone comfortable with the plan. This was acceptable to risk management, although they suggested better documentation.

Medical Approach

The "duty to protect and warn" is especially important in psychiatric practice, in which a practicing psychiatrist is often the recipient of patients' overt threats toward themselves or others. Depending on the formulation and the concrete nature of a patient's plan, the psychiatrist may have an obligation to report that threat to law enforcement.

Legal Analysis

The seminal "duty to warn" case is universally held to be *Tarasoff* v. *Regents of the University of California*.[1] Here an outpatient seeking voluntary care allegedly confided their intention to kill someone to their treating psychologist. The psychologist notified campus police, who briefly detained the patient, but he was released as rational and the police failed to warn the victim of the potential threat. Unfortunately, the patient completed his threat and the victim's family alleged a failure to commit and failure to warn. The Supreme Court of California held that plaintiffs have an ability to amend their complaint so that even though the attempt at commitment failed, the therapist's duty to warn was intact. Interestingly, they concluded the police had no special relationship with the assailant that mandated a duty to incarcerate.

In *Durflinger* v. *Artiles*, a psychiatric patient was discharged from the hospital after an involuntary commitment procedure. He returned home and allegedly killed his mother and brother.[2] The remaining family sued the physicians for alleged negligent release of the patient. The district court noted the

Table 35.1 Duty to protect and warn in 50 states and four territories

1.	Mandatory statute	22
2.	Permissive statute	19
3.	Caselaw guidance	4
4.	No guidance	6
5.	Foreclose warning statute	3
		54

Reference: National Conference of State Legislatures[3]

difficulty in predicting violent behavior by a patient, but held that should not be a reason to preclude recovery. The defendant's motion for a new trial was denied, but their motion to amend to decrease the amount of damages awarded as liability for premature discharge was affirmed by the court.

The National Conference of State Legislatures (NCSL) has defined the established obligations for mental health professionals to warn, balanced by patient confidentiality issues.[3] First, 22 states have a statutory mandatory duty to protect and warn, in which health-care providers are liable for failure to warn. Second, 19 states or territories have a permissive duty to warn, again guided by statute, permitting but not requiring reporting. Third, four states have no statutory authority, but warning is allowed, based on caselaw. Fourth, six states or territories have not clarified a state posting on the matter. Fifth, three states or territories have statutorily precluded the duty to protect or warn (Table 35.1).

Wettstein evaluated the ability to predict violent behavior in patients, noting the duality of the requirement to protect and warn balanced with the lack of clinical feasibility.[4] The first generation of violence prediction studies focused on long-term predictions in offending populations. The irony is that the focus population is non-offenders in an outpatient setting. Second-generation studies target imminent violence in non-criminal populations evaluated for involuntary commitment, demonstrating low levels of predictive accuracy and generalizability. Wettstein concludes that in a low-risk outpatient population there is likely to be a significant number of false positives, and suggests the antitherapeutic effects of confidentiality breach should be monitored.

Conclusion

Circumstances in emergency medicine are often similar to those in the psychiatric community. Typically, in the ED environment the patient often has a compounding factor of drug or alcohol use, but we also have a duty to warn based on the specificity of threat. Preemptive hospitalization to avoid any subsequent tragedy is frequently resorted to in the ED setting.

References

1. *Tarasoff* v. *The Regents of the University of California*, 17 Cal. 3d 425 (1976).

2. *Durflinger* v. *Artiles*, 563 F. Supp 322 (1981).

3. National Conference of State Legislatures (NCSL). Mental Health Professionals' Duty to Warn. January 1, 2013.

4. Wettstein RM. The prediction of violent behavior and the duty to protect third parties. *Behav Sci Law*. 1984;2(3):291–317. DOI:10.1002/bsl.2370020306.

Electronic Health Records

Case

The hospital was instituting a new electronic health record (EHR) system. The transition had gone as well as might be expected. There was some decrease in efficiency to begin with, but once people got used to the system it returned to about the same efficiency level as before. The promise of greater efficiencies would certainly take time to appear as the experience of the group matured.

The hospital quality improvement team contacted the emergency department (ED) staff to report there had been issues with the documentation system. There were selective problems in the system that seemed to disproportionately affect some of the ED patient care records. There appeared to be a systematic error that changed the physicians listed in the discharge instructions, as well as making errors in the patient's age and sex in the demographic section. In addition, there was some preprogrammed text that seemed to repeat itself in an illogical fashion, and seemed to be simply cut and pasted into the EHR.

This issue had come to the quality team's attention because they had received an attorney complaint attempting to file suit over a patient care matter. It did not seem to rise to the level of any harm to the patient or adverse outcome, but the attorney had been contacted by a number of patients who had errors in their discharge paperwork. He thought approaching the facility to settle out of court in light of the sloppy documentation practice would be successful. The group director's view was that this demographic download was not really related to any physician activity and suggested if there were concerns about the EHR the hospital should address this issue with the EHR vendor.

Medical Approach

Most, if not all, facilities will transition to an EHR system in the near future. Ideally, it is better for patient care, efficiency, and medicolegal documentation. In practice, however, we recognize that there is certainly a decrease in efficiency with some EHR systems and the promised improved medicolegal capabilities have not materialized in some settings.

The obvious question raised by the clinician is what is the effect of the EHR on medical malpractice liability. The four core functionalities of EHR systems include first, documentation of clinical findings; second, recording of testing and imaging results; third, computerized provider order entry (CPOE); and fourth, clinical decision-making support (Table 36.1).[1] Mangalmurti et al. reported the potential expansion of medicolegal liability in the implementation of an EHR.[2] The potential expanded liability includes violation of privacy and confidentiality laws, disputes of ownership of health data, and heightened vulnerability to fraud claims because of improved tracking of services billed and provided.

Health-care professional and provider organizations should stand ready to manage EHR-associated risks (Table 36.2).[3] First, they should decline to sign contractual provisions that immunize the system developer. Second, they must select a system designed to minimize the risk of error or misuse. Third, the system should maximize the ease of record retrieval. Fourth, organizations should provide adequate training and education. Fifth, organizations should define their expectations. Sixth, they should ensure that practice conditions allow the new technology to be maximized. Seventh, they should manage patients' expectations about secure messaging and accessing of the EHR. Eighth, they should serve as experts to

Table 36.1 Core functionalities of the EHR

1. Documentation of clinical findings
2. Recording of testing and imaging results
3. Computerized entry of provider orders
4. Support for clinical decision-making

Reference: Jha et al.[1]

Table 36.2 Managing EHR risks

1. Decline liability immunization of vendor
2. Minimize risk of error or misuse
3. Maximize ease of record retrieval
4. Provide adequate training and education
5. Define organizational expectations
6. Ensure practice conditions allow technology maximization
7. Expectations of secure messaging and records
8. Define limitations in legal realm

Reference: Mangalmurti et al.[2]

Table 36.3 Productivity analysis of the electronic medical record (EMR)

Work product	Proportion
	95% CI, %
1. Data entry	44
2. Direct patient contact	28
3. Colleague discussion	13
4. Review test results and records	12
5. Other	3

Reference: Hill et al.[6]

inform the judicial system of the limitations of clinical decision support systems and the appropriateness of departures from the norm.

Legal, ethical, and financial issues have also been raised.[4] The legal issues include the clinician's responsibility for reviewing the clinical synopsis from multiple clinicians and facilities, liability from overriding clinical decision support warnings, and alerts and mechanisms to publicly report potential EHR safety issues. The ethical dilemmas include opt-out provisions that exclude patients from electronic record storage, sale of deidentified patient data by EHR vendors, control of adolescent medical data stored, and permitted access to the financial data.

The advent of the integrated delivery system and the interface with the EHR allow commoditization of both the data and the technology delivery system.[4] The importance of secure collection, storage, and use of protected patient health data has become paramount in the industry. The risks of aggregation and dissemination of the associated metadata are formidable.

An interesting paradoxical safety effect has been noted in the setting of the preprogrammed monitoring and triggering systems designed to prevent clinical error. Kesselheim et al. described "alert fatigue," in which the sheer number of warning alerts may cause clinicians to become desensitized to this safety feature.[5] Overtly sensitive warning systems must commonly be overridden by practitioners. Kesselheim et al. recommend a more restrained and deliberate warning system, requiring input from the clinicians themselves.

Adverse effects on provider efficiency have been described as well. Hill et al. evaluated the impact of an EHR on physician efficiency in a community hospital ED (Table 36.3).[6] The majority of the time was spent on data entry (44%), followed by direct patient care (28%), discussion with colleagues (13%), reviewing test results and medical records (12%), and additional activities (3%). In a busy 10-hour shift, approximately 4000 mouse clicks were needed for the ED physician's charting functions. The key is to streamline the EHR to minimize excess steps, based on the recommendations of end users.

Legal Analysis

Caselaw in this area is a nascent industry, but it is starting to develop along two lines: liability for a data breach and rights to computerized information.

In *Paul v. Providence Health System – Oregon*, computer disks with information on 365,000 patients were stolen from the personal vehicle of an employee of a not-for-profit health system.[7] The trial court and appeals court held that the plaintiffs had failed to state a valid claim for negligence, or for violation of the Unlawful Trade Practices Act, which prohibits, "unfair or deceptive acts or practices in or affecting commerce."[8] The Supreme Court of Oregon held that short of evidence of any actual inappropriate use of this information, the plaintiffs have not suffered damages consistent with a negligence action, granting the motion to dismiss their complaint. Since there was no evidence of unapproved use of this information by unapproved third parties, there were no resultant damages at the test point in time.

In *Bowman* v. *St Luke's-Roosevelt Hosp. Ctr.*, the patient presented with a leg complaint, given a diagnosis of gastroenteritis, discharged, and eventually succumbed to necrotizing fasciitis. The emergency medicine resident testified that they were bound by the diagnostic system's templates that guided the diagnostic and treatment plans.[9] A medical malpractice action was filed seeking discovery of the treating ED physician's work product, including "screen shots of every stage of the data input process in the Emergency Department EM-STAT system as testified to." The discovery target, clinical care templates focused on fever used in ED practice, was felt to be "over-broad and oppressive" by the hospital. The Supreme Court of New York County held in a final disposition the request for protective order was denied. The request for review was not "overly broad," and the petitioner was allowed to view the computerized program available to the treating ED physician.

Conclusion

It is crucial that the physician review the documentation program on a periodic basis to ensure there are no systematic errors or discrepancies that could change their documentation and affect their liability in an adverse way. Most documentation programs are managed off site. It is crucial to establish an interface locally, with ongoing improvement provided by the service provider, to ensure the system at the individual facility is compliant.

References

1. Jha AK, DesRoches CM, Campbell EG, Donelan K, Rao SR, Ferris TG, et al. Use of the electronic health records in US hospitals. *N Engl J Med*. 2009;360(16):1628–1638. DOI:10.1056/NEJMsa0900592.

2. Mangalmurti SS, Murtagh L, Mello MM. Medical malpractice liability in the age of electronic health records. *N Engl J Med*. 2010;363(21):2060–2067.

3. Sittig DF, Singh H. Legal, ethical and financial dilemmas in electronic health record adoption and use. *Pediatrics*. 2011;127(4):e1042–e1047. DOI:10.1542/Peds.2010-2184.

4. Anderson JG. Security of the distributed electronic patient record: a case-based approach to identifying policy issues. *Int J Med Inform*. 2000;60(2):111–118. DO:10.1016/S1386-5056(00)00110-6.

5. Kesselheim AS, Cresswell K, Phansalkar S, Bates DW, Sheikh A. Clinical decision support systems could be modified to reduce "alert fatigue" while still minimizing the risk of litigation. *Health Aff*. 2011;30(12):2310–2317. DOI:10.1377/hlthaff.2010.1111.

6. Hill RG, Sears LM, Melanson SW. 4000 clicks: a productivity analysis of electronic medical records in a community hospital ED. *Am J Emerg Med*. 2013;31(11):1591–1594. DOI:10.1016/AJEM.2013.06.028.

7. *Paul* v. *Providence Health System-Oregon*, 273 P.3d 106 (2012).

8. Unfair Trade Practices Act, FTC Act, 15 U.S.C §45.

9. *Bowman* v. *St Luke's-Roosevelt Hosp. Ctr*, 2011 NY Slip Op 32738 (U), October 17, 2011.

Emergency Consent

Case

Emergency medical services (EMS) had brought the patient to the back door of the emergency department (ED) with the presentation of acute left-sided weakness. She had hemiplegia, as she could not move the left side of her body. She could barely speak, but seemed aware of her circumstances. However, after she arrived in the ED her respiratory status quickly declined, and required immediate endotracheal intubation for airway control.

The paramedics stated that the patient had met them at the door of her residence stating she had left-sided paresthesias or numbness, and then quickly lost control of the motor capability of that left side. They transported her rapidly to the hospital. She was otherwise healthy, had diabetes and hypertension, but was active. She worked as a teacher and had recently run a half-marathon, according to her next-door neighbor. Also according to this neighbor, she had no family or at least no close family to speak of.

A CT scan was performed quickly, showing no signs of intracranial hemorrhage or acute stroke. She was clearly within a time window for intravenous administration of tissue plasminogen activator (TPA) and the pharmacy prepared the medication for administration. They asked about the patient's or her family's informed consent. It was quickly recognized the patient could not consent, and no immediate family was present. A distant relative was listed with a phone number that was found to be non-functioning, and the ED staff clarified again with the neighbor that the patient had no other immediate family.

A quick consult with neurology recommended intravenous TPA administration. The time window was appropriate for treatment and the patient had no CT evidence of injury and no complications, making her an ideal TPA candidate.

After discussion with her primary care physician, neurology, and the radiologist, it was felt that TPA should be administered. The treating physician signed the emergency consent form and proceeded. Things seemed to go well; the patient woke up and started to move her left side, but then became unresponsive. A repeat CT scan showed a large intracranial hemorrhage and the patient was transferred to the neurosurgical referral center with a post-thrombolytic intracranial hemorrhage.

The hospital-based quality improvement committee evaluated this case and found the care to be appropriate within the current guidelines. The hospital legal department contacted the ED physician 3 months later, stating that a distant cousin had filed suit alleging battery as one of the issues as the patient had not given informed consent for the administration of this medication.

Medical Approach

Today, with rapidly changing emergency medicine diagnostics, procedures, and interventions, the requirement for informed consent is clear. However, cases in which informed consent cannot be obtained, typically due to the patient's lack of competence and the absence of any relative available to consent, other measures are required. Typically, there is consensus surrounding the "doctrine of emergency consent" that allows the physician to sign a consent form for the patient when the preponderance of evidence suggests an intervention is appropriate, as was clearly done with this case.

A more formalized presentation of this consent in an urgent situation is the "doctrine of implied consent," which again suggests that physician truly makes a balanced logical decision in the patient's stead. Here they balance the benefits and the detriments of a treatment, focusing on the patient's best interest.

However, most patients want to be informed about even minor procedures, or at least consent to them. Easton et al. performed an analysis of 174 patients asking them to estimate the amount of time required for procedural consent.[1] They rated simple procedures such as venipuncture to require a mean of 1.02 minutes of extra practitioner time and complex procedures, such as lumbar puncture, to require 7.78 minutes. Approximately half of patients (48–52%) felt no consent was required for drawing blood or starting an intravenous drip. They concluded that defining procedures amenable to implied consent may be difficult.

Lastly, in an attempt to preserve the concept of informed consent, the "doctrine of deferred consent" is often used in the research realm. Here, the patient or family is approached after the intervention has been administered and the risks and benefits discussed. If there is consent, the intervention continues; without it, the intervention is ended.

Legal Analysis

Shine v. *Vega* raises the question of the balance between the right of a competent adult to refuse medical treatment and the right of a physician to preserve life.[2] The patient had severe asthma, was in severe respiratory distress, and had repeatedly and vigorously declined intubation and mechanical ventilation. The ED physician intervened and intubated the patient, who eventually died 2 years later. Her father sued for alleged tortious conduct and wrongful death, as she was traumatized by this experience. The trial court instructed the jury that the patient did not have the right to refuse emergency treatment in an "emergency situation," nor could the physician commit battery in this situation. The Massachusetts Supreme Judicial Court vacated the trial court judgment, holding that the jury instruction was erroneous, remanding for a new trial.

In *Martin* v. *Richards*, the patient presented to the ED with a head injury after striking the back of an automobile while on a bicycle.[3] The patient's presentation consisted of a loss of consciousness at the scene, vomiting, and post-event amnesia. The patient was diagnosed with a concussion, admitted for observation, and went on to have an epidural hematoma and significant residual neurological deficit. The family filed suit alleging the emergency consent for admission should have discussed the availability of CT on the premises and the lack of neurosurgical

Table 37.1 Informed consent disclosure not required (Wisconsin §448.30)

1.	Detailed technical information
2.	Risks known to patient
3.	Extremely remote possibilities
4.	Failure to treat more harmful than treatment
5.	Patient incapable of consenting
6.	Alternate treatments for conditions not in differential

Reference: Wisconsin State Legislature.[4]

capability to address progression or complication. The issue raised was whether the physicians were obligated to discuss these matters with the family, citing the Wisconsin Informed Consent Statute §448.30 in which "any physician who treats a patient shall inform the patient about the availability of reasonable alternate medical modes of treatment, and about the benefits and risks of these treatments."[4] The disclosure standard would require information to be disclosed that a "reasonable" physician, in the same or similar medical specialty, would know and disclose under these circumstances. However, there are issues the physician is not required to discuss. First, detailed technical information the patient might not understand. Second, risks that are apparent or already known to the patient. Third, the presence of extremely remote possibilities that might falsely or detrimentally alarm the patient. Fourth, information in emergencies in which failure to provide treatment would be more harmful than the treatment. Fifth, information when the patient is incapable of consenting. Sixth, information about alternate modes of treatment, when that disease or condition was not included in the differential (Table 37.1).

The jury found the ED and admitting physician were not negligent in the care provided, but the ED physician was negligent in the failure to discuss the treatment alternatives, with a significant financial award. Following the verdict, the circuit court granted the ED physician's motion to dismiss the informed consent complaint, holding the likelihood of intracranial hemorrhage was "extremely remote." The appeal court reversed and remanded, taking issue with the "extremely remote" classification. The Supreme Court of Wisconsin affirmed the appeal court decision, allowing the jury verdict to stand and concluding emergency consent required discussion of treatment alternatives. They reversed the appeal court decision in that although the verdict did not have a causation question linking informed consent with causation, it was not a fatal flaw.

In *Baptist Memorial Hospital System* v. *Sampson*, a patient was bitten by an arachnid eventually identified to be a brown recluse spider.[5] She was taken to the ED, diagnosed with an allergic reaction, and discharged. She presented again a day later, was evaluated by a different physician, and similar treatment was continued. She then returned 14 hours later in a critical condition, and was correctly diagnosed and treated. She later filed suit with question raised concerning the "employment" status of the ED physicians and hospital responsibility. The hospital offered as defense a patient-signed "Consent for Diagnosis, Treatment and Hospital Care Form," that stated the hospital was not responsible for the ED physicians:

> "I acknowledge and agree that the hospital is not responsible for the judgment or conduct of any physician who treats or provides a professional service to me, but rather each physician is an independent contractor, who is self-employed and is not the agent, servant or employee of the hospital."

The Supreme Court of Texas held the plaintiff had not met her burden to prove vicarious liability or ostensible agency responsibility for the independent contractor physicians, although the patient alleged that at the time of her illness she did not remember signing the forms, seeing any signage, or choosing her doctor. The Texas Supreme Court reversed the appeal court verdict and rendered a decision that the plaintiff take nothing.

Conclusion

The emergency exception to the informed consent requirement is based on the premise that a reasonable person would not be denied necessary medical

Table 37.2 Emergency exception to informed consent

1.	Patient incompetent and unable to consent
2.	Treatment is lifesaving
3.	Default pathway for minors without parents
4.	Event is emergent or unexpected
5.	Precludes chronic condition or routine care
6.	Not used to counteract a patient decision

Reference: Richards.[6]

care because they were too incapacitated to consent to treatment.[6] There are legal requirements for the emergency exception. First, the patient must be incompetent and unable to consent. Second, the treatment is necessary to save their life or prevent permanent disability. Third, minors by default enter this pathway if the parent or guardian is not available. Fourth, event is emergent or unexpected. Fifth, this exception precludes intervening with chronic conditions or routine care. Sixth, it is not to be used as justification to intervene if the patient has declined treatment (Table 37.2).

References

1. Easton RB, Graber MA, Monnahan J, Hughes J. Defining the scope of implied consent in the emergency department. *Am J Bioethics.* 2007;7(12):35–38. DOI:10.1080/15265160701710196.

2. *Shine* v. *Vega*, 429 Mass. 456, 709 N.E.2d 58 (Mass. 1999).

3. *Martin* v. *Richards*, 531 N.W.2d 70 (1995).

4. Wisconsin State Legislature, §448.30:Informed Consent.

5. *Baptist Memorial Hospital* v. *Sampson*, 969 S.W.2d 945 (1998).

6. Richards EP. The Emergency Exception. Law and the Physician Homepage. biotech.law.lsu.edu/books/lbb/x268.htm.

Emergency Medical Services

Case

The emergency medical services (EMS) crew stationed at the football game received a response call for a patient who had fallen down an escalator. When they arrived they found an elderly woman in apparent cardiac arrest, with some bystanders performing CPR. The patient did not seem responsive and an external automated external defibrillator (AED) was used. The patient was defibrillated without response.

The EMS crew began to prepare for intubation, with the bag valve mask and endotracheal tube ready. A man emerged from the crowd and stated he was an anesthesiologist and that he was going to handle the airway. His responses seemed a little slow and the EMS crew had concerns that he might have been drinking. The crew told him that in this state paramedics work with field protocols under EMS direction that provides standing orders and protocols. This meant that online medical command was not necessary and they would handle this case. The volunteer's assistance could be helpful, but hopefully would not be necessary. They proceeded to care for the patient. The volunteer began to be argumentative, saying that he was a physician and they were only paramedics, so he was more qualified to perform the airway procedure.

The paramedic again reiterated that circumstances were capably in hand. Along with her partner she successfully incubated the patient. The volunteer physician's wife now arrived and advised him to come back to his seat. The intubation achieved a successful return of spontaneous circulation and the patient was transported to the hospital.

Medical Approach

Cases such as this occur far too frequently when there are multiple health-care providers at a scene, some have emergency and field training and others do not. Most states operate a paramedic-based field resuscitation system, working with medical direction and standing orders and protocols that typically does not allow intervention by bystanders even if they are qualified, unless they are asked to offer assistance by the first responders. Some EMS services, jurisdictions, and state agencies will offer an informational card to bystanders to explain this policy, aid in their understanding, and avoid any subsequent controversy at the scene that may impact patient care.

Information concerning EMS malpractice litigation has been sparse but largely consistent over time. Goldberg et al. reviewed prehospital care litigation in a large metropolitan EMS system, analyzing cases for a 12-year period from 1976 to 1987.[1] The EMS responded to two million calls and half were transported. Sixty claims were filed, equivalent to one lawsuit per 27,371 encounters or 17,995 transports, and 38% (26) of cases were either dismissed or settled for nominal amounts.

Morgan et al. evaluated a cohort from 1987 to 1992 and identified 76 cases, half of them cases of ambulance collisions, typically at intersections, and half relating to patient care issues.[2] Almost half the cases cited specific EMS personnel, either an emergency medical technician (EMT) or paramedic, with five claims settled for more than $1 million. Allegations in the patient care events included arrival delay, inadequate assessment, inadequate treatment, patient transport delay, and no patient transport (Table 38.1).

Wang et al. performed a more recent analysis of 326 EMS claims for a one-year period from 2003 to 2004.[3] Once again the most common claim was related to emergency vehicle crash in 37% (122), followed by patient handling 36% (118), clinical management 12% (40), other events 10% (33) and response or transport events 8% (25) (Table 38.2), analysis of patient outcome found death in 17% (54), and life-threatening or disabling injuries in 8% (25) of patients.

Table 38.1 EMS malpractice allegations

1. Arrival delay
2. Inadequate assessment
3. Inadequate treatment
4. Patient transport delay
5. No patient transport

Reference: Morgan et al.[2]

Table 38.2 Type of EMS claims

	Incidence (%)
1. Emergency vehicle crash	37
2. Patient handling errors	36
3. Clinical management	12
4. Other events	10
5. Response or transport events	8

Reference: Wang et al.[3]

Legal Analysis

One of the basic tenets of EMS care is the necessity of scene safety. In *Zepeda* v. *City of Los Angeles*, the plaintiff alleged no care was rendered by on-scene paramedics to a patient shot in the neck, even though allegedly there was no apparent danger, until law enforcement arrived.[4] The trial court felt the paramedics had no obligation to render assistance, and held no liability until that treatment was begun. The Superior Court of Los Angeles County concluded, as a matter of law, that the plaintiff's action is without merit and the trial court properly sustained the City's demurrer.

In *Wright* v. *City of Los Angeles*, the paramedic happened upon the patient at an accident scene, asked if they were all right, did a brief inspection in which the patient appeared normal, but obtained no vital signs.[5] The patient died 5 minutes after the paramedic left the scene. The trial court granted summary judgment for the defense on some counts, but held the paramedic accountable. The defense petitioned for "judgment non-obstante verdicto," judgment notwithstanding the verdict (JNOV), a motion in which the allegation is that the jury verdict is not supported by the evidence and the judge should overrule the verdict, which was granted in this case.[6] This motion has been replaced by "judgment as a matter of law," assuming no reasonable jury could find for the opposing party, but presented before the jury reaches a verdict.[7] However, on appeal of other pleadings, the defendant felt damages awarded to the plaintiff were excessive, and death was due more to a pre-existing medical condition than to the quality of the care provided. The Court of Appeals of California held that the paramedic was responsible since they had assumed care responsibilities, but had not upheld conventional standards of care in the evaluation. They reversed the JNOV and order granting a new trial, finding provider liability.

Another concern is evaluating and not transporting the patient, based on the patient's refusal of care. In *Hackman* v. *AMR*, paramedics responded to a motor vehicle accident (MVA) scene and talked with the driver, who declined treatment or transport, feeling she had no injury.[8] Bystanders felt she was confused, but she was standing talking to the police officer next to her vehicle when paramedics arrived. They stated they conducted a "visual and interactive" assessment, and allegedly felt she was not in need of additional care. The patient subsequently collapsed 20 minutes later, and the paramedics returned and transported her to the hospital. The trial court awarded the defendant's summary judgment motion holding that a contract for patient care was not entered. However, this decision was overruled by the appeal court, who held that indeed a care event was begun, and that standard of care duty was breached by the paramedics in their evaluation and decision-making.

In *Applewhite* v. *Accuhealth, Inc.*, a child was administered an antibiotic by a home health nurse and suffered an anaphylactic reaction. The family called 911. The initial response was by a Basic Life Support crew staffed by EMTs alone, a service provided by the city government.[9] They began CPR, while awaiting the Advanced Life Support (ALS) crew, which took another 20 minutes, declining the mother's request to transfer to a local hospital four minutes away. The mother stated she was not informed it would take 20 minutes for ALS support to arrive. The nurse settled and the home health agency dissolved in bankruptcy. The trial court held that the City defendant, responsible for the EMS and paramedic responders, did not owe a special duty of care, nor were they the proximate cause of harm. The New York Appellate Division reversed and reinstated the claim against the City, as the existence of a special duty to the patient is a justiciable issue for a jury to decide.

Table 38.3 EMS immunity

1.	Not gross negligence
2.	Within scope of employment and training
3.	Good faith and intent

Reference: Shin.[10]

Conclusion

Most EMS personnel are obviously concerned about their liability in these changing times. Generally speaking, the EMS immunity basis includes, first, the care provided need not be perfect, but not characteristic of gross negligence.[10] Second, the practitioner should act providing service within their scope of employment and training. Third, the care should be provided in good faith and intent (Table 38.3).

References

1. Goldberg RJ, Zautcke JL, Koenigberg MD, Lee RW, Nagorka FW, Kling M, Ward SA. A review of prehospital care litigation in a large metropolitan EMS system. *Ann Emerg Med.* 1990;19(5):557–561.

2. Morgan DL, Wainscott MP, Knowles HC. Emergency medical services liability litigation in the United States: 1987–1992. *Prehosp Disast Med.*1994;9(4):214–220.

3. Wang HE, Fairbanks RJ, Shah MN, Abo BN, Yealy DM. Tort claims and adverse events in emergency medical services. *Ann Emerg Med.* 2008;52(3):256–262. DOI:10.1016/j.annemergmed.2008.02.011.

4. *Zepeda* v. *City of Los Angeles*, 223 Cal. App. 3d 232 (1990).

5. *Wright* v. *City of Los Angeles*, 792 F.2d 145 (1986).

6. Motion for Judgment Notwithstanding the Verdict. www.law.cornell.edu. Accessed May 15, 2016.

7. Federal Rules of Civil Procedure. Title VI. Rule 50: Motion for Judgment as a Matter of Law in a Jury Trial.

8. *Hackman* v. *American Medical Response*, 2004 WL 823206 (Cal. App.4 Dist.) (Unpublished Opinion).

9. *Applewhite* v. *Accuhealth, Inc.*, N.E.2d, 2013 WL 3185185 (N.Y. 2013).

10. Shin RK. Protection against liability for emergency medical services providers. *J Emerg Manag.* 2010;8(3):17–21. DOI:10.5055/Jen.2010.0015.

Chapter 39

Emergency Medical Treatment and Labor Act

Case

The patient came in to the emergency department (ED) with a significant hand injury after using a chainsaw. The chainsaw had kicked back and the dorsum, or back of his hand, was lacerated by the saw blade. The patient had divided the extensor tendon of his second and third digits, and the skin laceration was complex but able to be closed. The ED physician asked about the patient's tetanus status, got a radiograph, ordered intravenous antibiotics, and contacted the physician who was on call for hand surgery that evening.

The orthopedist on call stated that although he was indeed on hand call, he was not prepared to deal with the hand laceration as he had not done a hand fellowship in his training. He suggested the ED physician should notify the on-call plastic surgeon. When plastic surgery was contacted they pointed out that there was an orthopedist on call. When the orthopedist was recontacted he suggested that this "trauma patient" should be transferred to another facility. Plastic surgery was notified once more and replied, "This is a constant problem and I'm not doing another hand case. They need to take responsibility." The ED physician called orthopedics back for the last time, saying the plastic surgeon felt the orthopedist should do the case. Once again, the orthopedist refused, and told the ED physician to transfer the patient. Arrangements were made with the tertiary care referral center and the patient was transferred to the hand surgery service after a discussion with the on-call hand surgeon.

Two weeks later the hospital risk management department received a request from the state health department concerning a potential EMTALA violation. The patient felt he had been transferred for financial reasons, because he did not have insurance. The ED physician assured risk management that at no point did any insurance discussion ever take place. The issue was that the orthopedics on-call physician, who

had not done a hand fellowship, felt uncomfortable with providing care, so the transfer to a higher level of care was appropriate and proper for this patient.

Medical Approach

EMTALA is a statute requiring medical screening and stabilization of a patient presenting for emergency care within the capabilities of the hospital facility and potential transfer when the capability of the facility is exceeded, irrespective of the patient's insurance status.[1] The statute specifies the requirements for the medical screening exam (MSE), the stabilization process, on-call systems, and the transfer protocol for unstable patients.[2]

Legal Analysis

EMTALA has been invoked to allege errors in medical screening and the diagnostic process.

In *Baber* v. *Hospital Corporation of America*, the patient presented to the ED with nausea and in a state of agitation. She was treated for alleged alcohol use and a pre-existing psychiatric illness.[3] Subsequently, she had a seizure; fell, suffering a head laceration; and was transferred for specialty care. She subsequently succumbed to a fractured skull and subdural hematoma. The trial court granted a summary judgment motion for the defendant, concluding the physicians could not be sued under an EMTALA theory, and it was not proven that the hospital failed to meet its screening and transfer obligations. This decision was affirmed by the United States Court of Appeals (USCA), Fourth Circuit, as no reversible errors were noted.

In *Power* v. *Arlington Hospital Association*, a patient presented to the ED with hip, abdominal, and back pain accompanied by fever and chills.[4] She was discharged home with pain medication and return instructions, but subsequently admitted with sepsis with catastrophic complications. The plaintiff filed suit alleging a failed medical screening procedure and being transferred in an unstable condition. The trial court awarded a $5 million verdict to the plaintiff concerning screening, but vindicated the hospital on the transfer. The hospital appealed to the USCA, Fourth Circuit questioning the interface of medical malpractice caps and tax-exempt status with EMTALA. The appeal court vacated the jury award and remanded to the district court to conform the verdicts to these financial limits.

In *Gatewood* v. *Washington Healthcare Corporation*, the patient allegedly died of a heart attack the day after being discharged from the ED with a diagnosis of musculoskeletal pain.[5] The claim was dismissed, with the district court holding that EMTALA did not provide a cause of action for fully insured patients who were misdiagnosed. The USCA, District of Columbia affirmed the dismissal of the complaint, stating that EMTALA did not provide a broad federal cause of action for medical malpractice. However, they felt the insurance status rationale of the trial court was not relevant and that EMTALA applied to "any individual" who presents to the ED.

EMTALA has also been used as a standard to allege deficient care relating to the transport process. In *Thompson* v. *Sun City Community Hospital Inc.*, a 13-year-old trauma patient suffered a partially transected femoral artery.[6] He was evaluated and stabilized by the ED physician, who consulted the orthopedic surgeon who evaluated the patient and then consulted vascular surgery by phone. The decision was made to transfer, presumably by the consultants, with the allegation that it was related to the patient's "charity care" status. The Supreme Court of Arizona found that the hospital breached its duty regarding this transfer and the initial favorable judgment was reversed. The directed verdicts exonerating the ED physician and the vascular surgeon were correct, while the orthopedic surgeon was not a defendant.

Clearly this case had no issues relating to the patient's insurance status. It was merely a question of the hospital's capability to care for that patient's specific health condition. EMTALA states if such a service is provided then a reasonable on-call system should be available with practitioners available to care for the patient.

Conclusion

A situation that often arises is when an on-call specialist suggests that the patient should be transferred because they have not done any additional specialized training for the medical issue at hand. Some aspects of medical practice have become so hyper-specialized that in some cases it is a reasonable contention that medicolegal risk may be increased by caring for these patients at the local site. Transfer of more complicated cases to a referral center is therefore becoming common. On the other hand, the patient does have the right to have a local hospital service provided within the capability of that institution, without having to go to another facility, if that service is routinely offered at the local facility.

References

1. Emergency Medical Treatment and Active Labor Act (EMTALA), 42 USCA §1395 (dd), (b) (1), (c) (1).

2. O'Rourke IK, Vukmir RB. *EMTALA: The Continued Evolution.* (Traverse City, MI: ECI Healthcare Partners, 2008).

3. *Baber* v. *Hospital Corporation of America*, 977 F.2d 872 (1992).

4. *Power* v. *Arlington Hospital Association*, 42 F.3d 851 (1994).

5. *Gatewood* v. *Washington Healthcare Corporation*, 933 F.2d 1037 (1991).

6. *Thompson* v. *Sun City Community Hospital, Inc.*, 141 Ariz. 597, 688 P.2d 605 (1984).

Employment Issues

Case

The physician was a long-time staff member. She had great clinical skills, was caring, and had great staff and patient relationships. She had won the "hospital physician of the year" award twice in the past. She had previously chaired the quality improvement committee, and had sat on the medical executive board. She was known as a passionate patient care advocate, and had an unwavering commitment to her work.

The facility had fallen on hard economic times, and after a number of interim solutions it was purchased by a larger hospital conglomerate. The transition took place rapidly, as there was significant institutional change with job cuts and personnel reassignment. In addition, there was a change in the hospital administration, as well as a change in the composition of the hospital board of directors. Previously sympathetic partners did not acknowledge the physician's concern and passion over patient care. They suggested that the same business strategy had been implemented at other institutions with success.

The physician was approached by the nursing staff from the unit in which she worked, who were concerned about the job cuts and an adverse effect on patient care. Together they drafted an evaluation that showed a worsening trend in hospital-based infections, length of stay, and hospital readmission rate. They had an opportunity at the next meeting of the board of directors for presentation of this data. Administration became aware of this plan, suggested a different format for presentation, and delayed the presentation time. The physician went ahead and presented the evaluation during the meeting under the "new business" section. The new administration was caught off guard and left to discuss their intervention, its untoward effect, and the correction plan.

Later, the physician's participation with hospital-based committees was ended and she was cycled off, ostensibly to add new members. On her annual contract renewal date, she found her contract was not renewed as she was a hospital-based employee.

Medical Approach

Cases such as this often are emotive, and can be the cause of considerable controversy. They are seldom resolved in the employee's favor. They rely on the legal concept of the "at-will" employee, in which either party is free to seek other opportunities for employment, so no party is bound to their present job. Essentially, there is no property right to their job. Under the "employ-at-will" doctrine, workers without an employment contract guaranteeing employment for a specific term can leave that position, or be terminated by their employer without cause.

However, more often than not, it is the employee who is disadvantaged as they are not likely to make a significant number of job changes in a stable work environment. The level of complexity is increased if academic tenure is involved, but typically this does not change the ultimate outcome.

Legal Analysis

In *Meeks* v. *OPP Cotton Mills*, the employee-at-will doctrine was utilized as rationale to terminate an employee ostensibly for filing a workers' compensation claim.[1] The Alabama Supreme Court held the employee could be fired for any reason, even the "wrong reason" or a retaliatory discharge, and declined to create a public policy exception to this practice. However, the Alabama legislature enacted a statute prohibiting a retaliatory discharge for filing a workers' compensation claim or safety complaints.[2]

The interface of management and employee requires constant attention. Discrimination, wrongful termination, and sexual harassment account for 60%

of all claims in employment litigation, often invoking the Civil Rights Act of 1964.[3,4] The employee selection process often begins with an interview, although its reliability is often questioned. Graves and Karren evaluated interviewers' selection decisions that have been demonstrated to be idiosyncratic. They concluded that variation in the interviewer's decision-making process may jeopardize organizational effectiveness.[5]

Pre-employment urine drug testing of potential hospital employees has significant implications. Levine and Rennie reviewed the literature and identified seven articles dealing with health-care pre-employment screening, where the incidence of positive tests was 0.25–12%.[6] They concluded that the testing was not always applied uniformly, and medical review was required to ensure the result truly correlated with illicit drug use. The goal is to develop a reliable program to achieve the stated purpose of decreasing absenteeism, employee turnover, workplace accidents, and medical errors.

Another area of controversy is the "honesty test," a test of integrity that assesses a job applicant's personality traits that may predict honesty and trustworthiness with secondary effect on productivity.[7] There have been legal challenges questioning the issue of privacy, discrimination, and effect on union activities.

Hospital administration is charged with monitoring the workplace for mistreatment at all levels of the organization. Harlos and Axelrod defined three dimensions of mistreatment: verbal abuse, work obstruction, and emotional neglect.[8] They defined the adverse work effects to be associated with diminished well-being, work satisfaction, organizational commitment, and higher rate of turnover. They recommend an interventional program to include improved communication, conflict resolution skills training, mentoring programs, and respect at work policies.

The caselaw has typically centered on employee termination. In *Swanson* v. *St John's Lutheran Hospital*, the plaintiff working as a nurse anesthetist was allegedly terminated for refusal to participate in a tubal ligation.[9] She initially brought action under Montana's Conscience Law providing, (1) it is unlawful to interfere with the right of refusal by duress, coercion, or other means and (2) the injured is entitled to injunctive relief and monetary damages.[10] The trial court judgment was entered for the defendant, then reversed and remanded. The district court then awarded financial damages to compensate for lost income.

In *Wagenseller* v. *Scottsdale Memorial Hospital*, the plaintiff was employed as an ED staff nurse with EMS responsibility, as an "at-will" employee without a specific contractual term.[11] The plaintiff alleged she did not participate in inappropriate activities at ED social functions, so administrative attitude changed toward her, which was corroborated by other staff. Although she had previously had excellent evaluations, she was allegedly asked to resign, whereupon she refused and was terminated. She filed suit, suggesting the termination was against public policy. The trial court granted summary judgment against the plaintiff on the wrongful termination "public policy" theory. The Supreme Court of Arizona held that in the absence of a contractual provision, an "at-will" employee may be terminated for "good cause, no cause, but not for bad cause." They reversed and remanded for review, adopting the "public policy" exception to "at-will" termination. She has the right to appeal to a jury on the premise of not participating in a behavior that is against public policy.

In *Reddington* v. *Staten Island University Hospital*, the plaintiff filed suit for breach of employment contract and violation of whistleblower protection law.[12] Her former duties at the hospital centered around service coordination for patients, including managing patient satisfaction surveys and managing personnel who provided language translation services. The trial court considered her claim, holding that even though one portion of the claim involving New York Labor Law was time barred, which was withdrawn, it did not concurrently bar the remaining action.[13] However, her claim was dismissed and affirmed by the United States Court of Appeals, Second Circuit as this action only applied to those who actually performed health-care service. This statute was meant to "safeguard only those employees who are qualified by virtue of training and/or experience to make knowledgeable judgments as to the quality of patient care, and whose jobs require them to make these judgments." Therefore, this whistleblower statute applies to "those that actually supply the service, but does not apply who merely coordinate those who do."

There are Protections for Employees supplementing the Fair Labor Standards Act of 1938, where they have, "objected to, or refused to participate in, any activity, policy, practice or assigned task that the employee (or other such person) reasonably believed to be in violation of any provision of this title (or amendment) of any order, rule, regulation, standard or ban under this title (or amendment)."[14]

Conclusion

The organization often uses some variant of the "business judgment rule," suggesting they are required to make the best decisions for the organization using all of the available data and industry standards to arrive at a viable business plan. Any employee is required to follow, within reason, the goals, mission, and objectives set by the business entity to participate in the corporate plan.

References

1. *Meeks v. OPP Cotton Mills, Inc.*, 459 So. 2d 814 (1984).

2. Alabama Code §25-5-11.1:Employee not to be Terminated Solely for Action to Recover Benefits nor for Filing Notice of Safety Rule Violation.

3. Doyle T, Kleiner BH. Issues in employment litigation. *Managerial Law.* 2002;44(1/2):151–155.

4. Civil Rights Act of 1964, Pub.L. 88–352, 78 Stat. 24, Employment Discrimination.

5. Graves LM, Karren RJ. The employee selection interview: a fresh look at an old problem. *Hum Res Manage.* 1996;35(2):163–180.

6. Levine MR, Rennie WP. Pre-employment urine drug testing of hospital employees: future questions and review of current literature. *Occup Environ Med.* 2004;61(4):318–324. DOI:10.1136/Orem.2002.006163.

7. Bergman TJ, Mundt DH, Illgen EJ. The evolution of honesty tests and means for their evaluation. *Employ Respons Rights J.* 1990;3(3):215–223.

8. Harlos KP, Axelrod LJ. Work mistreatment and hospital administrative staff: policy implications for healthier workplaces. *Healthc Policy.* 2008;4(1):40–50. DOI:10.1292/HCPOA.2008.20006.

9. *Swanson v. St John's Lutheran Hospital.* 615 P.2d 883 (1980).

10. Montana Code Annotated. MCA §59–5–504. Unlawful to Interfere with the Right of Refusal.

11. *Wagenseller v. Scottsdale Memorial Hospital*, 710 P.2d 1025 (1985).

12. *Reddington v. Staten Island University Hospital*, 543 F.3d 91 (2008).

13. New York Labor Law, Article 20-C Retaliatory Action by Employers, §§740, 741 Retaliatory Personnel Action by Employers;Prohibition; Prohibition, Health Care Employer Who Penalizes Employees Because of Complaints of Employer Violations.

14. Patient Protection and Affordable Care Act (ACA), P.L. 111–148: 18C Protections for Employees.

Expert Witness

Case

The physician had been in practice for over 20 years in a busy urban emergency department (ED). It was a highly litigious area, but she had always had a careful, conservative practice and had never had a lawsuit. However, a few months ago, she had received notice that she was the subject of a medical malpractice lawsuit. She had seen a patient with chest pain who met low-risk criteria according to the clinical decision rule. The patient stayed in the ED for 4 hours, had a negative EKG, negative chest radiograph, and two negative cardiac enzymes (troponins). Approximately one month later, after a visit with her primary care physician and cardiologist, she apparently had a myocardial event.

There were numerous discussions with the hospital-based attorney, and the ED group retained an attorney as well. They felt comfortable that the physician would prevail, and there were a number of court delays based on the fact that the plaintiff's attorney could not find an expert willing to provide a certificate of merit. On their last continuance they were able to produce an expert, who was not an emergency physician and did not work in an ED, but alleged that the standard of care was not met.

The provider questioned the attorney on how that would be allowed to proceed. The attorney suggested that in this particular state the expert witness criteria were lax and this testimony would be permitted. The case went to a jury trial with this physician providing a certificate of merit to qualify to provide expert testimony even though they were not certified in emergency medicine. Their suggested qualification was although not a full-time career, they had provided occasional "moonlighting" ED shifts earlier in their career, and spent time in the ED during their residency training.

Medical Approach

Some physicians have described medical malpractice litigation as the worst part of their practice experience. It is truly a life-changing event, with most physicians needing years to recover from the process itself. In addition, there can be significant costs and administrative time spent on the litigation process.

The Physician Insurers Association of America Data Sharing Project was examined by Carroll et al. who evaluated closed cases between 1985 and 2008.[1] The average medical malpractice claim costs more than \$27,000 to defend. The cost of taking a case to trial is significantly greater than for cases that are dropped, dismissed, or withdrawn. The cost is predominantly attorney fees (74%), with expert witness fees accounting for 26%. There is a strong correlation between the average case indemnity and defense cost. The goal should be to prevent lawsuits, not to defend them.

Legal Analysis

The use of expert witnesses, based on training and expertise, provides an authoritative interpretation of the facts and circumstances associated with the event that assists the fact finder in decision-making. The use of medical experts changed during the case of Daniel M'Naghten in 1843.[2] The defendant allegedly shot a man having mistaken his identity, and pled not guilty by reason of insanity. Prior to this, the physician expert had to have provided medical care for the patient to offer an opinion. Some of the witnesses who gave this evidence had previously examined the prisoner: others had never seen him until he appeared in court, and they formed their opinions on hearing the evidence given by other witnesses. The House of Lords decision was a verdict of not guilty, on the grounds of insanity.

In *Frye* v. *United States*, a murder trial in 1923, a medical expert for the defense offered an opinion on the "systolic blood pressure deception test," the precursor of the lie detector test, describing a more severe rise supposedly with deception.[3] The Frye test for admissibility of expert evidence held that the thing from which the deduction is made must be sufficiently established to have gained "general acceptance" in the particular field in which it belongs. The United States Court of Appeals (USCA), D.C. Circuit affirmed the conviction of the trial court, holding that the test had not yet gained standing and scientific recognition.

The Federal Rules of Evidence were codified in 1974, in which Rule 702: Testimony by Expert Witnesses states that:

> If scientific, technical, or other specialized knowledge will assist the trier of fact to understand the evidence, or to determine a fact in issue, a witness qualified as an expert by knowledge, skill, experience, training, or education, may testify thereto in the form of an opinion or otherwise.[4]

In *Daubert* v. *Merrell Dow Pharmaceuticals*, the petitioners were minor children with alleged birth defects due to Bendectin (a medication used for morning sickness), where again the court determined the standard for admitting expert scientific testimony.[5] The district court granted respondent's motion for summary judgment, as the petitioner's evidence did not reach the level of causation, agreed by the appeal court. The Supreme Court of the United States (USSC) granted certiorari to decide the proper standard for admission of expert testimony. They commented that nothing in Rule 702 establishes "general acceptance" as an absolute prerequisite to admissibility, minimizing the importance of the Frye rule.[4] The judge may adopt a gatekeeper role and the expert testimony should fit a multi-prong test: it should (1) rest on a reliable foundation, (2) that is relevant to the task at hand, and (3) is based on valid scientific principles. The appeal court decision was vacated for further decision-making concerning all evidence submitted.

In *Kumho* v. *Carmichael*, the court addressed the issue of how *Daubert* applies to experts who are not scientists.[6] The case centered on a blown tire and subsequent fatality. The USSC granted certiorari to decide whether a trial judge could consider the *Daubert* four-factor test to decide the admissibility of the engineering expert testimony. This four-factor test included appropriate testing, peer review, error rates, and acceptability to distinguish reputable from non-reputable science. They held that the judicial gatekeeping function applies to non-scientific expert testimony as well. The district court did not abuse its authority, and the appeal court verdict was reversed.

For physicians, the focus is mostly on the quality of the expert witness and can be addressed by professional societies. The American Academy of Neurology has formalized their requirements describing the elements of medical expert testimony (Table 41.1).[7] First, the purpose of the medical expert witness testimony is to assist the court or legal body to understand the medical evidence or to determine the medical facts in question. Second, when the testimony relates to a medical malpractice allegation the opinion should describe the relevant standard of care, specify violation of those standards, indicate whether those violations caused harm, and current clinical status and prognosis. Third, the medical expert testimony review includes: (1) the medical evaluation including interview, exam, laboratory, and imaging data; (2) formulation of an opinion based on this data; (3) communication of this opinion to attorneys, courts, licensing boards, and peer review bodies in the form of court testimony, deposition, answers to interrogatories, or affidavit.

The American College of Emergency Physicians (ACEP) concludes that if a physician claims to be a medical expert, this constitutes the practice of medicine.[8] ACEP's Expert Witness Guidelines were originally approved in 1990 and most recently revised in 2015. They include the following requirements. First, the expert witness must be currently licensed within the United States legal jurisdiction as a doctor of medicine or osteopathic medicine. Second, they must

Table 41.1 Physician expert witness guidelines (American Academy of Neurology)

1.		Assist in the understanding of medical evidence
2.		Medical malpractice allegation
	a	Relevant standards of care, specifying violations and harm
	b	Current clinical status and prognosis
3.		Medical expert testimony
	a	Evaluation of medical record for legal proceeding
	b	Formulate an expert opinion
	c	Communicate opinion in formal legal proceeding

Reference: Williams et al.[7]

Table 41.2 Physician expert witness requirements (American College of Emergency Medicine)

1.	Current medical license
2.	Certified by recognized emergency medicine body
3.	Active clinical practice 3 years previous to event
4.	If not in current practice, engaged during 3 years previous to event

Reference: ACEP.[8]

Table 41.3 Physician expert witness guidelines (ACEP)

1.	Possess current experience and ongoing knowledge
2.	Not provide information that is false, misleading, or without foundation
3.	Thorough review of medical record and contemporaneous literature
4.	Opinion contemporaneous with time of event
5.	Fair and objective review without exclusion
6.	Should not advertise false or misleading qualifications
7.	Willing to submit transcripts for peer review
8.	Cannot accept contingency fee
9.	Misconduct may expose to disciplinary action
10.	Adhere to state-specific negligence guidelines

Reference: ACEP.[8]

Table 41.4 Practical measures to minimize medical expert bias

1.	Testify for both plaintiff and defense
2.	Assess merits separate from testimony
3.	Review all records thoroughly
4.	Develop a solid medical posture
5.	Review in balanced critical manner
6.	Articulate in document, before legal proceeding

Reference: Boyarsky.[9]

be certified by a recognized certifying body of emergency medicine. Third, they must have been in the active clinical practice of emergency medicine for at least 3 years exclusive of training immediately preceding the occurrence of the event giving rise to the case. Fourth, if not currently in practice, they would have met the guideline if engaged during the 3 years immediately preceding the event in question (Table 41.2).

Once qualified, the medical expert must abide by guidelines (Table 41.3).[8] First, they must possess current experience and ongoing knowledge in the area of testimony. Second, they should not provide testimony that is false, misleading, or without medical foundation. Third, a thorough review of the medical records and contemporaneous medical literature is required. Fourth, opinion should reflect the state of the medical knowledge at the time of the event. Fifth, the facts should be reviewed in a fair and objective manner, and should not exclude relevant information to favor either plaintiff or defendant. Sixth, they should not engage in advertising or solicitation by misrepresenting their qualifications, experience, titles, or background. Seventh, the expert should be willing to submit transcripts of deposition and testimony for peer review. Eighth, they should never accept contingency compensation arrangements based on outcome. Ninth, misconduct as an expert, including the provision of false, fraudulent, or misleading testimony, may expose to disciplinary action. Tenth, they must strictly adhere to the state-specific definition of negligence, and be familiar with local state law, regulations, and practice of emergency medicine.

Six practical measures are recommended to minimize the potential for bias as a medical expert in professional liability cases (Table 41.4):[9] (1) testify for both plaintiff and defense; (2) assess the merits of the case, separate from the testimony; (3) insist on reviewing all the records thoroughly; (4) develop a solid medical posture for each case; (5) review in a balanced, critical manner; and (6) articulate the standard of care in a document before expressing in deposition or trial.

Interestingly, Milunsky surveyed 36 physician specialty organizations in 2003 by questionnaire to determine if they had proper guidelines, position statements, policies, or bylaws governing the disciplinary management of their members who allegedly testify falsely.[10] They found that over 80% had no definitive disciplinary policies to deal with this practice.

Eloy et al. made an interesting comparison of plaintiff and defendant expert witness qualifications by analyzing a legal database for otolaryngology expert witnesses (Table 41.5).[11] The plaintiff experts had less practice experience (31.8 vs. 35.4 years, $P = 0.047$) and lower scholarly impact in their publications (6.3 vs. 10, $P = 0.045$), while a higher proportion of those testifying for the defense were in an academic practice (49.3 vs. 31.7%, $P = 0.042$). However, no difference was found in post-residency fellowship training. In this medical discipline and study sample, those who repeatedly served as experts were more likely to be testifying for the plaintiff.

Table 41.5 Comparison of plaintiff and defense expert witness qualifications

	Qualification	Plaintiff	Defense
			P < 0.05
1.	Length of practice (yrs)	31.8	35.4
2.	Scholarly impact	6.3	10
3.	Academic practice (%)	31.7	49.3

Reference: Eloy et al.[11]

Table 41.6 Medical expert liability

Immunity
1. Proliferation and commercialization of experts
2. Inadequate testimony safeguards
3. Analogous to attorney malpractice
4. Deterrence function of tort law
5. Ineffectiveness of judicial gatekeeper
Accountability
1. Discipline by medical professional association
2. Discipline by state medical board
3. Prospect of tort liability

Reference: Binder[12]

The liability for medical experts has also increased, as suggested by Binder's analysis in the psychiatric community (Table 41.6).[12] English common law held the expert witness immune for broad policy reasons, but this premise has decreased in importance over time. The shift in the concept of immunity is due to (1) proliferation of experts and their commercialization, (2) inadequate safeguards to ensure honest testimony, (3) a parallel rise of attorney malpractice, (4) intent of tort to deter future misconduct, and (5) the ineffectiveness of the *Daubert* and *Kumho* judicial gatekeeper function. There are expanding areas of medical expert accountability and liability, including: (1) discipline by medical professional associations; (2) discipline by state medical boards; (3) the prospect of tort liability.

There are two clusters of caselaw that deal with the court's qualification of the medical expert from the patient perspective. In *Broders* v. *Heise*, the presenting patient had been found in an unconscious state on a sidewalk, refused to answer questions when she regained consciousness, and vomited.[13]

She was discharged with a headache attributed to a hangover, returned, had a CT that revealed skull fracture with brain injury, and died. The plaintiff offered an emergency medicine physician to be qualified as an expert witness, with a 16-year emergency medicine practice, and stated, "he had to understand and appreciate … what services can be provided by a neurosurgeon … in order to know what type of physician to recommend." The defense experts were two neurosurgeons who stated the injury was untreatable. The trial court excluded the emergency medicine expert testimony, holding that although his expertise was greater than that of the general public, the plaintiff did not establish expertise on the issue of cause in fact according to Rule 702.[4] The Supreme Court of Texas reversed the judgment of the appeal court, and rendered judgment in accordance with the trial court jury verdict that plaintiffs take nothing. They commented that the ruling did not mean only a neurosurgeon could comment on a neurosurgeon's care, and an emergency physician could not, but that "knowledge, skill, experience, training or education" are required regarding the specific issue before the court.[14]

In *Blan* v. *Ali*, the patient presented after slumping over at home, was seen in the ED, admitted to the medical service of his physician, a cardiologist, by phone consult with the ED physician. A neurology consult was scheduled for the next day.[15] The plaintiff expert was board certified in neurology with a 20-year practice and experience as chief of section. The expert acknowledged he did not know the standard of care for an emergency physician or cardiologist. The trial court struck the expert testimony. The plaintiff was left without an expert and summary judgment was awarded to the defense. The court cited Section 14.01 (a) of the Medical Liability Act specifying the expert witness qualifications to include:

1. Practicing medicine at the time testimony is given, or the time the claim arose;
2. Knowledge of accepted standards of medical care for the condition in the claim;
3. Qualified on the basis of training or experience to offer an expert opinion on the care standards.[16,17]

The Court of Appeals of Texas, Houston affirmed the judgment of the trial court, striking the expert report and awarding summary judgment for the defense.

In *Fields* v. *Regional Medical Center Orangeburg*, the patient presented to the ED with chest pain, with a smoking history, previous episodes of chest pain, and a normal EKG.[18] He then presented to another hospital, where he underwent an emergency cardiac catheterization and succumbed. The family filed suit and the defense expert opined the standards of care were met as the patient had numerous previous visits with negative testing. One of the plaintiff experts offered the explanation that his lack of certification was related to the fact that he helped design the test. Another plaintiff expert stated he failed to pass the certification exam by one point. The appeal court reversed the jury verdict and remanded for a new trial, since the trial court excluded part of the plaintiff emergency medicine expert explanation for their lack of board certification. The Supreme Court of Carolina felt that both parties presented experienced, well-qualified experts who offered opposing opinions, and this was a question for the jury, who decided in favor of the physician. They affirmed the appeal court's finding of trial court error in exclusion of explanation as inadmissible hearsay that resulted in potential detriment to the expert's opinion.

In *Pirdair* v. *Medical Center Hospital of Vermont*, the patient was involved in a motor vehicle accident, sustained multiple injuries, and had a head CT.[19] The scan was read 2 days later by an outside reading firm, and a subdural hematoma was allegedly not appreciated. Two days after this he collapsed. The CT was repeated, the patient was taken to surgery with a large hematoma, and died over a year later. The plaintiffs appealed to the Supreme Court of Vermont after a trial court verdict for the defense and a superior court affirmation. They allege the expert report concerning the repeat CT should be interpreted in light of newly discovered evidence, suggesting misinterpretation entitling them to a new trial.[20] The interpretation and treatment of the CT as heterogenous was in question. In addition, a plaintiff expert had treated a similar injury after the trial ended. The plaintiffs felt they should be able to present this information de novo to a jury in a new trial. The Vermont Supreme Court held there was no abuse of discretion, and the defense verdict stood.

The other caselaw cluster is related to expert physicians under scrutiny for their qualifications or testimony. In *Bd. of Reg. for the Healing Arts* v. *Levine*, an otolaryngologist was the subject of an attempt by the board to discipline his license for alleged false

testimony about his qualifications relating to successful exam completion details.[21] The board alleged violations of state law on the grounds of misrepresentation.[22] The Administrative Hearing Commission acknowledged the misrepresentation but dismissed the complaint, holding that it was not established that fees were obtained, and that expert testimony by a non-treating physician is not "the practice of medicine." The Missouri Court of Appeals, Western District held that there was no statutory evidence to support the validity for board oversight for expert witness testimony.

In *Joseph* v. *Board of Medicine*, the physician was censured with financial penalty for alleged false testimony and misrepresentations as an expert witness.[23] The board alleged this constituted a false report in the practice of medicine according to the D.C. Code.[24] The D.C. Court of Appeals heard the physician's contention that the board misconstrued their statutory authority in the definition of "the practice of medicine." The physician practiced emergency medicine and shock trauma, testified as an emergency expert, and was associated with a commercial medical expert search service. The medical case in question cited issues with alleged misrepresentation of thoracic surgery board certification, number one medical school class ranking, Phi Beta Kappa award, and society memberships that had lapsed being included in his CV. This issue was brought to the attention of the Commission on Medical Discipline, the information was not contested, and the physician was charged with "immoral conduct" and making false reports or records in the practice of medicine.[25] The court held that it is the practice of medicine, "when a medical expert in a malpractice case is retained to deliver an opinion based on a patient's records, as to the standard of care given, required and the damage caused by another physician's care." The appeal court affirmed the board decision.

In *Austin* v. *American Association of Neurological Surgeons*, the physician was suspended for 6 months by a voluntary professional medical association of which he had been a member, but had now resigned.[26] He filed suit alleging suspension "in revenge" for testifying for plaintiff against another member. As an aside, the plaintiff expert in the alleged medical malpractice case had allegedly performed the procedure in question 25–30 times, while the defendant was said to have performed it 700 times. The authoritative article he cited did not support his opinion, the defendant member complained, and a hearing was held followed by suspension. Ordinarily a dispute between a member and a voluntary membership association is governed by the law of contracts, with potentially legally enforceable obligations defined by charter, bylaws, and regulations.[27] The USCA, Seventh Circuit held that damages cannot be obtained by tort law for the dissemination of truthful information based on the testimony the expert witness provided under oath. As well, "an important economic interest" in his society membership had not been proven. The judgment affirmed the dismissal of the plaintiff's suit.

Conclusion

A typical malpractice case usually begins with a notification process, followed by interrogations, followed by a deposition, a formal court proceeding in which more questions are answered under oath, and finally the malpractice trial itself. A certificate of merit is required to have the court formally recognize the validity of the expert witness testimony and proceed to the litigation process.

The expert witness should be specially qualified to perform this duty, should have training and experience, and should provide an opinion that is different from that of the layman concerning the issue at hand. Regulations governing this process are state-based. In some states it is a fairly strict process with stringent requirements, and in others a plaintiff expert is given a wider scope with broader practice experience accepted for their qualifications.

References

1. Carroll AE, Parikh PD, Buddenbaum JL. The impact of defense expenses in medical malpractice claims. *J Law Med Ethics*. 2012;40(1):135–142. DOI:10.1111/j.1748-720X.2012.00651.x.

2. Daniel M'Naghten's Case. United Kingdom House of Lords Decisions [1843] J16, 8 ER 718.

3. *Frye* v. *United States*, 293 F. 1013 (D.C. Cir. 1923).

4. Federal Rules of Evidence, Article VII, Rule 702. Testimony by Expert Witnesses. Pub L. 93–595, §1, January 2, 1975.

5. *Daubert* v. *Merrell Dow Pharmaceuticals*, 509 U.S. 579 (1993).

6. *Kumho Tire Co.* v. *Carmichael et al.*, 526 U.S. 137 (1999).

7. Williams MA, Mackin GA, Beresford HR, Gordon J, Jacobsen PL, McQuillen MP, et al. American Academy of Neurology qualifications and guidelines for the physician expert witness. *Neurology*. 2006;66(1):13–14.

8. American College of Emergency Physicians. Expert witness guidelines for the specialty of emergency medicine. September 1990, June 2015.

9. Boyarsky S. Practical measures to reduce medical expert witness bias. *J Forensic Sci*. 1989;34(5):1259–1265.

10. Milunsky A. Lies, damned lies and medical experts: this abrogation of responsibility by specialty organizations and a call for action. *J Child Neurol*. 2003;18(6):413–419. DOI:10.1177/08830738030180060401.

11. Eloy JA, Svider PF, Patel D, Setzen M, Baredes S. Comparison of plaintiff and defendant expert witness qualification in malpractice litigation in otolaryngology. *Otolaryngol Head Neck Surg*. 2013;148(5):764–769. DOI:10.1177/0194599813481943.

12. Binder RL. Liability for the psychiatrist expert witness. *Am J Psychiatr*. 2002;159(11):1819–1825.

13. *Brodrers* v. *Heise*, 924 S.W.2d 148 (1996).

14. *Ponder* v. *Texarkana Memorial Hosp.*, 840 S.W. 2d 476.

15. *Blan* v. *Ali*, 7 S.W.3d 741 (1999).

16. Texas Medical Liability Insurance And Improvement Act, §14.01 (a).

17. Texas Revised Civil Statutes Annotated. art. 4590i, §14.01 (a) (1999).

18. *Fields* v. *Regional Medical Center Orangeburg*, 609 S.E.2d 506 (2005).

19. *Pirdair* v. *Medical Center Hospital of Vermont*, 173 VT. 411 (2002).

20. Vermont Rules of Civil Procedure V.R.C.P. §60 (b) (3).

21. *Bd. of Reg. for Healing Arts* v. *Levine*, 808 S.W.2d 440 (1991).

22. Missouri Revised Statutes §§334.100.2(4), (5) (1983) (1986) Denial, Revocation or Suspension of License, Alternatives, Grounds For – Reinstatement Provisions.

23. *Joseph* v. *Board of Medicine*, 587 A.2d 1085 (1991).

24. District of Columbia Code §2-3301.2 (7) (1989): Practice of Medicine.

25. Maryland Health Occupations Code Annotated §§14–504(3), (4) (1981).

26. *Austin* v. *American Association of Neurological Surgeons*, 120 F. Supp 1151 (N.D. Ill. 2000).

27. *Head* v. *Lutheran General Hospital*, 163 Ill. App. 3d 682 (1987).

Fitness for Duty

Case

She was a great surgeon and everyone liked her: the staff that worked in the operating room, the patients, and her peer physicians. She had been at the facility for years and had a very successful medical practice. She was effective as a practitioner, both in the operating room and in the clinical rounding scenario. She was always available for consultation to the other medical staff members. In addition to her hospital responsibilities, she maintained a number of staff hospital-based committees, contributing positively to the overall institutional goals.

Some of the staff noticed that she had periods when she seemed down and had some struggles with her clinical responsibilities, but she quickly rebounded, just noting that she was "having a bad day." There was never a time when she was unable to maintain her responsibilities in the operating room or the clinical floor units.

She requested some time off but came back within a week and attended to her patient care responsibilities. She informed the medical staff office that she had recently been diagnosed with bipolar disorder and she was self-reporting to make them aware although there was no impact on her hospital-based responsibilities. She returned to her job responsibilities and assignments without difficulty or concerns related to her patient care performance.

Her work status was that she was employed by the hospital as a hospital-based physician on an annual contract renewal basis. That next year her ever-renewing contract was not renewed. When she asked why, she was told there was a no-cause termination provision in her contract. The hospital chose to not have her continue to provide service at that facility, and they were within their rights and responsibilities to maintain the hospital's mission.

There were murmurings she had been released from her contract because of the diagnosis of bipolar disorder that she self-reported. This had come to the attention of some hospital board members who thought it was not appropriate for someone diagnosed with bipolar disorder to work in a high-stress specialty such as surgery.

Medical Approach

What should raise concerns in this case is that the physician self-reported a medical illness and shortly thereafter was released from a long-standing contract. There were no apparent issues with performance of job responsibilities, clinical capability, or patient care. This raises numerous concerns regarding the physician's right to practice with a disease state or condition that may be protected by the Americans with Disabilities Act (ADA).[1] As long as the condition had no adverse impact on the physician's workload, it is clear that if this rationale was used as the sole reason for discharge, she can probably contest this discharge decision and prevail.

The American Psychiatric Association's paper on "fitness for duty" evaluation defines impairment as "the inability to practice medicine with reasonable skill and safety as a result of illness or injury."[2] Illness may refer to disease, disability, psychiatric illness, or substance use disorder. Current estimates suggest that 15% of physicians will be impaired at some point in their careers.[3] This incidence is not greater for other professionals. However, there are predisposing factors to be found in the medical community. Physicians often possess a strong drive for achievement, exceptional conscientiousness, and an ability to keep personal problems separate from everyday work. These are considered positive career-building traits, but also predispose the practitioner to impairment.

Legal Analysis

In *Wachter* v. *United States*, the patient had coronary bypass surgery performed at a military hospital, in which a saphenous vein graft (SVG) was consented.[4] The SVG failed and a second procedure was performed by a different surgeon, also resulting in failure. The patient raised issues over physician qualifications, and the surgical alternatives such as an internal mammary artery graft not being discussed. The plaintiff alleged there was a lack of informed consent for cardiac surgery, negligence, lack of supervision, and negligent credentialing. These issues stemmed from a concern over the physician's alleged lack of competency, filing under the Federal Tort Claims Act (FTCA).[5] The district court dismissed with prejudice the bulk of the plaintiff's claims and granted summary judgment on the informed consent objection. The United States Court of Appeals (USCA), Fourth Circuit held that no mandatory disclosure of this consent information is required. The plaintiff must successfully plead the identity of an undisclosed risk, and that the risk materialized and caused a related injury. The court dismissed most of the plaintiff's complaints, and granted defendant's summary judgment motion on the informed consent provision for the defense, affirming the district court ruling.

In *Kroll* v. *White Lake Ambulance Authority*, the question raised is whether workplace directed counseling is a "medical examination" under the ADA.[6] An emergency medical technician (EMT) was asked to attend mandatory counseling in light of alleged workplace issues relating to relationship and behavioral issues. She did not comply and did not return to work, although the rationale was in dispute among the parties. She filed suit alleging the ADA prohibits "employers from requiring a medical examination, or inquiring about disability … unless such an examination or inquiry is shown to be job related and consistent with business necessity."[7] The USCA, Sixth Circuit vacated the district court decision, holding that psychological counseling indeed constitutes a medical exam under the ADA. For guidance, they relied on the Equal Employment Opportunity Commission (EEOC) statement on Disability-Related Inquiries and Medical Examination of Employees.[8] The EEOC defines medical examination as "a procedure or test that seeks information about an individual's physical or mental impairment or health." They define a seven-factor test to decide whether a request qualifies as a

Table 42.1 EEOC "medical examination" seven-factor test

1. Administered by health-care professional
2. Interpreted by health-care professional
3. Impairment of physical or mental health
4. Is the test invasive?
5. Measures task performance, not response
6. Administered in a medical setting
7. Is medical equipment used?

Reference: US Equal Employment Opportunity Commission[7]

"medical examination" (Table 42.1). First, whether the test is administered by a health-care professional. Second, whether the test is interpreted by a health-care professional. Third, whether the test is designed to reveal an impairment of physical or mental health. Fourth, whether the test is invasive. Fifth, whether the test measures an employee's performance of a task; or measures their physiological response to performing that task. Sixth, whether the test is normally administered in a medical setting. Seventh, whether medical equipment is used for the testing. If even one of these factors is met, it "may be enough to determine that a test or procedure is medical." Title I of the ADA prohibits employers from requiring a medical examination unless it is shown to be "job related" and consistent with "business necessity," quantified as a legitimate business purpose.[1] The USCA, Sixth Circuit held that the employer request was indeed a medical examination, but was undecided on the business necessity of this request so they remanded to the district court for reconsideration.

Conclusion

When a "fitness for duty" report is required, it should be adequately documented, with a clear relationship to job requirements and performance. It is key that the report must be specific to job requirements that may or may not be impacted by the employee's capability.

References

1. Americans with Disabilities Act of 1990, Pub. L. No. 101–336, §1, 104 Stat. 328 (1990).

2. Anfang SA, Faulkner LR, Fromson JA, Gendel MH. The American Psychiatric Association's resource document on guidelines for psychiatric fitness-for-duty evaluations of physicians. *J. Am Acad Psychiatr Law*. 2005;33(1):85–88.

3. Boisaubin EV, Levine R. Identifying and assisting the impaired physician. *Am J Med Sci.* 2001;322(1):31–36.

4. *Wachter* v. *United States*, 689 F. Supp.1420 (1988).

5. Federal Tort Claims Act (FTCA), U.S.C. §2671 et seq.

6. *Kroll* v. *White Lake Ambulance Authority*, Sixth Circuit Court, No. 10–2348 (August 22, 2012).

7. 42 U.S.C. §12112 (d) (4) (A). Discrimination.

8. US Equal Employment Opportunity Commission. Enforcement Guidance on Disability-Related Inquiries and Medical Examinations of Employees Under the Americans with Disabilities Act (ADA). July 27, 2000.

Chapter 43

Frequent User

Case

The triage nurse came back and said, "He's here again for his daily visit," and a groan went up from some of the staff members. This patient's complaints were numerous, including headache, back pain, chest pain, abdominal pain, and other pain complaints. He usually requested narcotic analgesics as part of the process. Sometimes the staff thought the purpose of his visit was to get out of the weather or to get a meal.

Extensive medical workups had been done and no pathology had been found at any time in the recent past. Recently, the patient had been through the hands of numerous primary care physicians (PCPs) as well as the medical clinic, and was non-compliant with most recommendations. He was typically the beneficiary of social service consults, sometimes pastoral care or the patient advocate depending on the circumstances. He would then ask for a final meal and transportation home, and the process would start over again the next day.

The patient had seen all the physicians on staff and usually tried to pick or choose physicians that he found more sympathetic, but gradually the group had become frustrated with his multiple presentations and non-compliance. It was estimated he had already had over 100 visits this year at this facility alone. It was rumored he had been seen at multiple other hospital locations that he could access by public transportation and had used their facilities as well.

Once again, his workup on this day was negative for any medical pathology and he was discharged home for follow-up with his PCP, now the primary care clinic.

Medical Approach

This is a common problem in the emergency department (ED) setting where patients use the ED as a resource not only for medical care but also for other psychosocial needs. A superuser is typically defined as a patient who uses the ED at least once a month; some accumulate hundreds of ED visits in their lifetime.

A relatively small subgroup of ED patients is responsible for a disproportionate number of visits and associated costs.[1] This "heavy user" group is felt to be medically and socially vulnerable, and perhaps representative of societal ills as well. The etiology is felt to relate to a complex series of interdependent problems including access to care, lack of primary preventive services, absent or inadequate social services, and fragmented service delivery (Table 43.1). Interestingly, the societal construction of the problem and the articulation of solutions are based on divergent and conflicting opinions.

The appropriateness of medical visits to the accident and emergency department of a university program were evaluated in 2980 patients using explicit criteria.[2] This study identified 29.6% (882) of visits as inappropriate, mostly associated with younger patients, own transportation, hospital referral, certain months of the year, and certain diagnoses of lower severity (Table 43.2). Commonly cited rationales for presentation include greater trust of the hospital than PCPs, 51.1% (451); inappropriate use of services by the patients, 18.1% (160); and inappropriate referrals by PCPs, 16.1% (142) (Table 43.3).[2] Interestingly, the patient rationale for this choice is a greater confidence, convenience, and accessibility of hospital-based services – all positives for the ED.

Althagafi et al. evaluated an observational cohort of 150,727 patients, where almost a third (31.4%) had four or more visits.[3] This group was further divided into occasional visitors (4–9 visits per year), moderately frequent visitors (10–19 visits), and very frequent visitors (>20 visits). This group had a mean age of 39 years, was 54% female, and had more cardiac

Table 43.1 "Heavy ED user" predisposition

1.	Lack of access to care
2.	Lack of primary care or preventive service
3.	Inadequate social service
4.	Fragmented service delivery

Reference: Malone[1]

Table 43.2 Frequent user profile

1.	Younger patient
2.	Own transportation
3.	Hospital referral
4.	Certain months of the year
5.	Diagnosis of lesser severity

Reference: Sempere-Silva et al.[2]

Table 43.3 Rationale for ED use

1.	Greater trust in the hospital	51.1%
2.	Inappropriate use by patients	18.1%
3.	Inappropriate primary care referral	16.1%

Reference: Sempere-Silva et al.[2]

disease, a higher incidence of accompanying diabetes and hypertension, longer ED stays, and more admissions.

Grover et al. evaluated a pilot intensive case management program to reduce ED visits.[4] In 2006–2008, 96 patients were enrolled for care by a multidisciplinary team of physicians, nurses, social services, pain management, and behavioral health specialists. Patients were enrolled if they had made five or more ED visits in the last month, if staff concern was raised, or if they were identified by the California prescription monitoring program. Prior to enrollment there were 2.3 ED visits per month. Analysis of early post-intervention decreased this to 0.6 visits per month, and late post-intervention to 0.4 visits ($P < 0.0001$). These patients averaged 25.6 CT images per month at a baseline, decreasing to 10.2 images initially ($P = 0.001$), then 8.1 images per month ($P = 0.0001$). A focused multidisciplinary group was able to decrease these patients' ED use by 83% and their radiation exposure by 67%.

Legal Analysis

The ability to cope with significant disease can be difficult for both patients and providers, often resulting in numerous care visits.

In *Payton* v. *Weaver*, a patient with end-stage renal disease on chronic hemodialysis had a 3-year relationship with a facility in which treatments were provided.[5] The physician notified the patient by letter that her treatment at the facility would no longer be permitted, citing numerous disruptive issues and persistent treatment non-compliance. She applied to another outpatient dialysis facility but was declined, while her current site continued to provide outpatient and emergency care over the next 5 months and sent another letter concerning the severance of the relationship. The patient then filed for a petition of mandate to compel her physician and the original dialysis center to continue treatment. The stipulated order called for continued treatment as long as the patient met certain conditions, including keeping appointments, restrictions on diet and drug or alcohol use, cooperation and compliance with physician recommendations, and seeking psychotherapy or counseling as appropriate.

However, by the next year she was again alleged to be non-compliant, was given other provider options, and helped to facilitate transfer. Once again, she filed for a writ of mandate to compel, naming all facilities and her physician as violating various rights to health and safety. She alleged violations of the Health and Safety Code (HSC) §1317 requiring provision of "emergency" treatment,[6] the Civil Rights Act of 1968,[7] and the Hill–Burton Act.[8] The trial court excluded the latter two claims as being unsupported and they were dismissed. The court concluded the patient had violated every one of the required stipulations, in a "knowing and intentional" way. As examples they offered a 15 kg weight gain between treatments, presenting in an intoxicated state, missing appointments, requiring 30 emergency treatments in a 1-month period, and "gross non-cooperation" with her treating physician. The Court of Appeals of California affirmed the trial court decision and acknowledged the emergent nature of the condition, but considered it did not fall within the scope of HSC §1317. "It is unlikely that the Legislature intended to impose upon whatever health-care facility such a patient chooses, the unqualified obligation to provide continuing preventive care for the patient's lifetime." They dispensed with her legal arguments, and recommended involuntary conservatorship but continued dialysis at the center until a final decision was made.

Visits can be closely grouped in sequence, typically with greater levels of accuracy with each repeat visit. In *Battle* v. *Memorial Hospital at Gulfport*,[9] a 15-month-old patient suffered from viral encephalitis resulting in extensive neurologic injury, the plaintiff citing the Emergency Medical Treatment and Labor Act (EMTALA).[10] The child was healthy and normal presenting to his pediatrician with fever and oral sores, was diagnosed with ear infection, treated with antibiotics, and developed a seizure at home. He was taken to the ED and evaluated, a lumbar puncture was performed and interpreted as normal, and he was discharged home with a new antibiotic. The next day he continued to have seizures. The family contacted their pediatrician and were instructed to return to the ED. The child was listed as self-pay on the second visit, was seen by a different ED physician, diagnosed with seizure disorder and pneumonia, and discharged on Dilantin (phenytoin). The mother alleged she was told not to bring the child right back to the ED "because Dilantin takes time to work." There was a counter-allegation relating to not wanting to be admitted, and it was over the Christmas holiday, complicating matters. The next day seizures continued. The child's primary care physician (PCP) was contacted and told the family to return to the hospital a third time. The child had a CT without contrast, which was normal, and an EEG, subsequently read as abnormal seven days later. The next day significant deterioration occurred, herpes simplex encephalitis was suspected and treated with acyclovir, and the child was transferred. The jury trial found unanimously in favor of the defendant emergency physicians, while the magistrate judge granted summary judgment for the hospital, finding no disparate treatment to justify an EMTALA claim. The United States Court of Appeals, Fifth Circuit found merit with the plaintiff's allegation of trial court error and judgment for defendants was vacated and remanded for further consideration by the lower court. They concluded that the second ED visit may not have met the stabilization prong of EMTALA, in which seizure was diagnosed and the child may not have been stabilized prior to discharge. Other plaintiff issues were validated with a comparative negligence instruction, involving parental decision-making, in which neither the infant nor the parent can be held culpable to decrease defendant liability.

Another concern may be previous visits for the same issue with the inherent potential for subsequent visits. In *Breckenridge* v. *Valley General Hospital*, the patient was evaluated in the ED for severe headache and suffered a massive occipital intracranial aneurysm.[11] She had a history of migraine headaches evaluated in the ED, experienced a sudden-onset event with neck pain that "worsened after a cigarette." She went to work, went shopping with a friend, and visited the ED that afternoon. The ED physician's chief complaint was "bad migraine," as vital signs were normal and the patient had similarly severe headaches in the past. The ED physician felt her physical exam involving neck pain with movement and equal grip strength ruled out hemorrhage, and a CT was not ordered as her headache improved. Two weeks later, she had an aneurysm rupture, and filed suit alleging a "herald bleed" on the initial presentation. The jury trial concluded unanimously that no medical malpractice was committed by the ED physician. The plaintiff moved for a new trial since two jurors interjected their personal experience with migraine as extrinsic evidence regarding the standard of care. The trial court ordered a new trial. This decision was reversed by the appeal court, as discussion of jury life experiences does not constitute misconduct. The Supreme Court of Washington affirmed the appeal court decision in that the post-verdict jury discussions cannot be included in appeal decision-making.

Conclusion

For patients who make repeated ED visits, defined medical issues are typically not found and psychosocial issues are more often in play. These may include needs relating to meals, transportation, and psychiatric issues. The key to most programs dealing with this difficult problem is typically to involve a multidisciplinary team. The process usually includes case management and social services to provide a proper care course that is both efficient and effective, but does not unduly burden the system.

References

1. Malone R. Heavy users of emergency services: social construction of a policy problem. *Soc Sci Med*. 1995;40(4):469–477. DOI:10:1016/0277–9536(94).

2. Sempere-Silva T, Piero S, Sendra-Pina P, Martinez-Espin C, Lopez-Aguilera I. Inappropriate use of an

accident and emergency department: magnitude, associated factors and reasons – an approach with explicit criteria. *Ann Emerg Med.* 2001;38(6):568–579. DOI:10.1067/mem.2001.113464.

3. Althagafi M, Alsolamy S, Alsaawi A, Alsuirmi K. Patterns and characteristics of frequent visitors to the emergency department. *Ann Emerg Med.* 2015;66(4S):s9. DOI:10.1016/j.annemerhmed.2015.07.053.

4. Grover CA, Close RJH, Villarreal K, Goldman LM. Emergency department frequent user: pilot study of intensive case management to reduce visits

and computed tomography. *West J Emerg Med.* 2010;11(4):336–343. PMCID: PMC2967685.

5. *Payton* v. *Weaver*, 131 Cal. App.3d 38 (1982).

6. California Health and Safety Code §1317 Emergency Treatment Provision.

7. Civil Rights Act of 1968, Fair Housing Act.

8. Hill-Burton Act 42 U.S.C. §291.

9. *Battle* v. *Memorial Hospital at Gulfport*, 228 F.3d 544 (2000).

10. EMTALA, 42 U.S.C §1395dd (1994).

11. *Breckenridge* v. *Valley General Hospital*, 75 P.3d 944 (2003).

Chapter 44

Futility

Case

The call from emergency medical services (EMS) stated the patient had presented with a seizure event. He had been given 5 mg of valium, and the seizure had stopped by that point. As they transferred him to the stretcher, they reported the blood glucose was normal at 85 mg/dl, and the patient had a complicated health history that included cancer. He was currently unresponsive, but was oxygenating well and maintaining his airway. At this point the physician ordered screening laboratory tests and quickly spoke with the family. The patient had stage IV small cell lung cancer with brain and bone metastases and was in the palliative care program. His oncologist had told the family he would survive only a few weeks.

The physician asked the wife if the patient had made an advance directive. She said that he had not decided, and had not yet signed an advance directive. The son and daughter spoke up at this point and said there had been a discussion, and that their father did not want to be uncomfortable, and did not want to be maintained on any "machines." On further discussion, his wife maintained the position he had wanted "everything done" but the son and daughter were sure that their father did not want any aggressive interventions. He had seen his brother suffer through a long, complicated disease course, and had told his daughter "he wouldn't have wanted to go that way."

The nurse asked the physician to come quickly from the counseling room as the patient had another seizure. This one was prolonged and he seemed to be losing his airway. In light of the family's uncertainty, it was decided that the proper course at this point was to go ahead and perform an intubation. After additional family discussions, involving the patient's oncologist, the patient was intubated. The appropriate standards were followed, to provide sedation and analgesia.

A call was placed to the patient's oncologist, who stated that the patient's prognosis was indeed very poor and she had told the family she thought he would not survive for more than a couple of weeks. The ED physician told the oncologist about the family disagreement concerning the different courses suggested by the patient's wife and his children. The oncologist was aware of this complex issue and knew the conflict had been going on for some time. She suggested the patient's outcome was so poor that the medical futility indication could be offered here to limit support, as the patient had literally no chance of survival. She thought extubation would be appropriate for the patient and he could go to the palliative care unit rather than the intensive care unit (ICU). This issue was put to the family again, but the wife was still adamant about wanting additional care done even in this circumstance, with the remainder of the family disagreeing and becoming quite frustrated.

The staff would do their best to accommodate the patient's wishes as soon as related by family members. The daughter asked again for a medical opinion and the ED physician pointed out that the oncologist's prognosis was dismal, with little or no chance of survival. The patient's long-term primary care physician (PCP) was contacted. The PCP was also a friend of the patient, and he reiterated what the oncologist had said, that the patient was not likely to survive. He had hoped the last few days would not be painful for his friend and patient, who had often confided this wish to him.

The nurse summoned the physician again, reporting that the patient was in cardiac arrest. The physician attempted to resuscitate him and provided one round of resuscitation medication. The family was approached yet again with the suggestion that at this point his physicians felt that his outcome was very poor, with little chance of survival. His wife initially objected, but finally said they were probably right.

Again, it was clarified that at some point medical care can provide no productive good outcome, and that we should cease these efforts to ensure the patient's end-of-life goals can be accomplished.

Medical Approach

We typically ask families to interpret the wishes of their loved one with regard to end-of-life care, but in some cases of medical futility, when there is no realistic chance of good outcome, the medical care system is under no obligation to provide ongoing care. Typically, this occurs when two physicians clarify that the patient's outcome is not survivable. Care can then be discontinued even against the family's wishes.

Early on, the critical care community felt that physicians did not have the responsibility to provide futile or unreasonable care.[1] They define "futile care" as that which does not benefit the patient on the whole, while "unreasonable care" is defined as an excessive treatment plan that is not generally agreed upon. The decision to not provide futile care is supported by the ethical principles of nonmaleficence – doing the least harm to provide the greatest benefit. Beneficence is when our goal is to produce the most good for the patient. Lastly, distributive justice attempts to allocate goods or beneficial effects in equal proportions.

Futility of care focuses on interventions with a low likelihood of expected benefit to the patient.[2] Decisions of care should be based on scientific evidence, societal consensus, and professional standards, not on individual bias concerning quality-of-life judgments. Decisions to withhold treatment should be carefully made after considering the scientific basis of medical benefit, intangible benefits, risks, and patient and family preferences. Special efforts should be directed toward effective communication, comfort, support, and counseling centered on the patient, family, and friends.

The ED, like the ICU, can often be the center of a discussion about the futility of care. Often the ED is the starting point for care that may be ultimately judged to be futile; treatment may be withheld, or the end-of-life communication process may begin with patient or family.[3] Thus, the ED physician has moral standing to both discuss and resist the implementation of futile treatment.

Table 44.1 Criteria for temporary restraining order

1. Likelihood of success on its merits
2. Significant threat of irreparable injury
3. Balance of hardships favor the appellant
4. Whether public interest favors granting an injunction

Reference: Raich.[7]

Legal Analysis

In practical terms the judicial predisposition is to continue to provide support when the family is supportive. In the *Matter of Baby K*, the hospital petitioned for a declaratory judgment that it was not required to provide treatment other than warmth, nutrition, and hydration to an anencephalic infant.[4] In this congenital anomaly portions of the brain, skull, and scalp are typically missing, resulting in a clinical condition of absent cognitive awareness and environmental interaction. The United States Court of Appeals, Fourth Circuit court affirmed the trial court ruling that the facility was obliged to provide respiratory support if the child presented in respiratory distress, according to EMTALA requirements.[5]

More recently, in *Winkfield v. Children's Hosp. & Research Ctr. at Oakland*, a minor patient allegedly sustained a cardiopulmonary arrest after a surgical procedure.[6] She was subsequently diagnosed with cerebral inactivity having fulfilled brain death certification by multiple providers. Her mother moved ex parte for a temporary restraining order (TRO) seeking to maintain cardiopulmonary support, and to place a tracheostomy and gastrostomy tube to allow transfer to another facility. The qualification for a TRO requires the moving party must demonstrate, "1. a likelihood of success on the merits; 2. a significant threat of irreparable injury; 3. the balance of hardship favors the applicant; and 4. is there a public interest that favors an injunction" (Table 44.1).

In *Raich v. Ashcroft*,[7] the district court deferred consideration of the motion to maintain current levels of therapy till a later hearing, but denied the request to compel an invasive procedure for tube placement. The patient was ultimately moved to a chronic care facility.

Conclusion

It is often difficult to go down this road and it requires significant support from hospital personnel including social service, clergy, a hospital-based ethics committee, and legal counsel. In some cases, our job is to provide care that extends the patient's productive life, and when the chance of a good outcome is completely eliminated, care should be withdrawn.

References

1. Luce J. Physicians do not have a responsibility to provide futile or unreasonable care. *Crit Care Med.* 1995;23(4):760–766.

2. Marco CA, Larkin GL, Moskop JC, Derse AR. Determination of "futility" in emergency medicine. *Ann Emerg Med.* 2000;35(6):694–612. DOI:101067/mem.2000.106991.

3. O'Connor AE, Winch S, Lukin W, Parker M. Emergency medicine and futile care: taking the road less travelled. *Emerg Med Australas.* 2011;23(5):649–653. DOI:10.1111/j.1742–6723.2011.01435.x.

4. In the Matter of Baby "K" (Three Cases), 16 F.3d 590 (1994).

5. EMTALA, 42 USCA §1395 (dd).

6. *Winkfield* v. *Children's Hosp. & Research Ctr. at Oakland.* No. C 13–5993 SBA (N.D. Cal. December 30, 2013).

7. *Raich* v. *Ashcroft*, 352 F.3d 1222, 1225 (2003).

Geriatric Abuse

Case

The patient was elderly and appeared frail, but her hair was nicely styled and she was dressed in her Sunday dinner finery. Her granddaughter had brought her in to the emergency department (ED) after a fall. The physical exam revealed a spiral humeral fracture, and a right-sided ecchymosis around her right eye was also noted. The history offered by the granddaughter was that she had fallen onto her left side and twisted her arm on the way down. However, the physician questioned the presence of both left- and right-sided injury. The granddaughter quickly responded that she had fallen last week as well, and that she had been falling a lot recently. The physician began to discuss the treatment plan and follow-up. The granddaughter excused herself from the room saying she had to make a phone call. She asked her grandmother for a credit card so that she could go to the cafeteria before she left.

The ED physician continued the discussion with the patient, including her need for pain control and immobilization of that left arm, as well as the result of a head scan, which was normal. They provided her with some literature and a referral concerning frequent falls. The ED physician also asked about her medication list and what her primary care physician (PCP) said about her falls. The patient thanked the physician for their attention and suggested she would follow up with her PCP and follow all of the care recommendations.

The physician was slightly concerned, as the patient seemed to have an odd collection of injuries. Her granddaughter leaving during an important health-care discussion, and asking for the patient's credit card to pay for her lunch, also seemed strange. Although each of these issues may not be significant on its own, sometimes combining individual clues into an identifiable pattern over time can help to identify an issue.

Although the ED staff had concerns, they did not have any definitive proof of any geriatric abuse.

The nurse then reported that while the patient was in the radiography suite the technician had asked her what happened, and she had given a different history concerning the fall than the one that was related to the physician. When the granddaughter returned she was asked additional questions concerning the patient's recent trauma, and seemed flustered. She said she had to go and that her mother would be there to stay with her grandmother. She then left abruptly. The path was now clear to consult social services and the geriatric service to ensure there was no elderly abuse in this case. The patient was admitted to the hospital for observation.

Medical Approach

Geriatric abuse is a more common problem in the ED than one might anticipate. The abuse can be more than simple neglect and may include physical abuse, sexual exploitation, and financial abuse. Most commonly, it is family members who are involved in abuse.

It is important to look for the signs and symptoms of geriatric abuse, and search for recognizable patterns: symptoms that would not be problematic individually, but when considered together illustrate the potential for abuse. There is an obligatory reporting requirement for geriatric patients, which will typically involve social service, Center for Aging, Adult Protective Services, and law enforcement if necessary.

It is helpful to define some terms to assist in screening:

- *Abuse* is the intentional infliction of physical, sexual, or emotional injury or harm including financial exploitation by any person, firm or corporation.[1]
- *Neglect* is the failure to provide services to an eligible adult by any person, firm, or corporation with a legal or contractual duty to do so, when such failure presents either an imminent danger

Table 45.1 Elder abuse: assessment and management plan

1. Supportive focus on patient and caregiver
2. Avoid assigning blame
3. Hospitalize or shelter those at risk
4. Suspected abuse should be reported to appropriate agency

Reference: Kleinschmidt[3]

to the health, safety, or welfare of the client or a substantial probability that death or serious physical harm would result.

- *Financial exploitation* of elderly or disabled people occurs when a person knowingly or by deception, intimidation, or force obtains control over their property with the intent to permanently deprive them of their property to their detriment and the benefit of another.

A survey performed by Jones et al. in 1988 estimated that annually in the US 1 million elderly people were battered, neglected, or exploited by family members or caretakers.[2] They reviewed 36 hospitalized elderly patients where 80% (29) suffered physical abuse and 44% (16) psychological abuse. In 1997 Kleinschmidt reviewed elderly abuse and estimated that 2.5 million elderly people were abused annually but less than 10% of abuse was reported.[3] The decreased reporting rates may be related to unfamiliarity with the reporting law or fear of offending patients or families. Staff in the ED may be concerned about time limitations and believe they do not have the appropriate evaluation skills.

The ED physician is placed in the critical role of identifying abuse, obtaining evidence, providing immediate treatment, and crisis intervention. The assessment and management plan should be formalized, with defined protocols. First, the intervention should be supportive focusing on the patient and caregiver. Second, assigning blame should be avoided, if possible. Third, those in immediate danger should be hospitalized, placed in a shelter, or otherwise protected. Fourth, suspected abuse should be reported directly to the appropriate state or local agency (Table 45.1).

Legal Analysis

In *Delaney* v. *Baker*, the elderly patient fell and fractured her ankle. She was placed in a skilled care facility and succumbed 4 months later with advanced decubitus ulcers.[4] The family alleged the patient was neglected, due to staff turnover and decreased routine staffing at the facility. The family had cited numerous concerns that were lodged over time concerning these issues before the suit was filed. The Superior Court of Lake County held the facility was liable under an elderly neglect theory, and was judged to be "reckless" but did not show "malice." Those who are licensed to care for elderly people are typically held to a higher standard than the general public. Therefore, a healthcare provider engaging in reckless neglect of an elderly patient has accentuated remedies that are specified by statute in the California Elder Abuse Act §15657.[5]

In *Gdowski* v. *Gdowski*, the elderly patient filed for a protective order citing the California Elder Abuse Act §15657 against his adult daughter with alleged verbal and physical abuse, while being cared for at home.[5,6] The California Court of Appeals, Fourth District held that a protective order should be issued. Their rationale was that a history of previous abuse was sufficient without the need to predict future events. As well, they recommended a "preponderance of evidence" rather than a "clear and convincing" evidence standard. This corresponds to a more likely than not, or a 51% likelihood standard, rather than a more absolute, highly probable requirement.

Conclusion

Most often we err on the side of caution. Even if there is further investigation the patient is admitted to hospital for care and observation, as well as involving the patient's primary care service, which often has a better history and understanding of family dynamics. Our goal is to protect the patient from any type of abuse, whether by friends, family, or strangers.

References

1. Missouri Revised Statutes (2005) – SS 570.145, 660.250 (1), (14).

2. Jones J, Dougherty J, Schelble D, Cunningham W. Emergency department protocol for the diagnosis and evaluation of geriatric abuse. *Ann Emerg Med.* 1988;17(10):1006–1015. DOI:10.1016/S0196-0644(88)80436-0.

3. Kleinschmidt KC. Elder abuse:a review. *Ann Emerg Med.* 1997;30(4):463–472. DOI:10.1016/S0196-0644(97)70006-4.

4. *Delaney* v. *Baker*, 20 Cal. 4th 23 (1999).

5. Elder Abuse and Dependent Adult Civil Protection Act, Welfare and Institutions Code, §15600 et seq.

6. *Gdowski* v. *Gdowski*, 175 Cal. App.4th 128 (2009).

Good Samaritan

Case

The physician was driving home from the end of a long shift in the emergency department (ED). It had been a busy day and he was tired. One more day left in the work stretch and he had the weekend off. But then he came upon a motor vehicle accident. A car was on its roof. A first responder was already there; it looked like a fire police vehicle, with blue lights flashing. An emergency medical technician (EMT) was calling for additional paramedic backup. The scene was horrific and the first responders seemed overwhelmed. The patient was still suspended in his seatbelt as he was removed from the vehicle, with the EMTs maintaining C-spine immobilization. A backboard and collar were applied. At that point the patient suffered a cardiac arrest and the EMTs began CPR. The physician asked the medics if they wanted him to intubate the patient, which he did successfully after the EMTs agreed. They established intravenous access and were ready for a quick "load and go." The physician offered to stay in the back of the ambulance to transport the patient to the hospital he had recently left. The patient was adequately ventilated, but had no pulse. CPR was again begun, while more fluid was administered.

The physician helped the EMTs to transport the patient to the ED entrance. CPR continued for another 15 minutes, while the trauma surgeon contemplated the plan. Quickly it was realized that on the basis of the patient's status, there was no chance of survival. The on-call physician stated she could manage the patient from here, and that the off-shift physician who had assisted in the field was free to go as his shift had ended long ago. He then headed back out of the ED to return home.

About 6 months later the physician who had responded at the accident scene received notification from the hospital's risk management department and legal office, telling him there was a lawsuit

concerning this patient and he was named along with the providers involved in the care delivered in the ED. The petitioner alleged improper diagnosis and care. The physician responded he had been off duty and responded to the accident as a "Good Samaritan" in the field. He questioned how he could be involved in a lawsuit.

Medical Approach

The Good Samaritan immunity presumption refers to the presentation of a patient in an emergency, in which care is rendered in good faith and typically without compensation. The provider should be immunized from medical malpractice allegations over time. Even if the provider responds in a fashion that is within the standards of care, allegations may be made suggesting the intervention was reckless and dangerous. The theory is that the absence of a contract or compensation should not absolve the provider of guilt, and that's where litigation has directed most of these cases.

A Good Samaritan law exists in all 50 states and the District of Columbia, providing blanket protection for anyone who provides assistance at the scene of an emergency.[1] The requirements of the law as it applies to EMS providers, EMTs, and paramedics include the following: first, they must act in good faith; second, they must act gratuitously, without expectation of remuneration; third, they must understand when, where, and how the law applies; fourth, the conventional standard of care must be applied to insure immunity (Table 46.1).

Legal Analysis

The caselaw as it applies to Good Samaritan immunity is critically dependent on venue and circumstance for analysis. In *McIntyre* v. *Ramirez*, a hospitalized patient with precipitous delivery was attended by an

Table 46.1 Good Samaritan law requirements

1.	Must act in good faith
2.	Must act gratuitously
3.	Proper time and place of applicability
4.	Conventional standard of care

Reference: Shin[1]

obstetrician who responded to a standardized hospital emergency call.[2] This obstetrician was not on call for the hospital, nor the patient's attending physician, but offered assistance to help. The delivery was successful but was accompanied by shoulder dystocia, with resultant arm nerve injury and paralysis. The trial court granted summary judgment to the physician, but this was reversed by the appeal court, suggesting he did not prove that no remuneration was expected for the service he provided. The Supreme Court of Texas reversed the appeal court's decision in that the physician satisfied the statutory requirements for immunity, and remanded to further proceedings consistent with this opinion.

In *Van Horn* v. *Watson*, the case involved a layperson who removed an accident victim from an automobile, and allegedly worsened a paraplegic state.[3] The plaintiff alleged the patient did not require removal from the vehicle, while the defendant stated she thought the car would "blow up." The trial court held the defendant was immune from liability. The California Court of Appeal, Second District reversed this decision and remanded for consideration under the theory that the immunity specified by the Health and Safety Code, §1799.102, applies only to the application of "emergency medical care."[4] The removal of the patient was not considered to come under that heading.

In *Home Star Bank & Financial Services* v. *Emergency Care & Health Organization, Ltd.*, the hospital's ED physician responded to an intensive care unit Code Blue event for a patient with a diagnosis of epiglottitis.[5] Code response was part of their normal job responsibility, but they did not routinely bill for this service. Initially, the circuit court ruled that the physician was immune from liability for alleged negligent care, citing the Illinois Good Samaritan Act (745 ILCS 49/25) and granted summary judgment to the defendant.[6] The plaintiff appealed and the appellate court reversed and remanded for reconsideration. An appeal to the Illinois Supreme Court affirmed, holding the Act was meant to apply to volunteers, not those compensated and acting within the scope of their employment.

Conclusion

The Good Samaritan common law understanding is that protection is afforded when one responds in good faith, to the limits of one's capability, without the expectation of payment. Physicians should recognize that today any patient care encounter puts us in the potential position of liability. We should act accordingly, while rendering care in a safe and effective manner within the bounds of our training, treatment, and practice to provide the best quality of care for the patient.

References

1. Shin RK. Protection against liability for emergency medical services providers. *J Emerg Manag.* 2010;8(3):17–21. DOI:10.5055/Jen.2010.0015.

2. *McIntyre* v. *Ramirez*, 109 S.W.3d 741 (Tex. 2003).

3. *Van Horn* v. *Watson*, 45 Cal. 4th 322, 197 P.3D 164, 86 Cal. Rptr. 3D 350.

4. California Health and Safety Code, Section 1799.100–112.

5. *Home Star Bank & Financial Services* v. *Emergency Care & Health Organization, Ltd.*, 985 N.E.2d 306 (Ill. 2013).

6. Civil Immunities Illinois Good Samaritan Act (745 ILCS 49/25).

Guidelines and Protocols

Case

The patient came to the emergency department (ED) with complaints of fever, nausea, and dysuria. She was an older woman, with hypertension and diabetes as part of her health history. She had previously been admitted a month earlier with a diagnosis of pyelonephritis and early sepsis. The physician further reviewed her symptoms at home, after her last hospital discharge. When she had presented to the ED her blood pressure was initially slightly decreased, but improved with fluid. Her temperature did not decrease with the acetaminophen (Tylenol) that had been ordered. She was admitted as a hospital inpatient for intravenous antibiotic therapy and fluid resuscitation.

The treating ED physician prescribed an antibiotic regimen that was consistent with the hospital-based guidelines directed toward pyelonephritis, including vancomycin, in light of the patient's hospital stay the previous month. Ciprofloxacin was administered and she was admitted to the medical ward for additional care by her primary care physician (PCP).

When the ED physician returned for his next shift 2 days later, he was informed that the patient had done poorly while admitted to the hospital medical ward. The vancomycin that the ED physician had prescribed was discontinued by the admitting physician, under the rationale of using a single quinolone intervention instead. The patient's subsequent course was rocky and she was admitted to the intensive care unit (ICU). She subsequently required intubation, and received vancomycin while she was in the ICU. She slowly recovered, and subsequent laboratory testing showed enterococcus bacteremia, which was also identified in her urine.

About 6 months later the hospital was contacted by the patient's attorney suggesting alleged misdiagnosis and mistreatment. The attorney emphasized that the hospital-based clinical guidelines were not followed.

In this particular case, the ED physician responded that he had indeed treated the patient according to clinical guidelines, but there must have been a change later in the patient's hospital course. This apparently occurred after the patient left the ED for admission to the floor.

Medical Approach

The use of clinical guidelines is well founded in all aspects of medical care practice. This approach clearly provides a definitive pathway that allows improved documentation, archiving, and analysis of the care provided, comparable to an industry benchmark or standard.

The Joint Commission on Accreditation of Healthcare Organizations (JCAHO), in the 2004 Clinical Practice Guidelines, proposed the new Performance Improvement (PI) standard PI.2.21, consolidating and replacing the Comprehensive Accreditation Manual for Hospitals Leadership Standards.[1] Clinical Practice Guidelines have been used to ensure consistency in the evaluation and treatment of people with a specific diagnosis, condition, symptom, or risk factor, or undergoing a high-risk procedure. The guidelines are evidence-based or are at least based on expert consensus.

The Joint Commission then went on to reformulate this guideline as Standard Quality Patient Safety (QPS) – QPS.2.1 Clinical Guidelines and Clinical Pathways Are Used to Guide Clinical Care (Table 47.1).[2] The measurable elements include: first, deciding on an annual basis the institutional priority and focus; second, following a precise process in implementing clinical guidelines, pathways, and clinical protocols; third, the institution shall implement at least two guidelines for each identified priority area annually; fourth, clinical leaders should demonstrate how the guidelines have reduced variation in process and outcome.

Table 47.1 Standard QPS.2.1 clinical practice guidelines

1.	Clinical leaders determine focus areas annually
2.	Process to implement clinical guidelines, pathways, and protocols
a	Incorporate mandatory national guidelines and select facility services
b	Evaluate relevance to identified patient populations
c	Adapt technology, drugs and process to national professional norms
d	Assess their scientific evidence
e	Should be formally approved or adopted by the organization
f	Measure for consistent use and effectiveness
g	Support staff should be trained to apply the guidelines
h	Periodic update based on evidence and evaluation of process
3.	Organization implements two guidelines for priority area annually
4.	Clinical leaders demonstrate program reduced variation in processes and outcome

Reference: Joint Commission on Accreditation of Health Care Organizations.[1]

Table 47.2 Clinical practice guidelines: interventional strategies

Weak	
1.	Didactic
2.	Traditional continuing medical education
3.	Direct mailings
Moderate	
4.	Audit and feedback
5.	Especially concurrent
6.	Target specific providers
7.	Delivered by peers and opinion leaders
Strong	
8.	Reminder systems
9.	Academic detailing
10.	Multiple interventions

Reference: Davis and Taylor-Vaisey.[5]

The most important issue regarding the use of guidelines is that if they exist, they need to be followed. Failure to do so is more likely to impose secondary medicolegal liability. Hyams et al. in their seminal work reported on a sample of 259 obstetric, anesthesia, and other claims, in which 6.5% (17) involved practice guidelines.[3] The attorneys reported that guidelines were used over twice as often in an inculpatory fashion (54% of cases) as in an exculpatory fashion (23% of cases). However, if the guidelines supported the physician's care, this often induced the attorney not to file suit. The importance of adherence to clinical guidelines therefore cannot be overstated.

Ransom et al. evaluated the influence of clinical pathways on subsequent medicolegal risk.[4] They compared obstetric malpractice claims for 290 cases with delivery-related complications compared to 262 control deliveries. Non-compliance with the clinical pathways was significantly more common among claims than in control patients (42% vs.11.7%, $P < 0.001$, OR = 5.76, 95% CI 3.59–9.2). In cases of deviation, the majority of claims (79.4%, 81) were based on departure from the clinical pathway as the cornerstone of the case. The excess malpractice risk attributed to pathway non-compliance directly explained one-third (104 of 290) of claims filed, with an attributable risk of 82.6%. The course is clear: if a clinical pathway exists, it must be followed.

Davis et al. studied the implementation of clinical practice guidelines, with mixed results.[5] The variables that affect the adoption of guidelines include the quality of the guidelines and the characteristics of health-care professionals. The characteristics of the practice setting, specifically incentives, regulation, and patient factors, can also influence pathway success. The specific interventional strategies fell into two categories: primary approaches, including publication and dissemination of guidelines, and secondary strategies to reinforce the guidelines. Davis et al. further rated the interventions as weak (didactic, traditional medical education, and mailings); moderately effective (audit and feedback, especially concurrent, targeted to specific providers and delivered by peers or opinion leaders); and relatively strong (reminder systems, academic detailing and multiple interventions) (Table 47.2).

Legal Analysis

In *Hutchinson* v. *Greater Southeast Community Hospital*, the patient was transported by ambulance to the ED, complaining of posterior headache, foam in his mouth, and weakness.[6] He was assessed by the on-duty ED physician, who had administrative responsibility, and diagnosed with a "non-emergent" condition. He was then placed in a cab and sent to a tertiary care referral hospital. He was found wandering the streets, partially clothed, and taken to the hospital. He was admitted to the hospital with a subarachnoid hemorrhage, and died there 4 days later. His family filed suit, alleging EMTALA violation for improper medical screening.[7] The ED group and facility defended by their policy that an uninsured patient designated "routine" would need to provide a cash deposit for care or is:

> To be seen by an emergency physician for a screening exam to determine if a medical emergency exists. Those patients whom the physician determines may have a medical emergency will be treated. Those patients whom the physician determines do not have a medical emergency will be denied care, but will be offered transportation to other treatment sites.

The Vice President of Medical Affairs of the hospital stated that "there were no hospital policies, protocols or procedure specifying any required content of an emergency screening exam, or describing what comprises an adequate or inadequate screening exam." Likewise, there was to be proper documentation of the screening exam including, "aspects of the history, observations, or the physical exam the physician performs, conclusions whether it is an emergency case or not, and the advice to the patient." However, he acknowledged that interpretation of a separate documentation policy could represent a "minimum standard" for a screening exam. The defendants filed a motion to dismiss, and in the alternative summary judgment. The defendant's summary judgment motion was granted and remaining plaintiff claims dismissed.

In *Ma* v. *City and County of San Francisco*, appellants appealed from a summary judgment in favor of the city and county.[8] The patient presented to the ED, where she died allegedly from an acute asthma attack. However, some time prior to the presentation, she had placed a call to the San Francisco CCSF 911 emergency service center. The appellants claimed that duty was breached in that the dispatcher on duty at the time was not trained in emergency protocols, and the dispatcher was negligent in failing to respond using these protocols. At that time, the 911 center used two protocols: Medical Priority Dispatching (MPD), which required answers to a series of questions that had to be asked of each caller regardless

Table 47.3 Factors establishing tort duty to given patient (Rowland)

1.	Ability to foresee harm to injured party
2.	Degree of certainty that injured party suffered harm
3.	Connection between defendant's conduct and injury
4.	Moral blame to defendant's conduct
5.	Prevent future harm
6.	Burden to defendant
7.	Duty to exercise care with potential liability

Reference: Rowland.[10]

of whether some of the questions were relevant, and Criteria Based Dispatching (CPD), based on a series of uniform criteria applied seeking pattern matches. The former is better suited to paramedic-based programs, and the latter to firefighter-based programs. The CPD program was instituted at this location and all dispatchers were trained, and would use written guidelines or protocols without exception. The program offered standardized responses to problem-based complaints, but did not distinguish between shock caused by trauma or infection. However, it triggered immediate dispatch for emergency conditions, through a "default principle" allowing detail resolution later. When in doubt, "better to send faster, than slower." CCSF filed a motion for summary judgment, contending no tort duty of care was owed the patient, or alternatively that if a duty was owed, the claim was barred by "discretionary immunity."[9] The trial court agreed on both counts, and entered judgment accordingly. The appeal court reversed the trial court decision. They held that a duty of care was indeed owed, not with regard to the design or structure of the 911 call center, but as to the manner in which call procedures were implemented citing the Rowland multi-prong tort analysis (Table 47.3).[10] The Rowland decision is a multi-element duty assessment in determining whether a particular defendant owes a tort duty to a given plaintiff. These factors include: (1) ability to foresee harm to the injured party; (2) degree of certainty that the injured party suffered harm; (3) closeness of the connection between the defendant's conduct and the injury suffered; (4) moral blame attached to the defendant's conduct; (5) policy of preventing future harm; (6) extent of the burden to the defendant; (7) consequences to the community of imposing a duty to exercise care, with the resulting potential liability.[3]

Table 47.4 Summary elements of clinical guidelines

1. Written by multidisciplinary group with broad expertise
2. Evidence-based development
3. Reviewed every one to two years
4. Published and available to all providers
5. Clear, concise algorithmic pathway
6. Functional efficiency and ease of operation

There is an established standard tort duty of ordinary due care obligation. However, the qualified statutory immunity offered to EMTs and paramedics under Health and Safety Code §1799.107 does not extend to 911 dispatchers at this point in time.[11] The appeal court found a duty, but rejected the argument that the dispatcher's duty was limited to providing service in a manner not grossly negligent or in bad faith. The tort duty owed is that of "ordinary care."

Conclusion

In summary, well-conceived and implemented guidelines include the following aspects (Table 47.4): first, they are written by a multidisciplinary group providing broad expertise; second, they should be evidence-based in their development; third, they should be re-reviewed every one to two years for accuracy and continuity; fourth, they should be published and available to all health-care providers at the institution; fifth, they should be unambiguous and concise, offering clear decision-making algorithmic choices; sixth, they should provide functional efficiency and ease of operation.

References

1. Joint Commission on Accreditation of Health Care Organizations. Comprehensive Accreditation Manual for Hospitals Proposed Changes to the Standard for the Use of Clinical Practice Guidelines. ED Quality Solutions, Inc. www.ed-qual.com>JCAHO_2004_ClinicalPracticeGuidelines. accessed April 20, 2015.

2. Chapman IJ (ed.). *Failure Mode and Effects Analysis in Health Care: Proactive Risk Reduction*, 3rd edition. (Oakbrook Terrace, IL: Joint Commission Resources, 2010), pp. 1–17.

3. Hyams AL, Brandenberg JA, Lipsitz SR, Shapiro DW, Brennen TA. Practice guidelines and malpractice litigation: a two-way street. *Ann Intern Med*. 1995;122(6):450–55 DOI:10.7326/0003-4819-122-6-199503150-00008.

4. Ransom SB, Studdert DM, Dombrowski MP, Mello MM, Brennan TA. Reduced medicolegal risk by compliance with obstetric clinical pathways: a case-control study. *Obstet Gynecol*. 2003;101(4):751–755.

5. Davis DA, Taylor-Vaisey A. Translating guidelines into practice: a systematic review of theoretic concepts, practical experience and research evidence in the adoption of clinical practice guidelines. *Can Med Assoc J*. 1997;157(4):408–416.

6. *Hutchinson* v. *Greater Southeast Community Hospital*, 793 F. Supp.6 (1992).

7. EMTALA, 42 U.S.C. §1395dd.

8. *Ma* v. *City and County of San Francisco*, 95 Cal. Rptr.2d 544 (2002).

9. California Government Code Article §820.2 (1963) Liability of Public Employees.

10. *Rowland* v. *Christian*, 443 P.2d 561 (1968).

11. California Health and Safety Code §1799.107: Liability Protection for Dispatching Available under Health and Safety Code.

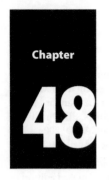

Health Insurance Portability and Accountability Act and Health Information Technology for Economic and Clinical Health Act

Case

It was an extremely busy day in the emergency department (ED). The department was short-staffed that day, and outside consultants were visiting to evaluate the operation of the ED. The consultants were there for hours asking numerous questions, beginning in the waiting room, and inspecting the clinical work areas, equipment, and storage areas. They were interviewing staff members and asking questions concerning the operation of the ED. One of the reviewers glanced at the electronic tracking board and noted the information contained there, as well as various times of service and patients' ultimate disposition (discharge versus admission). One of the reviewers asked a question about primary care physicians (PCPs), whose names were listed at the side of the patient care tracking board.

They subsequently reviewed the tracking board, asking for the specialty representation of a couple of the PCPs. They were told that one of these physicians was an infectious disease specialist. The reviewer asked if that physician had any other subspecialty and the answer was that he ran the immunology service as well as the HIV clinic at the hospital.

The following week the department received the written evaluation, which was largely supportive. However, it stated that there was a violation of the Health Insurance Portability and Accountability Act 1996 (HIPAA). Apparently, it is a HIPAA violation if a patient could potentially be identified by the specialty of their physician, rather than by the disease condition itself. Their health history and their disease state might be identified by the type of physician who was listed on a publicly visible patient tracking board. This outcome was especially likely in a small facility, where there are fewer physician treatment options.

Medical Approach

HIPAA mandates that protected health information (PHI) should not be revealed in an inappropriate fashion, or without the patient's explicit consent. In this particular situation, electronic patient care tracking boards are often overzealous in offering information that is visible in the public space. One must be cautious to not reveal too much PHI in the information-sharing environment, such as the patient's name or initials, information involved in the patient's chief complaint, or identification of their physician as one who only cares for a particular disease type. It is often helpful to have an objective third-party evaluation to help to elicit subtle violations of the HIPAA.

HIPAA, most recently updated in 2013, embodies the current privacy standards. It addresses the privacy and security of PHI, as well as reviewing requirements for reporting breaches of unsecured health information.[1] The Health Information Technology for Economic and Clinical Health Act (HITECH), part of the American Recovery and Reinvestment Act of 2009, also has an impact on practice.[2] HITECH promotes the adoption and meaningful use of health information, clarifying and expanding HIPAA and implementing new notification requirements for health information breaches.

The HIPAA Privacy Rule first focuses on the protection of all PHI in any format – paper, electronic, or oral transmission (Table 48.1).[3] It also defines the circumstances in which PHI may be disclosed to covered entities. The covered entity provides the individual or their representative with a procedure to obtain their health information, as well as an accounting methodology. The federal Privacy Rule supersedes state law, unless state law provides more stringent protections, which remain in effect.

One of the most critical questions is what PHI can be released without the patient's consent. The Privacy

Table 48.1 HIPAA Privacy Rule

1.	Any format – paper, electronic, or oral
2.	Define circumstances of disclosure
3.	Procedure and accountability of release
4.	Supersedes state law

Reference: OCR[4]

Table 48.2 Twelve national priority release purposes

1.	Required by law
2.	Public health activities
3.	Victim of abuse, neglect, or domestic violence
4.	Health oversight activities
5.	Judicial and administrative proceedings
6.	Law enforcement purposes
7.	Decedent's cause of death
8.	Organ, eye, or tissue donation
9.	Research
10.	Serious threat to health or safety
11.	Essential government functions
12.	Workers' compensation

Reference: C.F.R.[5]

Table 48.3 Law enforcement release purposes

1.	Required by law – court order
2.	Locate suspect, fugitive, or witness
3.	Victim or suspected victim of crime
4.	Injury caused by suspected criminal activity
5.	Evidence of crime on premises
6.	Notification of off-premises crime

Reference: C.F.R.[5]

Seventh, for a decedent the manner and cause of death can be released to the medical examiner or coroner. Eighth, information can be released to facilitate organ, eye, or tissue donation. Ninth, in response to a research request, as long as proper consent, protocol, and Institutional Review Board approval had been obtained. Tenth, clearly if there is a threat to public health or safety, a potentially violent individual could be reported. Eleventh, essential government functions are supported with release for military, intelligence or security purposes. Twelfth, pertinent information related to a work-related injury and subsequent workers's compensation claim can be released.

Legal Analysis

In *Maier* v. *Green*, a female patient presented to the ED as a victim of a domestic violence assault, and was admitted to the hospital.[6] The nurse called 911 to report the incident, which was then to be investigated by law enforcement as a domestic violence incident. In the interim the hospital case manager interviewed the patient, and denied law enforcement access to the patient for an interview. The plaintiff alleged for the patient that she had asserted her right to privacy for her medical condition. The case manager was the subject of an arrest warrant for obstruction of justice, but the district attorney declined to pursue. The court granted the defendant's motion for summary judgment, dismissing them from all claims relating to this arrest. Typically, law enforcement has broad power in relation to official civil and criminal investigations, but may be somewhat limited in domestic violence situations. Here, the victim and/or patient must usually consent to reporting unless certain violence or injury triggers are met in the alleged assault.

There is little tolerance for health-care professionals who access a patient's PHI without proper authorization or consent. The US Attorney's Office cited

Rule permits the use and disclosure of PHI without the individual's authorization for "twelve national priority purposes" striking the balance between individual and societal rights (Table 48.2).[4] First, those that are specified statute, regulation or court order. Second, those that compelled by public health sources, state, or federal agencies. Third, if a victim of abuse, neglect, or domestic violence, this information can be released to the appropriate governmental authorities. Fourth, standard health-care oversight activities that are routinely performed as audits or investigations are authorized to receive PHI. Fifth, as a part of a formal judicial or administrative proceeding a court subpoena may be honored. Sixth, requests made for valid law enforcement purposes, often complex, are honored including: (1) as required by law in order, warrant, or subpoena; (2) identify or locate a suspect or fugitive; (3) in response to an official request concerning a crime victim; (4) alert law enforcement of patient death if felt to be related to a crime; (5) PHI is evidence of crime occurring on the premises; (6) necessary to inform law enforcement of evidence of a crime not occurring on the premises (Table 48.3).[4]

a physician, an account representative, and an ED coordinator for inappropriate, unauthorized access to patient records.[7] The PHI was allegedly accessed from a home computer in one case, and from facility computers on multiple occasions on the basis of "curiosity." All defendants had undergone HIPAA training, and accepted responsibility by pleading to misdemeanor charges. This intervention was meant to deter health-care professionals from accessing patient PHI for inappropriate reasons.

This issue is often prominent in law enforcement requests for information. In *State of Wisconsin* v. *Straehler*, the issue arises whether suppression of evidence is a proper remedy for the alleged violation of health-care privacy laws, specifically HIPAA and Wisconsin Statute §146.82.[8] The patient, who was alleged to have run a red light, was in the driver's seat with the smell of intoxicants noted by law enforcement, and was air-evacuated to the hospital. When the detective attempted to interview the patient she was incoherent, so he contacted one of the nurses to determine the etiology of her current condition. The nurse stated that the patient smelled of alcohol, as noted by her and the other staff, and had told the staff that she had consumed alcohol prior to the event. A criminal complaint was filed, and the circuit court denied the patient's suppression motion, because even assuming a health-care privacy violation, the remedy of suppression of evidence is not appropriate. This decision was affirmed by the Court of Appeals of Wisconsin. HIPAA's Privacy Rule states in relevant part that a "covered entity" may not use or disclose PHI, except as permitted or required by regulations (45 C.F.R. §164.502 (a)). "Covered entities" include health plans, health-care clearinghouses, and providers who transmit any health information electronically (45 C.F.R. §§160.102 (a), 164.104 (a)).[9] Wisconsin Statute §146.82 states that confidentiality of patient health records provides that all patient health-care records shall remain confidential. Patient health-care records may be released only to persons designated in this section or with informed consent of the patient.[10]

In *State of Indiana* v. *Eichhorst*, the defendant was the driver in a one-car accident which resulted in the death of a family member, and was transported to the hospital with significant injuries.[11] An officer was dispatched to the hospital to request a blood sample for forensic testing. At the hospital the patient was noted to be loud, uncooperative, not aware of her surroundings, and smelling strongly of alcohol. The

ED physician ordered a blood alcohol test, among the other testing, so the patient would, "be able to be treated in the best possible way." He noted that intoxication may impair the patient's ability to describe pain and to consent to treatment. The nurse was told a law enforcement officer had called and requested a blood draw, and drew a vial for the police sample. She informed the officer he could not talk to the patient at this time. The patient stated she was drinking, and smelled of alcohol, but later denied that statement. The state filed a Motion for Issuance of a Subpoena Duces Tecum for her medical records, including the blood alcohol test. The trial court granted the defendant motion to suppress the blood alcohol test result. The Court of Appeals of Indiana reversed and remanded. The appeal court held that:

> To an extent a defendant does have an expectation of privacy in his medical records generally, we conclude that in Indiana at least, society does not recognize a reasonable expectation of privacy in blood alcohol test results and recorded by the hospital as part of its consensual treatment of a patient, where the results are requested by law enforcement for law enforcement purposes only in the setting of an automobile accident.

In *Allen* v. *Highlands Hospital*, the plaintiffs sued their employer for age discrimination under the Age Discrimination in Employment Act (ADEA) and the Kentucky Civil Rights Act (KCRA) implementing the statute locally.[12-14] Their employment had allegedly been terminated for violating the facility's confidentiality policy by breaching the confidentiality of one of its patients. Radiographs of the minor granddaughter of one of the employees were removed from the hospital, allegedly without the mother's authorization. The radiographs were removed by the grandmother at the mother's request for a follow-up appointment. The mother remembers asking the grandmother to pick the X-rays up. However, the grandmother, who worked at the hospital, was alleged to have "signed her daughter's name on the release form, backdated the document and put it in the X-ray jacket." The plaintiffs alleged the reason for firing the employee was a pretext to hide age discrimination. Both cases were removed to federal court and consolidated for trial. The defendant's motion for summary judgment was granted, and affirmed by the United States Court of Appeals, Sixth Circuit. Under both the ADEA and KCRA, employers are prohibited from discharging or otherwise discriminating against any employee with respect to compensation, terms, conditions, or privileges of employment because of the individual's age. New cost-cutting measures resulted in an increase in the annual turnover rate from 2% to 28%. Plaintiffs allege this initiative manifested a higher turnover in older employees, but this contention was not borne out in the data. There was apparently no written policy on this issue, but all administrators involved in the disciplinary process felt the breach of confidentiality was a group I (high-priority) offense resulting in termination.

Conclusion

The key is to ensure proper written policy, procedure, and education concerning patient confidentiality issues. These processes should be regularly reviewed, and timely updates communicated to all employees and consultants.

References

1. Health Insurance Portability and Accountability Act of 1996 (HIPAA), Title XI, Pub. L. 104–191, 110 Stat. 1936 (August 21, 1996), codified as 42 U.S.C. 1301 et seq.

2. O'Rourke IK, Vukmir RB. HIPAA – The Health Insurance Portability and Accountability Act of 1996/HITECH – The Health Information Technology for Economic and Clinical Health Act of 2009. *Emergency Consultants (ECI)*, revised November 2014: 1–8.

3. Health Information Technology for Economic and Clinical Health Act (HITECH), Title XIII of Division A and Title IV of Division B of the American Recovery and Reinvestment Act of 2009 (ARRA), Pub. L. No. 111–5, 123 Stat. 226 (February 17, 2009), codified at 42 U.S.C. §§300jj et seq.; §§17902 et seq.

4. OCR Policy Brief: Summary of the HIPAA Privacy Rule. United States Department of Health and Human Services, May 2003: 1–23.

5. 45 C.F.R. §164.512 (a): Security and Privacy.

6. *Maier* v. *Green*, 485 F. Supp.2d. 711 (2007).

7. Federal Bureau of Investigation: Little Rock Division. Doctor and two former hospital employees plead guilty to HIPAA violations (press release). US Attorney's Office, Eastern District of Arkansas, July 20, 2009.

8. *State of Wisconsin* v. *Straehler*, 745 N.W.2d 431 (2007).

9. 45 C.F.R. §164.502 (a):Uses and Disclosures of Protected Health Location.

10. Wisconsin Statutes §146.82: Confidentiality of Patient Care Records.

11. *State of Indiana* v. *Eichhorst*, 963 N.E.2d 1117 (2012).

12. *Allen* v. *Highlands Hospital*, 545 F.3d 387 (2008).

13. Age Discrimination in Employment Act (ADEA), 29 U.S.C. §623 (1967).

14. Kentucky Civil Rights Act (KCRA) Ky.Rev.Stat.Ann. §344.040 (1).

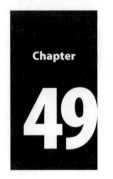

HIV

Case

The emergency department (ED) physician had sent off a fairly broad array of laboratory screening tests from triage. The patient's complaint was weight loss, diarrhea, and fatigue for the last eight weeks. She had a slight fever early on, but had improved significantly in the last couple of weeks. She had no previous health problems and did not have a primary care physician (PCP). The workup included standard screening laboratory tests: a complete blood count, Chem-7 metabolic tests, pregnancy test, urinalysis, thyroid functions, and an HIV screen. The patient's laboratory results were all essentially normal, although she was slightly neutropenic, and her sodium was a little low.

The provider suggested that her initial laboratory screening was normal, except for a couple of abnormalities that would require subsequent testing. The results would come back over the next few days, and they established a primary care referral for her to follow up the laboratory results with a PCP. Stool cultures were ordered, and the patient was going to take the specimen kit home and return that to the hospital when complete.

The quality assurance nurse with the ED reported 48 hours later that the HIV test was positive and asked what the patient's follow-up schedule was to discuss this result. The ED physician had designated a PCP and follow-up visit to establish a continuity plan with this physician. The laboratory testing was discussed with a call to the physician's office, stating that the patient had been referred for their care. Referral to the infectious disease unit for an additional care resource was also discussed.

A call from the patient advocate questioned the necessity for ordering the HIV test. The patient stated that she would not have wanted to know the test result, and was not involved in the decision-making. The patient stated that she should have been asked and needed to give consent for the HIV test to be done.

Even though she appreciated the fact that the diagnosis had been made, she would have preferred not to know in the first place.

Medical Approach

The use of HIV screening has become a highly emotive issue and has evolved from a patient mandatory consent requirement for screening testing. Testing requirements have changed, with the goal of improving individual and societal health, as HIV infection is a reportable communicable disease. A conventional testing strategy is to screen high-risk patients depending on their presentation, or if they present a blood contamination risk to others. The patient's consent is no longer required for HIV testing, as long as the testing is medically appropriate for the patient, or someone affected by the patient. It is important, however, to let the patient know the overall care plan and that communication needs to be optimized.

Another ostensible rationale invoked for not doing the test is that the patient has no PCP to discuss results. However, this is not a relevant argument here as primary care was not involved in this case initially and creating an opportunity for the patient to establish a relationship with a new physician will have overall health benefits.

In Pisculli et al.'s analysis of 1959 ED patients the rate of refusal of HIV testing is approximately one-third (29%).[1] Multivariate analysis suggests the cohort most likely to refuse testing are women, annual income >$50,000, reportedly not engaging in high-risk behavior, previous HIV testing, and early morning presentation.

Another area of controversy is unconsented HIV patient testing, typically in the setting of health-care provider exposure, evaluated by Cowan and Macklin.[2] They summarized the various state statutes to find that 36 states allowed unconsented HIV testing in

Table 49.1 HIV testing: requirements for counseling

1. Coping with emotional consequences of result
2. Discussion of discrimination problems of disclosure
3. Behavior change to prevent transmission
4. Informing of available medical treatment and services
5. Local or community-based HIV/AIDS support
6. Work toward involving a minor's parent or guardian
7. Discussion of need to notify partners

Reference: Connecticut General Statutes.[4]

Table 49.2 Emergency medical services personnel exposure law: blood available for testing

1. Documented exposure has occurred
2. Exposure was significant and results needed for treatment
3. Exposed patient provides blood sample
4. Source patient declines to provide consent
5. Source patient provided adequate information for decision-making
6. Consent for testing not required if hospital has made reasonable attempts to obtain consent

Reference: Minnesota Statutes.[5]

the setting of occupational exposure of health-care providers rendering care in the hospital setting. The remaining states either have laws that are not compatible, or no statute addressing this issue.

It is critically important to understand the statute and requirements specific to the state of practice. Washington State compels laboratory reporting of positive HIV test results within 3 days that include confirmatory testing (Western blot, p24 antigen, viral culture), viral load (detectable and undetectable), and CD4+ (T4) lymphocyte result of any value.[3]

The Connecticut General Statutes state that a person who has provided consent for general medical procedures and tests is not required to sign a specific consent for HIV testing.[4] However, the general consent states "you may be tested for HIV, but it is voluntary" and must be declined at that time and documented in the record. More importantly, if the test is ordered the "person ordering the performance" must stand ready to communicate those results to the patient and provide an extensive, comprehensive array of support and counseling services (Table 49.1). Therefore, a prudent course for the ED provider is to follow up personally with the patient if an HIV test is ordered.

The Minnesota Department of Health has advanced the Emergency Medical Services Personnel Exposure Law (Table 49.2).[5] The protocol requires that, if blood is available, testing can be performed without the patient's consent if the following criteria are met: first, a documented exposure has occurred; second, the evaluating hospital decides the exposure was significant and test results are needed to determine appropriate treatment course; third, the exposed person provides a blood sample for bloodborne pathogen testing; fourth, the hospital asks the source patient to consent and they do not; fifth, the source patient has been provided with all information required, including confidentiality and penalties for

disclosure; sixth, consent for testing is not required if the hospital has made reasonable attempts to obtain consent (Table 49.2).

If there is no blood available and the source patient refuses consent, then an alternate protocol is instituted (Table 49.3).[5] First, the hospital will inform the exposed patient of the source patient refusal. Second, the emergency medical services (EMS) agency or the exposed person may petition the court to compel a blood draw. Third, the hospital will cooperate with the submission of affidavits, and personnel will provide witness and oaths as necessary. Fourth, if petition is filed the source individual has the right to legal counsel.

The court may order a source individual to provide a blood sample if, first, there is probable cause to believe the exposed has significant exposure from the source individual;[7] second, the court imposes significant safeguards against unauthorized disclosure and specifies the official disclosure pathway; third, a licensed physician participating in the care of the exposed patient requires the test result to determine the appropriate treatment; fourth, the court finds a compelling need for the test result (Table 49.4).

Legal Analysis

Historically, the caselaw has involved alleged discrimination in the care of patients with HIV infection, or breaches in confidentiality. In *Lee* v. *Calhoun*, the patient filed a medical malpractice action for emergency surgery to repair a perforated bowel.[6] When the suit was filed, the defendant physician was approached by a reporter, and revealed the patient's disease status in the explanation and defense of his position. These details then appeared in the local newspaper. The facts were not in dispute, as the patient presented

Table 49.3 Emergency medical services personnel exposure law: blood not available for testing

1.	Hospital inform exposed patient of refusal of source patient
2.	EMS or exposed patient may petition court to compel
3.	Hospital will cooperate with petitioner
4.	Source individual has right to legal counsel

Reference: Minnesota Statutes.[5]

Table 49.4 Court order for source patient

1.	Probable cause to believe significant exposure
2.	Impose appropriate safeguards against unauthorized disclosure
3.	Test result is necessary for medical care
4.	Court finds compelling need for test result

Reference: Minnesota Statutes.[5]

to the ED with abdominal pain, was diagnosed with appendicitis, and surgery was consulted. The operation was performed, revealing a bowel perforation, a colostomy was performed, and additional blood testing revealed abnormalities that were not disclosed in the medical history. The patient filed suit for medical malpractice and then defamation, invasion of privacy, and breach of doctor–patient confidentiality and intrusion upon seclusion. The malpractice claim was dismissed, and summary judgment motions entered for the defendant, holding he waived his physician–patient privilege, and had not established his right to proceed on the others. The United States Court of Appeals, Tenth District found no error and affirmed the trial court decision. They held the subject of the defamation claim failed as it was true. The plaintiff's claims were embodied in the Restatement (Second) of Torts (§625A) involving invasion of privacy (§652D),[7] in which "One gives public information concerning the private life of another, that would be highly offensive to a reasonable person and not of legitimate concern to the public." However, there is no liability when the defendant merely gives further publicity to information the plaintiff has already made public. There is liability if there is public disclosure of a private fact not of "legitimate public concern." [8] Waiver of physician–patient privilege is exempt from liability in any legislative or judicial proceeding, proper discharge of an official duty, or fair report of any legislative or judicial

proceeding.[9] Likewise, there is a conditional privilege in Restatement §594 that allows publication of matter that is of sufficient interest to the publisher, and recipient's knowledge of defamatory matter will be of service to the lawful protection of that interest. In addition, the conditional privilege extends to one who feels their own reputation is being defamed or invaded by another and is analogous to self-defense, which is permitted.

In *Robinson* v. *Henry Ford Health Systems*, the patient was brought to the ED by city EMS complaining of shortness of breath, dizziness, and headache.[10] During this visit she disclosed a previous positive HIV test result. She was diagnosed with an upper respiratory infection after normal blood work, chest radiograph, and an 11 hour ED stay. The next day she presented in cardiac arrest, and she was pronounced dead. Representatives filed a lawsuit alleging medical malpractice, a breach of EMTALA, and three separate counts of discrimination, alleging inadequate treatment because of her pre-existing condition.[11] These include: (1) the Michigan Handicappers Civil Rights Act,[12] established to prevent discrimination in those with disabilities; (2) the Detroit City Ordinance established to prevent AIDS discrimination;[13] (3) the Federal Rehabilitation Act,[14] in which "no otherwise qualified individual … solely based on their disability … be denied the benefits of, or be subjected to discrimination under any program or activity receiving federal financial assistance." The district court held that the plaintiff did not meet the required elements of a legally cognizable claim, and the defendant's summary judgment motion was granted. The plaintiff failed to establish a discriminatory motive, a lack of medical screening exam, or the production of an emergency medicine expert witness, only a pathologist.

There is another cadre of cases that deal with notification. In *In re Sealed Case* the appellant states she contracted HIV from her husband, and filed suit against a physician contracted to review laboratory results and perform "quality control" data reviews.[15] The consultant reviewed six pages of patient laboratory results and returned them to the physician with some notes that the physician countersigned. The plaintiff filed suit, alleging this laboratory review required review of her husband's complete medical file, which demonstrated a positive test for blood-borne disease and informing her she was at risk. The trial court defined a narrow scope of consultant relationship that did not give rise to an obligation to review. The consultant did not have a duty to the plaintiff and therefore could not have breached that duty. There was no obligation for the consultant to review the entire file of every patient whose laboratory data was reviewed at the doctor's request.

Conclusion

HIV infection and its associated testing requires one of the highest levels of confidentiality and protection. All health-care providers should be most cautious of their own privacy practice, as it relates to patient confidentiality. They should also monitor the practice of colleagues in relation to patient confidentiality.

References

1. Pisculli ML, Reichmart WM, Losina E, Donnell-Fink LA, Arbelaez C, Katz JN, Walensky RP. Factors associated with refusal of rapid HIV testing in the emergency department. *AIDS Behav.* 2011;15(4):734–742.

2. Cowan E, Macklin R. Unconsented HIV testing in cases of occupational exposure: ethics, law and policy. *Acad Emerg Med.* 2012;19(10):1181–87. DOI:10.1111/j.1553–2712.2012.01453.x.

3. Washington Administrative Code, Title 246, Chapter 246-101.

4. Connecticut General Statutes – General Consent Required for HIV Related Testing. Counseling Requirements. Exceptions. Title 19a, Chapter 368x, 19a-582.

5. Minnesota Statutes. Minnesota Department of Health Emergency Medical Services Personnel Exposure Law. 144.7401 – 2015.

6. *Lee* v. *Calhoun*, 948 F.2d 1162 (1991).

7. Restatement of the Law Second, Torts, §504–707A (1977).

8. *McCormack* v. *Oklahoma Publishing Co.*, 613 P.2d 737 (Okl. 1980).

9. Oklahoma Statutes, Title 12 1991 §1443.1.

10. *Robinson* v. *Henry Ford Health Systems*, 892 F. Supp. 176 (1994).

11. EMTALA 42 U.S.C. §1395dd.

12. Michigan Handicappers Civil Rights Act (MHCRA):M.C.L.A. §37.1103 (b).

13. Detroit City Ordinance, AIDS Discrimination 33–88, September 12, 1988.

14. Federal Rehabilitation Act, 29 179 U.S.C §794.

15. In re Sealed Case, 67 F.3d 965 (1995).

Hospital Medicine

Case

The patient came in to the emergency department (ED) with a complaint of weight loss and cough, which had been present for the last month. She appeared to be quite thin. She said she had been spending a lot of time at work, and had not been eating well. There had been a little extra stress in her life as well. She thought she might have had a fever at night and some nausea. After questioning, she agreed that maybe her appetite had decreased a little.

The ED physician did a complete workup and the patient's laboratory results showed slight anemia. There was no white blood cell count elevation but her chest radiograph showed an infiltrate that seemed a little denser than it should be. The physician started the patient on intravenous antibiotics, then notified the hospitalist, who admitted her and signed off. The ED physician reminded the hospitalist to evaluate the patient for cancer with a contrasted CT scan since she had a significant smoking history. The hospitalist agreed with the CT, and suggested they would contact the patient's primary care physician (PCP) on discharge for additional follow-up.

Two years later the hospital attorney informed the ED that a legal case had been filed concerning this patient. Apparently, the patient went on to succumb allegedly to lung cancer, which was not diagnosed for another 9 months after her ED visit. The ED physician responded that she had discussed this with the hospitalist, suggesting additional follow-up to ensure there was no malignancy. This was indeed the case, but apparently the hospitalist had not performed a CT scan during the hospital visit. He had intended to discuss the scan with the PCP in the follow-up plan, but omitted that part of the process and told the patient to report it to their PCP. Apparently, the PCP did not receive any record of the visit or of the chest radiograph findings. The hospital-based electronic health record did not offer any additional automatic process of record referral to the PCP, or an automated discharge plan referred by the hospitalist.

Medical Approach

The transition of care between health-care providers is often a problematic area for medicolegal reasons and patient safety concerns. In this particular case, there were two transitions, one between the ED physician and the hospitalist and the second between the hospitalist and the PCP. Clearly, information was available to both providers. With conditions such as cancer that require mandatory follow-up, appropriate documentation is essential. The ED physician should make a clear record of contact with the admitting physician, as well as discussion with the patient. In addition, the hospitalist should ensure that all salient points related to the patient's visit are communicated to the PCP and clearly documented.

The key legal principles from the hospitalist's perspective are to define the responsibilities of the ED physician, admitting physician, and PCP in the transition of care process. The hospitalist is responsible, first, for providing information concerning diagnosis, treatment, and ongoing therapy.[1] Second, they are responsible for the process of relating completed, pending, or changing test results. Third, often small incidental findings are encountered in an evaluation, so the need arises to discuss these findings, which may take one out of the comfort zone of an established patient–physician relationship. Fourth, the information communicated must be clearly documented in the medical record (Table 50.1).

Overall, the key recommendations for the effective hospitalist interface include: first, both the hospitalist and the PCP assuming responsibility for the discharged patient;[1] second, the hospitalist must emphasize the importance of follow-up with the

Table 50.1 Hospitalist key responsibilities

1. Provide information concerning diagnosis, treatment, and therapy
2. Relate completed, pending, or changing test results
3. Address incidental findings that are encountered
4. Communicate and document

Reference: Alpers.[1]

Table 50.2 Patient, hospitalist, and PCP interface

1. Both hospitalist and PCP assume responsibility for discharged patient
2. Hospitalist must emphasize importance of PCP follow-up
3. Both patient and PCP must be informed of important findings
4. Both hospitalist and PCP are responsible for coordinating care

Reference: Alpers.[1]

Table 50.3 Malpractice claims rate

	Specialty	Incidence (Claims/100 PCYs)
1.	Hospitalist	0.52
2.	Internal medicine	1.91
3.	Emergency medicine	3.50
4.	General surgery	4.70
5.	Obstetrics-gynecology	5.56
		($P < 0.001$)

Reference: Schafer et al.[2]

patient; third, both the patient and the PCP must be informed of important or changing diagnoses or test results; fourth, both the hospitalist and the PCP are responsible for coordinating care when a follow-up appointment is missed (Table 50.2).

Although it is a relatively new medicolegal exposure model, the hospitalist care model has a defined liability impact. Schafer et al. performed a retrospective observational analysis of the claims data of 52,000 filings (Table 50.3).[2] Hospitalists have a malpractice rate of 0.52 claims per 100 patient coverage years (PCYs), significantly lower than their counterparts in other specialisms. The incidence for non-hospitalist internal medicine physicians was 1.9 claims per 100

PCYs, emergency physicians 3.50 claims, general surgeons 4.70 claims, and obstetrician-gynecologists the highest of the evaluated specialities at 5.56 claims. Although hospital medicine is a lower-risk specialty, vigilance is required. Focusing on the hospitalist claims, Schafer et al. reported the most common allegations were for errors of medical treatment (41.5%) and diagnosis (36.0%). The most common contributing factors were deficiencies in clinical judgment (54.4%) and communication (36.4%). These related to higher acuity claims, with 50.4% of cases involving patient death.

Legal Analysis

The case precedent seen suggests the hospitalist is held up to scrutiny in their consultative care. In *Osonma and IPC* v. *Smith*, the patient was admitted from the ED with a traumatic thumb amputation and surgical reimplantation.[3] The nursing assessment documented risk factors for deep venous thrombosis (DVT) and pulmonary embolism (PE) as "surgery, trauma, and more than 40 years of age." The surgery failed, heparin was stopped, the thumb was amputated, and the patient was transferred to a ward bed with medical consult. Allegedly, there was no DVT/PE prophylaxis in the surgical order sent. The patient developed chest pain and dyspnea, the hospitalist was consulted, and an EKG and sequential cardiac enzymes were ordered. Allegedly, the diagnosis was musculoskeletal chest pain. The patient's oxygen was discontinued and he succumbed the next day with an autopsy-proven PE.

The provider and employer appealed the trial court's interlocutory order denying their motion to dismiss the health-care liability claims brought against them. The appeal court affirmed the order of the trial court, denying the dismissal of the case against the defendants.

In *Luna* v. *Diverse and Hamilton County Hospital*, the patient had a surgical procedure removing vocal cord polyps with the hospitalist monitoring the postoperative recovery.[4] The patient was transferred to the post-anesthesia recovery unit, evaluated by the hospitalist, had a normal exam, was taking orally, and was felt to be stable for discharge home. The patient allegedly did not want to be discharged, and did not have transport home. Subsequently, transport was found and she was discharged. The patient then filed a pro se lawsuit representing herself, alleging "premature discharge" resulted in her suffering a heart attack and a stroke, and falling into a diabetic coma. The trial court granted the defendant's summary judgment motion to dismiss. The Court of Appeals of Tennessee affirmed the dismissal motion of the trial court.

In *Cunningham* v. *Thomas Memorial Hospital*, the patient was admitted with an unspecified medical condition to the hospitalist physician after an ED stay.[5] Care was transferred from the admitting hospitalist while she was on vacation to another hospitalist physician, who then consulted surgery. A surgical procedure was performed, an infection developed, and the patient alleged postoperative complications. The patient filed suit against the hospitalists, the surgeon, and the hospital in an agency relationship with vicarious liability for this alleged physician negligence.[6] In the alternative, the vicarious liability theory was directed at this physician–hospital described "joint venture." Summary judgment was awarded to the defendant by the trial court. This decision was affirmed by the Supreme Court of Appeals of West Virginia.

Conclusion

The ED physician has a particular requirement for effective communication. In addition to communicating with the hospitalist, the same discussion should be had with the PCP concerning the patient's discharge. An automatic referral system, with a mandatory triggered electronic health record report that would be referred to the accepting physician for care, could prevent such significant errors of omission. This is especially important with findings that are either critical or otherwise incidental.

References

1. Alpers A. Key legal principles for hospitalists. *Am J Med.* 2001;111(9B):5S–9S.

2. Schafer AC, Puopolo AL, Raman S, Kachalia A. Liability impact of the hospitalist model of care. *J Hosp Med.* 2014;9(12):1–6.

3. *Osonma* v. *Smith*, No. 04-08-00841-CV, 2008-CI-00951, Fourth Texas Court of Appeals of Texas, San Antonio, July 1, 2009.

4. *Luna* v. *Deversa*, No. E2009-01198-COA-R3-CV, Tennessee Court of Appeals, Knoxville, June 17, 2010.

5. *Cunningham* v. *Thomas Memorial*, 737 S.E.2d 270 (2012).

6. W Va. Code §55-7B-9 (g) (2003) (Repl. Vol. 2008).

Immigrant Care

Chapter

51

Case

The patient was an elderly woman, frail and of slight build. She smiled pleasantly, but didn't speak. Her family related the history: she was visiting the area and had run out of her medications for her congestive heart failure and chronic obstructive pulmonary disease (COPD). When she presented for care to the emergency department (ED) her family related that she had no insurance, nor was she a US citizen. Her family asked for consideration, so that she could get care in the ED. The ED staff reassured the family that they cared for patients regardless of their circumstances. There was more discussion with registration, but care was already being delivered at the hospital facility.

The ED evaluation went well. She indeed had long-established congestive heart failure, but she felt better with administration of some intravenous furosemide, as well as a breathing treatment for her chronic lung disease. Initially, it was thought she might have to be admitted, but over time her clinical condition improved, and she and her family were pleased with the response. The ED staff offered to dispense the medicines that they could and wrote for additional prescriptions at a low-cost pharmacy, as well as providing some hospital vouchers to get her prescriptions filled. The patient was given this information, which was translated by a volunteer interpreter and her family. Everyone seemed comfortable with the outcome and response. She was discharged home, with follow-up with one of the local primary care physicians (PCP) while she remained in the area.

The next day the ED received a call from a family member asking about this care event. The caller alleged the patient had truly required admission, but the hospital had declined to admit her ostensibly because of her lack of insurance and citizenship status. The ED responded that the decision was a purely

medical one. All patients are treated in the ED regardless of insurance status. The patient had clinically improved, the family was happy with her care, and she was discharged with the appropriate medicines. The medications were prescribed in a way that ensured they could be filled without financial encumbrance. In addition, the staff ensured that she did indeed receive her medicines prior to her discharge from the ED. The non-emergent medications were to be filled locally, using the pharmacy services provided.

Medical Approach

The question of how a hospital provides care to an undocumented immigrant, who may be uninsured as well, is one that often arises. Most hospital facilities go out of their way to provide charity care and would never turn a patient away on the basis of these criteria. Although this is often alleged, it is typically not substantiated.

> Immigrants' rights to health care present some of the most difficult and controversial problems of all health care issues facing the poverty population in the United States. The language, the environment and cultural differences that immigrants bring with them make it harder for them to overcome the barriers to health care that face all poor people.

Although this quote could be taken from today's headlines, it is actually from a 1986 paper entitled "Immigrants' right to health care."[1] Obviously, this is not a new issue, nor is it any less emotive or problematic an issue today than it was 30 years ago.

In 2007, it was estimated that there were 12 million undocumented immigrants in the United States, and these non-citizens accounted for 20% of the 45 million uninsured Americans.[2] At that time they did not typically qualify for federal health-care programs, and clinics and hospitals relied on state, local, or charitable contributions to deliver much-needed care.

143

Study of this problem is limited by difficulties in the collection of data, for a number of inherent reasons. Siddharthan and Ahern reported on the utilization of inpatient care by undocumented immigrants without insurance in a large South Florida county hospital.[3] They monitored disease severity as Case Mix Severity Index (CMSI) and resource use, reported as average length of stay, procedures, and/or diagnostic tests performed. They then compared the native-born population and those with permanent residency status, insured by Medicaid or uninsured, to the undocumented immigrant population. The undocumented immigrants had more severe illness with a higher CMSI, but a lower adjusted average length of hospital stay. The undocumented immigrants had a similar number of adjusted procedures or tests performed compared to uninsured US residents, but less than Medicaid beneficiaries.

Chan et al. reported on their experience with an undocumented immigrant population evaluated in an academic ED located in the western US, 20 miles from the US–Mexico international border.[4] They evaluated 2721 patients in a single month, where 8.6% (227) of patients were identified as undocumented immigrants. From this group, 104 patients consented to a telephone survey. This population was predominately Hispanic (89.4%), where 83% intended to remain in the US permanently and 80% (83) cited lack of funding as the reason to seek ED care. At the time, the highest uninsured rate was in the undocumented Hispanic population (64%) compared to the Hispanic (32%) and non-Hispanic (30%) documented population. When asked about their use of the ED, 36% (38) of the survey group stated they had difficulty obtaining care elsewhere, 51% (53) knew of no other sources of care, and 44% (46) said it was their preferred source of care. Although this study is now dated, we recognize that the ED is a crucial part of the health-care delivery system for undocumented immigrants residing in the US.

Jacobs et al. analyzed the care provided to an immigrant population in a large urban academic ED in the eastern US.[5] They prospectively surveyed 896 immigrant patients, from 80 different countries, and 394 non-immigrant control patients. Multivariate logistic regression was used to eliminate the confounding variables in the analysis (Table 51.1). At this time, the immigrant population was more likely to be less educated, have a lower income, and not have health insurance. The women were less likely to have had a Pap smear or breast self-examination, the men less likely to use condoms. They were less likely to have received a PPD test (to screen for tuberculosis) or a tetanus immunization, or to have visited a dentist. These are clear differences in education, economic standards, and preventive health measures that may affect the health of an immigrant population.

The immigrant population has lower rates of health insurance, uses less health care, and has been suggested to receive lower-quality health care than US-born populations, according to Derose et al.[6] This vulnerability is related to socioeconomic status,

Table 51.1 Characteristics of immigrant and non-immigrant ED populations

	Characteristic	Immigrant n = 896 %	Non-immigrant n = 354 %	Comparison
1.	Not reached high school	28.9	8.5	$P < 0.001$
2.	Annual family income <$20,000	73.8	64.5	$P < 0.01$
3.	No health coverage	51.7	30.8	$P < 0.001$
4.	Never had Pap test	16.1	1.4	OR11.24 CI 2.7–46.8
5.	No breast self-exam	20.8	7.5	OR 2.03 CI 1.29–3.20
6.	No condom use	63.4	42.8	OR 1.61 CI 1.20–2.15
7.	No dental car	21.2	7.8	OR 2.54 CI 1.60–4.04
8.	No PPD skin test	30.3	9.1	OR 3.85 CI 2.56–5.80
9.	No tetanus immunization	48.1	13.5	OR 3.09 CI 2.17–4.42

Reference: Jacobs et al.[5]

recognized immigration status, English proficiency, welfare reform, residential location, stigma, and marginalization.

The operative question is the availability of health care to undocumented immigrants in the US.[7] Undocumented immigrants are not typically eligible for federally funded public health insurance programs, including Medicare, Medicaid, and the Child Health Insurance Program. Emergency care is available as mandated by EMTALA, mandating stabilization and transfer in emergency conditions.[8] There are selective coverage opportunities through the healthcare safety net, from recognized "disproportionate share hospitals" receiving additional funding for uncompensated care, as well as public, private, and charitable clinic centers. The Patient Protection and Affordable Care Act does not specify undocumented immigrants as "qualified individuals" to receive benefits, but they may purchase their own health-care insurance through an exchange.[9]

Legal Analysis

The issue began with the provision of emergency care to undocumented immigrants. In *Greenery Rehabilitation Group* v. *Hammon*, the defendants, representatives of the state and federal government, appealed the bench trial declaratory judgment for the plaintiff-appellee health-care facility.[10] The district court held that undocumented immigrants who suffered serious traumatic brain injury were suffering from an "emergency medical condition" within the meaning of 42 U.S.C. §1396b (v) (3), defining Medicaid criteria, 42 C.F.R. §440.255 (b) (1) defining limited services available to immigrants, and corresponding New York State regulations.[11,12] The patients were now stable, but had chronic debilitating conditions requiring daily care, following their initial treatment. The court ordered payment to the rehabilitation group pursuant to Medicaid.

Undocumented immigrants or those not permanently residing in the US under the color of law generally are not entitled to full Medicaid coverage.[13] The only exception to this exclusion is payment for medical assistance that is "necessary for the treatment" of an emergency medical condition (EMC) as defined in EMTALA 42 U.S.C. §1396b (v) (114):

> As a medical condition, including emergency labor and delivery, manifesting itself by acute symptoms of sufficient severity, including severe pain, such that

the absence of immediate medical attention could reasonably be expected to result in:

a. Placing the patient's health in serious jeopardy
b. Serious impairment to bodily functions
c. Serious dysfunction of any bodily organ or part.

This EMTALA description was adapted as a corresponding regulation in 42 C.F.R. §435.406,[13] entitling immigrants to Medicaid coverage in emergency conditions. The obvious question presented to the United States Court of Appeals, Second Circuit was whether chronic debilitating conditions resulting from sudden serious injury are emergency medical conditions. The appeal court held that a literal reading of the EMTALA statute requires an emergency condition and not "ongoing and regimented care," so payment is not indicated and the trial court decision was reversed.

In *Diaz* v. *Division of Social Services*, the question was the scope of coverage and reimbursement for a non-qualifying immigrant's medical treatment under state and federal Medicaid law.[15] The patient presented to the ED with a sore throat, nausea, vomiting, bleeding gums, and lethargy and was later diagnosed with a form of leukemia requiring chemotherapy. The patient authorized the hospital to seek Medicaid coverage through the Division of Medical Assistance. They approved all emergency care, but denied all subsequent non-emergency services such as chemotherapy, surviving the highest level of administrative appeal. The superior court reversed the respondent's decision, holding that Medicaid shall pay for all care and services medically necessary for the treatment of an emergency medical condition. Respondent appealed to the Court of Appeals, which unanimously affirmed the trial court decision denying payment. The Supreme Court of North Carolina allowed discretionary review, and reversed the appeal court decision.[16]

Conclusion

Every facility should have a protocol in place that addresses this common scenario by providing medical care of an urgent nature to uninsured undocumented immigrants. This often requires a multidisciplinary approach that may involve local resources involving standard insurance networks, as well as community-based, governmental, or religious charitable organizations.

References

1. Drake SB. Immigrants' rights to health care. *Clgh Rev.* 1986 Summer;20(4):498–510.

2. Okie S. Immigrants and health care – at the intersection of two broken systems. *N Engl J Med.* 2007;357(6):525–529. DOI 10:1056/NEJMp078113.

3. Siddharthan K, Ahern M. Inpatient utilization by undocumented immigrants without insurance. *J Health Care Poor Underserved.* 1996;7(4):355–363. DOI:1.1353/hours.2010.0068.

4. Chan TC, Krishel SJ, Bramwell KJ, Clark RF. Survey of illegal immigrants seen in an emergency department. *West J Med.* 1996;164(3):212–216.

5. Jacobs DH, Tovar JM, Hung OL, Kim M, Ye P, Chiang WK, Goldfrank LR. Behavioral risk factor and preventive health care practice survey of immigrants in the emergency department. *Acad Emerg Med.* 2002;9(6):599–608. DOI:10.1197/aemj.9.6.599.

6. Derose KP, Escarce JJ, Lurie N. Immigrants and health care: sources of vulnerability. *Health Aff.* 2007;26(5):1258–1268. DOI:10.1377/hlthaff.26.5.1258.

7. Gusmano MK. Undocumented immigrants in the United States: US health policy and access to care. The Hastings Center. October 3, 2012.

8. EMTALA 42 U.S.C. §1395dd.

9. Patient Protection and Affordable Care Act (Public Act 111–148), 42 U.S.C. & 18001 et seq. (2010).

10. *Greenery Rehabilitation Group* v. *Hammon*, 150 F.3d 226 (1998).

11. 42 U.S.C. §1396b (v) (3): Payment to States.

12. 42 U.S.C. §440.255 (b) (1): Limited Services Available to Certain Aliens.

13. 42 U.S.C. §435.406.

14. EMTALA 42 U.S.C. §1396b (v) (1).

15. *Diaz* v. *Division of Social Services*, 615 S.E.2d 409 (2005).

16. *N.C. Dep't of Env't & Natural Res.* v. *Carroll*, 358. N.C. 649, 659, 599 S.E.2d 888, 894–95 (2004).

Impaired Physician

Case

Murmurings among the nurses suggested some concerns involving a physician employed in the emergency department (ED). He had been falling asleep at his desk, and had recently started to make medical errors of judgment. There had been some family stressors lately, a divorce and difficulty with his children. The physician was asked to discuss the behavior in question with the medical director. He pointed out he had been through a stressful time, but things were back on track and would improve.

The medical director received a call from a local pharmacy, concerned the physician had written for a significant amount of narcotic medication for a number of patients well known to the system, for whom the pharmacy had filled multiple narcotic prescriptions recently. Additionally, the physician failed to show up for work, and a backup physician had to come in to cover the shift. The medical director called the physician at home. He apologized and said he had the flu, but would be in for his next scheduled shift and that he would cover the shift at a later point on the schedule that month.

During his next shift, there was a call from nursing suggesting that he was slow in seeing patients, and remained in the call room for most of the day. At that point, the medical director came in and relieved the physician. She asked him to go home and take care of his health for the day. He was notified that on his next shift he would have to come to the office to discuss his recent performance, and that his shifts would be covered until this issue could be satisfactorily resolved.

He did not show up to that meeting, stating once again that he had the flu and that he had a doctor's appointment that day. The director requested a fitness evaluation from his physician stating that he was ready to come back to work.

Medical Approach

This issue comes up with some regularity. Physicians estimate that approximately 10% of the general public has an issue with drug or alcohol: unfortunately, that same ratio extends to our physician colleagues as well. The markers are clear, including erratic work performance, job absenteeism, and personality changes typically noted by the staff. When these issues occur, it is incumbent upon us to help our physician partners ideally to self-report and refer themselves to physician help agencies, often through the state medical board and standard drug and alcohol rehabilitation programs. Some states have mandatory reporting requirements, if impairment is suspected.

The areas of concern for a potentially impaired physician include drug or alcohol abuse, psychiatric illness, chronic medical conditions, acute illness, sexual boundary issues, and age-related decline (Table 52.1). It is recommended that all facilities have an established protocol to deal with this issue. This protocol is best framed in relation to patient safety and should discuss education, reporting, evaluation, intervention, remediation, referral, correction, termination, and legal or law enforcement interface (Table 52.2).

There are numerous moral, ethical, or legal quandaries concerning the impaired provider issue. There is typically a mandatory reporting requirement that physicians report a potentially impaired colleague, as mandated by professional societies and state medical boards. Most states have a self-report pathway, which should be encouraged as a more desirable path.

The system relies on peer review and reporting of the impaired physician. However, physicians are often reluctant to report colleagues. DesRoches et al. reported on a sample of 1891 physicians, in which 64% (1120) agreed with the professional commitment to report, 69% (1208) felt prepared to report an impaired

Table 52.1 Physician impairment: categories

1. Drug and alcohol abuse
2. Psychiatric illness
3. Chronic medical conditions
4. Acute illness
5. Sexual boundary issues
6. Age-related decline

Table 52.2 Impaired provider protocol

1. Patient safety focus
2. Education
3. Reporting
4. Evaluation
5. Intervention
6. Remediation
7. Referral
8. Correction
9. Termination
10. Legal, law enforcement interface

Table 52.3 Criteria for interlocutory appeal

1. Outcome would be conclusively determined by the issue
2. Matter collateral to the merits
3. Matter unreviewable if appeal not resolved

Reference: Lauro.[6]

colleague, and 64% (1126) were prepared to deal with an incompetent colleague.[1] However, although 17% (309) of the physicians had direct personal knowledge of a colleague who was incompetent to practice, only 67% of them (204) had actually reported this colleague. Their rationale for inaction was that someone else would address the issue (19%, 58), that nothing would happen as a result of the report (15%, 46), and fear of retribution (12%, 36).

Legal Analysis

In *Cronin* v. *Strayer*, the plaintiff, an orthopedic physician, accused the defendant, another orthopedic physician, of defamation by falsely informing the Impaired Physicians Committee (IPC) of the state medical society that he was impaired.[2] The issue at hand was a motion by the reporting physician and medical society to quash a subpoena requesting information concerning this filing. The superior court denied the request for a protective order. They cited Massachusetts General Laws (G.L.c. 231, §85N), which grants immunity to a professional society or committee for good-faith actions, but not for discovery.[3] The Supreme Judicial Court of Massachusetts dismissed the appeal as discovery orders are interlocutory so

therefore are not appealable, and confirmed the trial court's judgment.

In *Sharpe* v. *Worland*, the plaintiff alleged an anesthesiologist negligently supervised a postoperative pain control procedure.[4] As part of this discovery, they requested the hospital produce "all documents related to all complaints and incident reports," and "all minutes of any meeting or hearing of the Board of Trustees" relating to this physician. The hospital's position was that documents relating to the physician's participation in the Physician's Health Program were privileged and should be protected from disclosure. The trial court denied this protective motion, and the appeal court dismissed the defendant's appeal as an interlocutory order. However, the Supreme Court of North Carolina reversed, blocking the release so as not to interfere with a "substantial right."

The overall judicial strategy with interlocutory judgment is to prevent the piecemeal use of the appeal process to delay the final disposition of the matter. The appeal right is codified in federal statute (28 U.S.C. §1291) based on *Lauro Lines s.r.l.* v. *Chasser*, 490 U.S. 495 (1989).[5,6] The appeal is permitted only if (1) outcome would be conclusively determined by the issue, (2) appealed matter was collateral to the merits, (3) matter is unreviewable if immediate appeal is not allowed (Table 52.3).

In *Kees* v. *Medical Board of California*, a physician allegedly exhibited unusual and erratic behavior noted by patients, and was compelled to have a psychiatric evaluation, in which he was alleged to have performed poorly.[7] As a result, the medical board revoked his license for 10 years, stayed the revocation, and placed him on probation with conditions instead. He filed a petition for writ of mandate for further decision review, which was denied by the trial court. The Court of Appeals of California felt that there was substantial evidence to support this order, and upheld the lower court decision.

In *Guttman* v. *Khalsa*, a physician with a history of complaints and denials of staff privileges was referred to the Impaired Physicians Committee (IPC) for evaluation, in which he allegedly misrepresented his work history.[8] The medical board revoked his medical license, raising public safety concerns regarding his practice relating to demeanor and adverse interactions. The physician brought suit under Title II of the Americans with Disabilities Act (ADA).[9] The United States Court of Appeals, Tenth Circuit concluded that the Eleventh Amendment protects the state from a money damages claim, invoking sovereign immunity.[10]

Sometimes these issues may appear in the setting of a workplace dispute, in whole or part. In *Serry* v. *Yale-New Haven Hospital*, a nurse anesthetist brought suit alleging that a physician colleague was impaired in the midst of a workplace dispute, in which retaliation was alleged.[11] The impairment allegation appeared to have some factual basis, but appeared in the context of a dispute with ongoing discussion with the facility and requests for action concerning a confrontation. The trial court granted the motion for directed verdicts for the defense, and precluded pain and suffering damages. The Appellate Court of Connecticut upheld the trial court verdict.

Conclusion

It is crucial that an impaired physician be removed from the practice environment so that they may better return to a state of health. This should be done with the assistance of human resources and the potential for hospital counsel in problematic cases. The process may involve random drug testing, focused drug testing, or referral to an external addiction specialist for use, misuse, or addiction. It is important to protect the physician's confidentiality, but it is more important to protect patients and other staff members from impaired performance and return the physician to productive, healthy practice.

References

1. DesRoches CM, Rao SR, Fromson JA, Birnbaum RJ, Iezzoni L, Vogeli C, Campbell EG. Physicians' perceptions, preparedness for reporting and experiences related to impaired and incompetent colleagues. *JAMA*. 2010;304(2):187–193. DOI:10.1001/jama.2010.921.

2. *Cronin* v. *Strayer*, 467 N.E.2d 143.

3. Massachusetts General Laws. Chapter 231, Section 85N.

4. *Sharpe* v. *Worland*, 522 S.E.2d 577 (N.C. 1999).

5. U.S. Code, Title 28, Chapter §1291. Final Decisions of the District Courts.

6. *Lauro Lines s.r.l.* v. *Chasser*, 490 U.S. 495 (1989).

7. *Kees* v. *Medical Board*, 7 Cal. App.4th 1801 (1992).

8. *Guttman* v. *Khalsa*, 466 F.3d 1027 (2006).

9. Americans with Disabilities Act (ADA), Title II, 42 U.S.C. §§12131–65.

10. U.S. Const. Amend. XI, Judicial Limits.

11. *Serry* v. *Yale-New Haven*, Court of Appeals of CT, February 28, 1989.

Indigent Care

Case

The elderly patient's chief complaint when she presented to the emergency department (ED) was "breast infection." When the ED physician asked her what was wrong, she said, "I have a little infection in my breast." Having asked the usual historical questions concerning fever and other systemic complaints, he asked her to let him look at the infection itself. Asking where it was, she motioned and said it was on the outer aspect of her left breast. As he went to take down the gown, he noticed that she was still wearing her bra, with a wad of paper towel padding that had to be pried away.

The physician quickly realized that he was looking at a case of advanced breast cancer. He asked the patient how long her breast had been like that. She replied, "For a little while, but it just got infected in the last week or so." The physician commented that it looked like she had this problem for some time, and she responded that she was waiting for her husband's insurance, which was just about to kick in when he reached the age of 65. The physician suggested that she should not worry about that, and that they would take care of everything they could and admit her to the hospital to get this problem addressed by the surgeons and oncologist.

Once again, she tried to decline the admission, and was informed that it did not matter whether she had insurance or not. The hospital had an indigent care program that would take care of her, and would work on getting her enrolled in an insurance program. One way, or another she would be cared for. She seemed reassured by that. The ED physician recommended that if she ever had medical concerns in the future, she should present to the ED who would find a way to get things taken care of, just as they did today.

Medical Approach

Most hospitals have some sort of indigent care program, in which free care is provided for both outpatient and inpatient care. It is not mandatory, but it is typically expected that most hospitals will provide some charity care to the community, funded either by the hospital itself or by directed charitable donations. It is important to realize, however, that a significant number of hospitals in all parts of the country have become insolvent because of the large proportion of charity care provided to indigent patients in their community.

One category of indigent patients is those who are homeless. D'Amore et al. evaluated a homeless population with 252 homeless individuals, compared to 88 control patients.[1] The homeless population was more likely to be younger, male, with a history of TB, HIV, penetrating trauma, depression, schizophrenia, alcoholism, dental issues, social isolation, and a higher number of annual ED visits (6.0 vs. 1.6, $P < 0.01$) (Table 53.1). This population has obvious needs, which are addressed with directed programs.

The Centers for Medicare and Medicaid Services has published an informational bulletin to reduce non-urgent use of the ED.[2] It is recommended that access to primary care services should be broadened. It also focuses on frequent ED users, defined as people making more than four ED visits per year. The needs of people with behavioral health problems should also be targeted.

The hospital financial structure is often questioned as it relates to charity care, especially the tax-exempt offset. Kennedy et al. studied Texas facilities to evaluate their compliance with a statutorily based standard of 4% of net patient revenue to be spent on charity care.[3] They found that less than 20% of the not-for-profit hospitals spent less than this threshold percentage.

Table 53.1 Health-care associations with homelessness

Factors N = 88	Comparison (P < 0.01)
1. Younger	
2. Male	
3. History of TB	
4. History of HIV	
5. Penetrating trauma	
6. Depression	
7. Schizophrenia	
8. Alcoholism	
9. Dental issues	
10. Social isolation	
11. Annual ED visits	6.0 vs. 1.6

Reference: D'Amore et al.[1]

Legislation compelled the lower-spending facilities to meet the threshold, but some higher-margin facilities decreased their contribution.

Another area of focus is uncompensated care provided by public hospitals. Thorpe and Brecher analyzed access to uncompensated care for poor patients in public hospitals.[4] Multiple regression analysis indicated that public hospitals provided 31–34 uncompensated adjusted admissions per 100 uninsured poor patients. This was greater than the 24 admissions on average in cities without a public hospital. Therefore, the tax exemptions and financial support provided are necessary to maintain care access.

Legal Analysis

In *Simon, Secretary of the Treasury* v. *Eastern Kentucky Welfare Rights Organization*, several indigent patients and organizations filed suit alleging the Internal Revenue Service violated the Internal Revenue Code of 1954 (Code) and the Administrative Procedure Act by issuing a Revenue Ruling allowing favorable tax treatment to a non-profit hospital that offered only emergency room services to indigent patients.[5-7] The intent was that hospitals that receive a tax-exempt status provide health care in addition to emergency services. The Supreme Court of the United States ruled that the plaintiffs did not have adequate standing to bring this suit. However, they reiterated the premise of the IRS ruling of 1956, Revenue Ruling 56–185 stating that for a hospital to be considered a charitable entity,

the 501 (c) (3) code establishes "four general requirements."[8,9] The most important of these requirements states, "it must be operated to the extent of its financial ability for those not able to pay for the services rendered and not exclusively for those who are able and expected to pay."

In *Thornton* v. *Southwest Detroit Hospital*, the patient was admitted through the ED for a ten-day stay in the intensive care unit (ICU) and an 11-day inpatient stay.[10] There was a plan to transfer her for post-rehabilitative care, but the transfer institution declined allegedly on the basis of insurance issues, and she was discharged to home care, where she worsened and required readmission. The plaintiff brought action citing The Emergency Medical Treatment and Labor Act (EMTALA), alleging her emergency medical condition was not stabilized prior to discharge.[11] The district court granted summary judgment to the defendant, which was affirmed by the United States Court of Appeals, Sixth Circuit. They concluded no genuine issue of material fact existed, as her condition had stabilized.

Conclusion

It is our responsibility to ensure the patient will be provided for, and to do our best to use all social support networks, charitable care, and health-care resources available to accomplish this worthy and necessary goal.

References

1. D'Amore J, Hung O, Chiang W, Goldfrank L. The epidemiology of the homeless population and its impact on an urban emergency department. *Acad Emerg Med*. 2001;8(11):1051–55. DOI:10.1111/j.1553-2712.2001.tb01114.x.

2. Center for Medicare and Medicaid Services. Reducing Nonurgent Use of Emergency Center Departments and Improving Appropriate Care in Appropriate Settings. CMCS Informational Bulletin, January 16, 2014.

3. Kennedy FA, Burney LL, Troyer JL, Stroup JC. Do non-profit hospitals provide more charity care when faced with a mandatory minimum standard? Evidence from Texas. *J Accounting Public Policy*. 2010;29(3):242–258. DOI:10.1016/j.jaccpubpol.2009.10.010.

4. Thorpe KE, Brecher C. Improved access to care for the uninsured poor in large cities: do public hospitals make a difference? *J Health Polit*

Policy Law. 1987;12(2);313–324. DOI:10.1215/
03616878-12-2-313.

5. *Simon* v. *Eastern Kentucky Welfare Rights Org.* 426 U.S.
26 (1976).

6. 26 C.F.R. 1.0-1 – Internal Revenue Code of 1954 and
Regulations.

7. Administrative Procedures Act. 5 U.S.C. §704.

8. Internal Revenue Service 1956 Revenue Ruling
56–185.

9. 26 U.S.C. §501 (c) (3) – Exemption from Tax on
Corporations, Certain Trusts, etc.

10. *Thornton* v. *Southwest Detroit Hospital*, 895 F.2d 1131
(1990).

11. EMTALA 42 U.S.C. §1395dd.

In-Flight Emergencies

Case

This was the last leg of a long flight home. Everyone on board was tired and ready to get off the plane, get their baggage, and get home. The plane was beginning its descent when the captain asked if there was a physician on board. A physician looked toward the back of the plane and saw some commotion there. He could see a young woman who was belted upright but looked like she was ready to pass out. He unbuckled his seatbelt and headed back.

The woman was traveling with her husband. The physician checked with her husband that she had no chronic medical conditions, and quickly recommended that they get her unbelted and lying flat on the floor. There was some discussion among the flight attendants, who were concerned about the approach and landing, but they decided that it was the right thing to do. Another passenger with medical experience stated that she was probably OK sitting upright. The husband decided it would be better to get her out of her seat as the first physician suggested.

When she was laid down in the aisle, her color gradually returned and she said that she felt better. She had recently had a bout of gastroenteritis, and had not eaten anything that day. The husband and crew thanked the physician, but on the way out the other provider again suggested that she was fine and she should have stayed in her seat for safety reasons.

Medical Approach

The likelihood of an in-flight emergency is relatively low, but they can still occur. These cases are often complex because the crew has some training and there is often a health-care professional on the flight. Things get especially complicated when there is more than one health-care professional on the flight and a difference of medical opinion arises. It is important to remember that the captain is in charge of everything

that is done on the plane, including the decision to divert or whether any medical care is provided.

In 1989, Cummins and Schubach made one of the first studies of airline-related emergencies.[1] They analyzed emergency personnel response to 1107 people, where 68% (754) were travelers, 21% (232) were airport or airline employees, and 11% (118) were area residents. Of the 754 travelers, 25% (190) had an in-flight emergency, and an unscheduled landing occurred in 3.6% (7) of these flights. The predicted incidence of in-flight emergencies was 0.133% or 1 in 753 inbound flights, or 1 in 39,600 inbound passengers. The most common emergencies encountered were abdominal pain, chest pain, shortness of breath, syncope, and seizures, and 25% of the incidents were related to minor trauma. The majority of air traveler emergencies (75%, 564) occurred within the terminal, and the vast majority (84%, 633) were handled by emergency medical technicians (EMTs).

In 2009, there were 2 billion commercial airline travelers annually. Flight issues are becoming more common.[2] The environmental conditions and physiologic changes at altitude include mild hypoxemia and gas expansion, which can exacerbate chronic medical conditions that may incite acute in-flight emergencies. Post-flight emergencies can be associated with venous thromboembolism in long-haul flights, exposure to cosmic radiation, jet lag, and suboptimal cabin air quality. The recommendations include training, equipment, and telemedicine ground support systems.

The Aviation Medical Assistance Act of 1998 specifies the placement of medical equipment, personnel training, death report requirements, decision on automatic external defibrillator (AED) implementation, and limits of carrier liability.[3] Perhaps the most important addition is the "Good Samaritan" law, in that there is no liability in an in-flight response unless gross negligence or reckless behavior occurs. As the system has matured there have been advances in

Table 54.1 Good Samaritan Act immunity

1.	Ethical, not legal obligation
2.	Not for compensation
3.	Excludes gross negligence
4.	Only emergencies
5.	Scene-based care
6.	No established relationship

Reference: Stewart et al.[5]

Table 54.2 In-flight medical command

1.	Conventional standards of care in force
2.	Liability if commercial enterprise
3.	Conventional confidentiality standards for documentation
4.	Telemedicine ground support assist flight crew and health-care providers
5.	Health-care providers are a covered entity
6.	Secure system to provide and document care

equipment, typically including EKG monitor, AED, oxygen, and medications; crew training; and remote medical control.[4]

Good Samaritan legislation has been enacted in all 50 states, typically establishing an ethical but not a legal obligation for health-care professionals to provide care, not for compensation, to someone not in their care, at the scene of an emergency (Table 54.1). The only exception is Kentucky, which requires a state license for immunity, but provides an exception for American Heart Association (AHA)-trained CPR providers.[5]

Similar to maritime law, the prevailing law for aircraft in flight is historically based on the "flag right," i.e., where the plane is registered. The captain and crew are in charge in any medical emergency; the health-care provider should be viewed as an invited consultant. The provider is not necessarily a Health Insurance Portability and Accountability Act (HIPAA)-covered entity, but normal confidentiality protocol should be followed.

In 2005, it was estimated that 0.01% of all airline passengers may fall ill during the flight, resulting in 14,000 emergencies, 2.9% (400) of which may result in onboard deaths.[6] It is also estimated that 65–70% of flights have a physician on board. The question that arises is whether they are qualified to respond in an emergency.

Another large survey estimated one medical emergency per 10,000–40,000 passengers on commercial aircraft. Graf et al. analyzed in-flight emergencies at one international carrier over a one-year period.[7] They encountered gastrointestinal conditions (diarrhea, nausea, vomiting), circulatory collapse, hypertension, stroke, and headache. The majority of annual "emergencies" were psychiatric in nature (79.4%, 81), followed by in-flight death (11.8%, 12), cardiac arrest (7.8%, 8), and delivery (1%, 1). They concluded that given the estimate of one event per 10,000 passengers

with an average of 400 passengers per flight, at least one medical incident occurs per 24 intercontinental flights flown.

The use of emergency call centers for in-flight telemedicine assistance has become more common. Baltsezk presented a one-year retrospective study of a major international airline that fielded 191 flight-to-ground consultations.[8] The most common complaints were gastrointestinal issues or a simple faint in half the calls (50.2%), of which 12% (23) were pediatric patients. Antiemetics were the most common administered medication. There was a physician on board in almost half the emergencies (45.5%). The decision to divert the flight was made in only a small minority of cases (3.1%, 6). The remote telemedicine in-flight emergency call center is typically a commercial enterprise and distinct from immunity protection (Table 54.2).

Legal Analysis

In *Abramson* v. *Japan Airlines*, the patient was traveling with his wife and had an attack of gastrointestinal distress that would improve if he could lie flat. This was denied, and he was hospitalized at his destination.[9] The plaintiff filed suit in New Jersey, presenting a physician statement that the "self-help" treatment would have prevented surgery. The district court awarded summary judgment to the defendant. The United States Court of Appeals, Third Circuit held that the event was not an "accident" within Article 17 of the Warsaw Convention and the claim was properly dismissed as stated in *DeMarines* v. *KLM Royal Dutch Airlines* (1978).[10,11]

In *Somes* v. *United Airlines*, the suit was commenced after a passenger suffered a cardiac arrest and died in flight.[12] The family alleged the flight was not equipped with the proper medical equipment including an automatic external defibrillator (AED), or else he would have survived. They filed suit under the Massachusetts wrongful death statute.[13] The defendant moved to dismiss on the grounds that the plaintiff claim was preempted by federal law including the Federal Aviation Act of 1958 (FAA) and Airline Deregulation Act of 1978 according to Federal Rules of Civil Procedure.[14–16] The district court denied the defendant's motion to dismiss, holding that the preemption theory in which the federal mandate would preclude state requirement for a medical kit was not meritable. There was no indication that the FAA would have denied the need, and other airlines had already installed these devices on board.

In *Olympic Airways* v. *Husain*, the patient suffered from asthma and was exposed to secondhand smoke. He asked for a seat change that was initially denied, but then accommodated once he became symptomatic.[17] He was treated with epinephrine from the emergency kit by an onboard physician, but eventually succumbed to respiratory distress. The family filed suit invoking Article 17 of the Warsaw Convention,[10] which "imposes liability on the air carrier for a passenger's death or bodily injury caused by an 'accident' that occurred in connection with an international flight."[18] The airline contended that the passenger's reaction was his internal response to expected operations. The Supreme Court of the United States held that the Article 17 "accident" criterion was satisfied by the passenger request and carrier response. There is a link of causation between the passenger's medical condition, and aggravation by a "normal" part of aircraft operations.

In *Tobin* v. *AMR Corporation*, because of a flight delay a passenger had to rush to the next flight, with his wife in a wheelchair. This exertion was followed by a devastating medical event.[19] The crew and medical volunteers attempted to resuscitate him using an AED, just before paramedics arrived, and he succumbed. The family filed suit, with failure to train the crew in the proper use of the AED as one of their theories. The district court held the defendant was not immune under the Illinois AED Immunity Statute for AED use, in which:

> The AED user is not liable for civil damages as a result of any act or omission involving the use of an AED in an emergency situation, except for willful or wanton misconduct, if the requirements of the Act are met;[20]

nor for the Illinois Good Samaritan Act for CPR attempt in which:

> Any person currently certified in basic cardiopulmonary resuscitation who complies with generally recognized standards, and who in good faith, not for compensation, provides emergency cardiopulmonary resuscitation to a person who is the apparent victim of acute cardiopulmonary insufficiency shall not, as a result of his or her acts or omissions in providing resuscitation, be liable for civil damages, unless the acts or omissions constitute willful and wanton misconduct.[21]

Likewise, they rejected the defense's federal preemption claims by the FAA or Deregulation Act.[14,15]

Conclusion

There is significant nuance and sometimes debate concerning the effectiveness of Good Samaritan protections from liability. They require very specific provisions to be applicable. However, in an emergency situation physicians are urged to offer helpful intervention and assistance to the extent of their capabilities.

References

1. Cummins RO, Schubach JA. Frequency and types of medical emergencies among commercial air travelers. *JAMA*. 1989;261(9):1295–1299. DOI:10.1001/jama.1989.03420090059031.

2. Silverman D, Gendreau M. Medical issues associated with commercial flights. *The Lancet*. 2009;373(9680):2067–2077. DOI:10.1016/S0140-6736(09)60209-9.

3. Aviation Medical Assistance Act of 1998. 49, U.S.C §§44701–50105. PL 105–170, April 24, 1998.

4. Rayman RB, Zanick D, Korsgard T. Resources for inflight medical care. *Aviation Space Environ Med*. 2004;75(3):278–280.

5. Stewart PH, Agin WS, Douglas SP. What does the law say to Good Samaritans? A review of Good Samaritan statutes in 50 states and on US airlines. *Chest*. 2013;143(6):1774–1783. DOI:10.1378/chest.12-2161.

6. Becker H, Buhrle E. Preparing for and handling of in-flight medical emergencies. Patent Application US 20050240423 A1. April 27, 2004.

7. Graf J, Stuben U, Pump S. In-flight medical emergencies. *Dtsch Arztebl Int*. 2012;109(37):591–602. DOI:10.3238/arztebl.2012.0591.

8. Baltsezak S. Clinic in the air? A retrospective study of medical emergency calls from a major international airline. *J Travel Med*. 2008;15(6):391–394. DOI:10.1111/j.1708-8305.2008.00233.x.

9. *Abramson* v. *Japan Airlines*, 739 F.2d 130 (1984).

10. Warsaw Convention, 49 Stat. 3000; 137 LNTS 11 (1929): Article 17 – Liability of the Carrier.

11. *DeMarines* v. *KLM Royal Dutch Airlines*, 580 F.2d 1193 3rd Cir. (1978), 435, 436

12. *Somes* v. *United Airlines*, 33 F. Supp.2d 78 (1999).

13. Massachusetts General Laws, Chapter 229, §2 Wrongful Death Statute.

14. Federal Aviation Act of 1958, P.L. 85–726, 72 Stat. 731. Approved 1958-08-23.

15. Airline Deregulation Act, Pub.L. 95–504, 49 U.S.C. §1371 et seq. Approved October 24, 1978.

16. Fed.R.Civ.P. 12 (b) (6).

17. *Olympic Airways* v. *Husain*, 540 U.S. 644 (2004).

18. *Air France* v. *Saks*, 470 U.S. 392 (1985), 435, 443.

19. *Tobin* v. *AMR Corporation*, 637 F. Supp.2d 406 (2009).

20. Illinois AED Immunity Statute, 410 Illinois Comprehensive Statutes §4/30 (d) (2007).

21. Illinois Good Samaritan Act, 745 Illinois Comprehensive Statutes §49/10 (1998).

Informal Consultation

Case

The patient came in to the emergency department (ED) with a presenting complaint of chest pain. It was a classic presentation: substernal location, radiation to the left arm. She was short of breath, the EKG was abnormal, and borderline ST elevation myocardial infarction (STEMI) was diagnosed. The ED physician was going to call cardiac alert, activating the cath lab team. However, a cardiology attending physician was actually in the ED seeing another patient. He was asked to review the EKG. He said he wasn't sure, it might be a myocardial infarction (MI) or it might not, and they should wait until the troponin result came back.

The ED physician stated that she was concerned there was an early STEMI, affecting the inferior wall of the heart with 1 mm ST elevations in the inferior leads to II, III, and avf. The cardiologist said he saw that change, but still wanted to wait for the troponin result before activating the lab. The cardiac troponin came back at <0.01 and the cardiologist recommended admission to the medical service with a cardiology consult.

The patient's admission was upgraded to a telemetry-focused floor and the patient was admitted with aspirin, nitroglycerin, and low molecular weight heparin to be administered. Cardiology was asked to complete a consult and they said that they would. They were advised that a "curbside consult" would not be appropriate here, since they were going to have to see the patient anyway.

The next day there was discussion that the patient had gone to the cath lab and the interventional cardiologist attending for that day felt that perhaps she should have had a cardiac catheterization the day before. The subsequent treating cardiologist also felt that she had an early STEMI, as suggested by the ED physician. The ED physician's decision had been to consult cardiology emergently, but the consult was changed to routine by the admission team, allowing a greater delay in consult timing. The quality review finding, however, suggested there was no documentation of an emergent cardiology consult performed in the ED. Later that evening the official routine consult was requested. However, it was clear it was by no means a curbside consult, as the patient was seen "officially" by the cardiologist attending in the ED, when assistance was requested by the ED physician and treatment recommendations offered.

Medical Approach

This is an example of the infamous "curbside" consult, with a physician participating in a patient care event due to availability of a fellow practitioner. Without documentation and billing of the visit it is not an official consult. It is clear that for a proper consult it is necessary that the request be declared and documented as an order. This then sets realistic expectations for all parties involved in the system – the patient, the requesting provider, and the consulting provider.

The assessment of consulting physician liability, as the result of an informal curbside communication, finds that courts examine all facts and circumstances to determine if a relationship exists.[1] Physicians should encourage formal consultation, when a specialty opinion is needed for more reliable and effective information exchange. It is acknowledged that an informal interchange can provide education to the provider team, but it has disadvantages as well. The consultant should avoid providing specific recommendations about patients not examined, and provide general information as appropriate.

In a survey of the available literature and caselaw, Olick and Bergus concluded that no physician–patient relationship exists in the "informal consultation" situation.[2] In the absence of this relationship, the courts have found no grounds for a medical malpractice claim. They concluded that the malpractice risk associated with informal consultation appear to be minimal irrespective of the method of communication of the request.

Legal Analysis

In *Clanton* v. *Von Haam*, the patient presented to the ED with back pain, and while in the department allegedly developed leg numbness and difficulty walking. She was discharged home on pain medication.[3] She felt worse at home, called the ED, was told the treating physician had left, and then called a physician she had seen previously. This physician returned the call immediately, but was unable to see her in the hospital that day although he could see her the next morning. The patient subsequently worsened further and returned to the hospital with paralysis. The trial court granted the appellee's motion for summary judgment, concluding that no physician–patient relationship had existed. The Court of Appeals of Georgia affirmed again, concluding that the phone conversation between patient and physician was not a "consensual transaction" establishing a care relationship.

In *Reynolds* v. *Decatur Memorial Hospital*, a pediatric patient was evaluated in the ED after a 2-foot fall from a couch. An abnormal breathing pattern was found,[4] standard laboratory screening was ordered, and a cervical radiograph was normal. The child was admitted and evaluated by a pediatrician, who found a fever. She phoned an at home consultant and discussed the case findings. A lumbar puncture was performed. The specialist was not asked to consult by phone, but the nurse was asked to leave a consult for the morning. The child was transferred with a diagnosis of Guillain–Barré syndrome and was subsequently diagnosed with a spinal cord injury. The trial court ruled that there was no established physician–patient relationship with the consultant and no duty owed in this circumstance, and this finding was affirmed by the Appellate Court of Illinois.

In *Majzoub* v. *Appling*, the patient presented to the ED with difficulty breathing and was diagnosed with pharyngeal inflammation and exudate with stridor.[5] The on-call otolaryngologist was paged, returned the call, and spoke with the ED physician. There was a prolonged discussion about treatment with antibiotics, breathing treatment, observation, and to return a call with worsening. The patient had a respiratory arrest with intubation attempt, ENT notification, and tracheostomy. He was transferred to the intensive care unit (ICU), where he died 3 days later. The trial court ruled that no patient–physician relationship was established, and that the Court of Appeals of Texas, Houston affirmed. Their rationale was as follows:

> Although a physician–patient relationship may be established by the implied consent of the physician, the on-call status of the physician does not automatically impose a duty. *St John* v. *Pope*, 901 S.W.2d at 424.[6] Further, we hold that a duty is not automatically imposed when an on-call physician consults with an emergency room physician regarding a patient. Nor is a duty necessarily imposed when a doctor agrees to see the patient at a future time. Rather, as we have noted before, without the express consent of the physician or prior physician-patient relationship, there must be some affirmative action of the physician to treat the patient to create such a relationship. *Day* v. *Harkins*, 961 S.W.2d at 280.[7]

In *Bessenyei* v. *Raiti*, the patient had a thumb injection injury, was evaluated in the ED, had a phone consult with a specialist, and was told to report to a specialty hand clinic.[8] The timing of the call to the specialist was uncertain: he was not technically on call for the ED and the ED physician relayed the consult recommendation to the patient. The patient was discharged with an instruction to present to the hand clinic if worsening. The condition worsened due to a high-pressure injection injury and required amputation. The court again concluded this consultation did not constitute a physician–patient relationship, and the ED physician was responsible for the decision-making.

Another area of concern is the informal consult that may take place between the patient and physician in a non-health-care setting. In *O'Rourke* v. *Nakamura*, the patient had a discussion in the parking lot about his chest pain.[9] His physician of 20 years prescribed nitroglycerin and scheduled an outpatient stress test, but the patient died before this could take place. The Appellate Division of the Supreme Court of New York denied the motion alleging care deviation.

Conclusion

There is a clear recommendation for physicians to avoid patient care events outside a medical setting. If this is inevitable, then refer the patient to a conventional care setting, avoid writing prescriptions, document the encounter if you can, involve family in the

Table 55.1 Informal consultation in a non-health-care setting

1.	Avoid consultation in a non-health-care setting
2.	Refer to conventional care setting
3.	Avoid writing prescriptions in a non-health-care setting
4.	Document the encounter in the proper setting
5.	Involve family when appropriate
6.	Encourage compliance with the plan

discussion, and encourage patient compliance with the plan (Table 55.1).

The worst-case scenario from a medicolegal perspective is believing a consult was performed when in fact it was not, suggesting that the decision-making was focused on one practitioner rather than being a group decision-making process, as most consultations are in complex disease states.

References

1. Fox BC, Siegel ML, Weinstein RA. "Curbside" consultation and informal communication in medical practice: a medicolegal perspective. *Clin Infect Dis*. 1996;23(3):616–622.

2. Olick RS, Bergus GR. Malpractice liability for informal consultations. *Fam Med*. 2003;35(7):476–481.

3. *Clanton* v. *Von Haam*, 340 S.E.2d 627 (1986).

4. *Reynolds* v. *Decatur Memorial Hospital*, 660 N.E.2d 235 (1996).

5. *Majzoub* v. *Appling*, 95 S.W.3d 432 (2002).

6. *St. John* v. *Pope*, 901 S.W.2d 424 (1995).

7. *Day* v. *Harkins and Munoz*, 961 S.W.2d 280 (1997).

8. *Bessenyei* v. *Raiti*, 266 F. Supp. 2d 408 (2003).

9. *O'Rourke* v. *Nakamura*, 2009 NY Slip Op 66171 (U).

Informed Consent

Case

The patient came to the hospital with an acute onset of substernal chest pain. He was very short of breath. The prehospital EKG showed acute inferior wall elevation and that was consistent with the EKG recorded in the emergency department (ED). He had pain onset 3–4 hours before calling emergency medical services (EMS) and had taken an aspirin at home prior to transport.

The ED physician called the cardiology referral center and they accepted the patient for a percutaneous interventional (PCI) procedure. However, the referral center called back to say the weather was so bad there was no flight capability and it would take more than 2 hours for the patient to get there by ground transfer. The interventional cardiologist at the referral center commented that it would be best to give the patient an intravenous thrombolytic agent in the ED where he was and they would catch the patient on arrival.

This chain of events was shared with the patient and family, discussing the risks and benefits of the "clot busting" agent, tissue plasminogen activator (TPA). The treating physician told the family that this was an acute inferior wall myocardial infarction with ST elevation (STEMI). The vessel had to be reopened soon, the patient was more than 2 hours away from any interventional facility, and the cardiologist there had also recommended administering the thrombolytic agent intravenously. If it was to be administered there was a risk of intracranial hemorrhage, as well as malignant arrhythmia. The patient said that he would go ahead with the treatment, stating he just wanted to be better. He signed a consent form with his family in agreement.

They administered the TPA and the patient immediately had a ventricular arrhythmia and required CPR for 15 minutes. He was eventually resuscitated

and by then the ground transport crew had arrived. The patient was transferred to the referral facility and again rearrested during the catheterization procedure.

A little less than 2 years later the physician was contacted by the hospital attorney, who had received a pleading and summons alleging medical malpractice. They alleged that an informed consent was signed under duress and not understood by the family, alleging a battery claim for the administration of the intravenous TPA. The physician replied that the informed consent was indeed signed, with the proper discussion of risks and benefits, as well as being in agreement with the receiving physician at the cardiology referral center.

Medical Approach

Informed consent requires that the patient be competent, or have the capacity to make a medical decision, fully understand the risks and benefits, be given an explanation of alternatives to care, and able to ask any questions concerning the procedure or medical interventions themselves. Often in an emergency setting we are forced to obtain this consent quickly when the circumstances may be dire.

Multiple issues may arise with informed consent for patients seen by the ED physician, balancing autonomy and optimal patient care.[1] Recommendations include individualizing the consent to the particular situation based on the clinical circumstances. Although general rules apply, no strict rules can guide every case. Documentation of both consent and refusal of treatment are required for quality initiatives and legal liability concerns. "Appropriate" legal consent follows from good medical care and strict concern for the patient's health and rights (Table 56.1).

According to the emergency care exception, if immediate care is required to prevent death or serious harm to the patient, then treatment is provided

Table 56.1 Informed consent in the ED

1. Individualize the consent to the particular situation
2. General rules apply, no strict rules can guide
3. Documentation is required for quality and liability concerns
4. Appropriate legal consent accompanies good medical care
5. Strict concern for patient's health and rights

Reference: Siegel.[1]

Table 56.2 Informed consent provisions

1. Discussion of diagnosis or procedural intervention
2. Specifics of the intervention to be informed
3. Likelihood of success or failure
4. Explain alternative approaches
5. Define the risks and benefits
6. Options if the patient declines

Table 56.3 Informed consent in minors

1. Medical care should not be withheld pending consent
2. Provider should be familiar with EMTALA regulations for minors
3. Written policies and guidelines for minor consent are necessary
4. All efforts at obtaining consent should be documented
5. Consent should be discussed with minor commensurate with understanding

Reference: AAP.[3]

guidelines regarding minor consent. Fourth, all efforts at obtaining consent and aspects of the discussion should be documented. Fifth, consent should be discussed with the minor, commensurate with their age and understanding (Table 56.3).

Legal Analysis

Canterbury v. *Spence* was the seminal case defining the reasonable patient standard for informed consent.[4] Here, a 19-year-old patient presented with midthoracic pain after suffering a disk herniation. The procedure was explained to the patient and his mother by phone. His mother asked if it was serious, and the physician replied, "not any more than any other operation." A laminectomy was performed. On the first postoperative day the patient fell, and underwent reoperation due to lower extremity weakness. The patient alleged that the physician had not disclosed the risk of serious disability inherent in the operation.

The United States Court of Appeals for the District of Columbia held that there were issues requiring jury resolution, reversed and remanded to the district court for a new trial. The complex decision focuses on the right to know from the patient perspective, rather than the physician's.

> In our view, the patient's right of self-determination shapes the boundaries of the duty to reveal. The scope of the patient's communications to the patient, then, must be measured by the patient's need, and that need is the information material to the decision. Thus, the test for determining whether a particular peril must be divulged is its materiality to the patient's decision: all risks potentially affecting the decision must be unmasked.

In *Cobbs* v. *Grant*, the patient had refractory peptic ulcer disease, and had a surgical procedure after discussion with his primary care physician.[5] The

without informed consent.[2] However, some emergency physicians may rely on this exception, at the expense of the doctrine of informed consent. This doctrine implies that the patient is competent and has the capacity to make a medical decision once their options are discussed. Typically, informed consent involves first, discussion of diagnosis or procedural intervention; second, the specifics of the intervention to be performed; third, the likelihood of success, or alternatively probability of failure; fourth, explaining the alternative approaches; fifth, defining the risks and benefits of the procedure or intervention; sixth, the pathway and options if the patient declines the recommended intervention (Table 56.2).

Consent for pediatric patients can be especially problematic. There are numerous issues regarding informed consent involving uncertainties of confidentiality, financial reimbursement, responsibility, and compliance. The American Academy of Pediatrics (AAP) Committee on Pediatric Medicine offered a list of recommendations focused on always providing appropriate care.[3] First, medical care for minors in emergent or urgent conditions should not be withheld or delayed pending consent. Second, the provider should be familiar with The Emergency Medical Treatment and Labor Act (EMTALA) regulations applying to consent for minors. Third, every clinic, practice, and ED should develop written policies and patient went on to have multiple operations related to the initial disease and subsequent complications. The jury decided there was a failure to disclose the inherent risks of surgery, the Supreme Court of California reversed and remanded for a new jury trial. They again emphasized that the information to make a decision required by the "reasonable patient" must be delivered by the provider. They concluded that battery applies to circumstances in which the patient did not consent. If a procedure is performed and then an undisclosed, low-probability complication occurs, there is no intentional deviation from consent.

In *Sard* v. *Hardy*, the "doctrine of informed consent" was reviewed for the first time.[6] Here, the patient underwent a tubal ligation procedure. She alleged she was not informed that the procedure might not succeed in preventing future pregnancies, or there were alternative ways of performing the procedure. The doctrine of informed consent requires that "a physician treating a mentally competent adult, under non-emergency circumstances, cannot properly undertake to perform surgery or administer other therapy without the prior consent of the patient."[7] The trial court directed a verdict for the physician appellees and affirmed by Court of Special Appeals. The Court of Appeals of Maryland granted certiorari, reversed and remanded for consideration to the jury to decide whether the material disclosure was sufficient to make an informed decision.

In *Harvey* v. *Strickland*, the patient had a carotid endarterectomy performed after signing the operative consent, but declined to receive blood as he was a Jehovah's Witness.[8] The patient had postoperative bleeding and his mother was approached to consent to blood transfusion. She consented, he was transfused, and recovered. The physician was sued for medical malpractice and battery. The Supreme Court of South Carolina held that the trial court erred in a directed defense verdict, and the case was remanded to the jury to decide whether the transfusion was indicated.

In *Shinal* v. *Toms*, it was alleged that the surgeon failed to provide "adequate" prospective informed consent prior to a neurosurgical intervention.[9] The theory alleged that the physician assistant provided the consent explanation, which violated the Medical Care Availability and Reduction of Error (MCARE) Act.[10] The plaintiff alleged the physician owed a duty to "give a description of the surgery, risks or alternatives, that a reasonably prudent patient would require to make an informed decision concerning that procedure." The trial court instruction allowed this physician assistant to be considered "qualified staff" as part of the informed consent process. The trial court found in favor of the surgeon, and this decision was upheld by the Superior Court of Pennsylvania.

Conclusion

We must recognize that having the patient sign the form is not enough. They need to truly understand the alternatives and all their options before making the decision. In medicolegal situations it is often alleged retrospectively that the patient did not truly understand the risks and benefits, or was under duress, or the information was not explained properly by the health-care provider.

References

1. Siegel DM. Consent and refusal of treatment. *Emerg Med Clin North Am*. 1993;11(4):833–840.

2. Moskop JC. Informed consent in the emergency department. *Emerg Med Clin North Am*. 1999;17(2):327–340.

3. American Academy of Pediatrics Committee on Pediatric Emergency Medicine. Consent for emergency medical services for children and adolescents. *Pediatrics*. 2003;111(3):703–706. DOI:10.1542/peds.111.3.703.

4. *Canterbury* v. *Spence*, 464 F.2d 772 (1972).

5. *Cobbs* v. *Grant*, 8 Cal.3d 229 (1972).

6. *Sard* v. *Hardy*, 379 A.2d 1014 (1977).

7. *Mohr* v. *Williams*, 95 Minn. 261, 104 N.W. 12, 15 (1905).

8. *Harvey* v. *Strickland*, 566 S.E. 2d 529 (2002).

9. *Shinal* v. *Toms*, 122 A.3d 1066(2015).

10. Medical Care Availability and Reduction of Error (MCARE Act), Act 13 of 2002.

Insurance

Case

The patient had cut her finger while preparing dinner and presented to the emergency department (ED) with a laceration. The cut was deep, but thankfully spared the nerves and tendons. The laceration was repaired quickly. She received a tetanus shot and was advised to return to the ED for a wound check in 3 days if necessary and have the sutures removed by her physician at 7–8 days. The ED physician felt good about the care, the patient was in and out quickly, and he went on to the next patient.

Registration staff then approached the medical director with concerns expressed by the patient, who was now disgruntled. The patient advocate discussed the issue with her. She said that she was indeed happy with her care, but was unhappy with the fact that she had to make a co-payment for the emergency care that had been delivered, stating that all emergencies "were covered" under her plan. Registration and patient billing discussed the matter with her, but she was still unhappy. The director suggested that the proper care had been provided independent of her insurance status. She was evaluated, her laceration was repaired, and they indeed asked for co-payment on discharge from the ED, which was completely appropriate after care was completed. The patient advocate had offered an explanation of financial responsibility, but the patient was still unhappy. She left stating that "If you have insurance, emergencies should be covered." She refused payment, and posted these complaints as patient feedback on the hospital website.

Medical Approach

The proper approach to any patient, whether they have insurance, or not is to perform a medical screening evaluation and provide definitive care that is appropriate within the confines of the patient's disease state and the facility's capabilities. Insurance information can be obtained only after the care process is substantively complete. In some facilities there is a preliminary "preregistration" step that obtains information to get the patient logged into the system before the complete registration process is performed. Typically, insurance information is requested at this point, but it is not a requirement for the provision of care. Hospital facilities then deliver the care required. Whether the patient has a co-pay is discussed by registration upon discharge, when it is entirely permissible and indeed required.

Medicare hospitals have well-defined special responsibilities in emergency cases, referencing 42 C.F.R. 489.24, the primary Emergency Medical Treatment and Labor Act (EMTALA) subchapter.[1] If the patient "comes to the emergency department," whether eligible for Medicare benefits or having the ability to pay, the hospital must provide a medical screening exam by a qualified staff member as described in hospital bylaws, 42 C.F.R. 482.55, provide necessary stabilizing treatment and appropriate transfer for further treatment if required. The mandate is clear in "true emergencies" with obligatory care provided through the ED, but is more uncertain with cases of urgent or routine care.

Legal Analysis

In *Gatewood* v. *Washington Healthcare Corporation*, the patient succumbed to a myocardial infarction (MI) after being discharged allegedly with a diagnosis of musculoskeletal strain.[2] His surviving spouse raised an EMTALA claim, which was dismissed by the district court, concluding that EMTALA does not provide a cause of action for fully insured patients who may be misdiagnosed. The United States Court of Appeals, District of Columbia found the district court erred by injecting the insurance status into the analysis. Whether the patient is insured or not is not critical to an EMTALA claim, and the Emergency Act covers "any individual" who presents to the ED. However, the appeal court agreed that this statute does not create a broad federal cause of action for alleged medical malpractice. Therefore, the standard of analysis focuses on the diagnostic, treatment protocols, and likelihood of medical malpractice alone. However, the appeal court affirmed the complaint dismissal for failure to state a claim for which relief can be granted.

In *Correa* v. *Hospital San Francisco*, the elderly patient presented to the ED with dizziness and nausea, and the family stated she also complained of chest pain.[3] The family alleged the staff scrutinized her insurance card and had them wait. They stated they tired of waiting and drove to a physician's office. Here, the physician started treatment and tried to transfer the patient to the hospital but she died before she could be transferred. The family alleged an EMTALA violation and medical malpractice claims and were awarded damages. The district court denied the hospital's post-trial motions for judgment as a matter of law, ordering a new trial and remission of damages. The United States Court of Appeals, First Circuit heard the appeal and affirmed the trial court jury's award. They concluded that the hospital's inaction amounted to a de facto denial of medical screening, absent additional mitigating circumstances. They held that EMTALA should be interpreted to proscribe both actual and constructive "dumping" of patients.

Questions are often raised concerning a hospital's ability to care for the uninsured. Norton evaluated the correlation between hospital ownership and access to care for the uninsured.[4] They found that when for-profit and not-for-profit hospitals are in the same area, they provide care to an equivalent number of uninsured patients. However, they theorized that for-profit facilities relocated to areas that had more patients with insurance.

Likewise, from older data there was a correlation between parent's insurance coverage and access to care for low-income children. Davidoff et al. analyzed the National Survey of America's Families database and reported that having an uninsured parent decreases the likelihood of any medical provider visit by 6.5%, and well-child visit by 6.7%.[5] If the parent was uninsured, but the child had insurance, there was a 4.1% decrease in medical visits and a 4.2% decrease in well-child visits. Efforts to increase insurance coverage

Table 57.1 Patient Protection and Affordable Care Act emergency care

1. Prudent layperson standard for ED evaluation
2. No prior authorization required
3. Formalized appeal process to challenge insurer decision
4. No distinction between in-network and out-of-network care

Reference Patient Protection and Affordable Care Act.[6]

of parents was postulated to have a positive spillover effect on children as well.

The Patient Protection and Affordable Care Act memorialized a number of state- and plan-based provisions.[6] First, health plans are required to abide by the "prudent layperson standard" and to pay for ED visits for which the average person believes their health would be threatened. Additionally, the final discharge diagnosis does not modify the insurer's requirement to cover the ED visit. Second, no prior authorization is required for the ED visit. Third, the Act affords the patient greater ability to challenge their insurer's decision with a formalized appeal process. Fourth, there is no distinction between "in-network and out-of-network" ED care, and they must be reimbursed at the same rates (Table 57.1).

Interestingly, as patients gain more power in negotiation with insurers, the medical community may be placed in a more difficult situation. In *Prospect Medical Group* v. *Northridge Emergency Medical Group*, the focus was on a narrow issue on appeal, whether an ED group can "balance bill" if the health maintenance organization (HMO) reimburses less than the payment required for emergency services.[7] After a billing dispute arose between Prospect and the emergency physicians, the care network alleged that the emergency group has the right to "reasonable" compensation they felt was equivalent to the Medicare rate, and that the practice of balance billing was unlawful. The trial court sustained the emergency physicians' demurrers without leave to amend. The appeal court concluded that balance billing was not statutorily prohibited and there is no requirement that the Medicare rate be imposed, but concluded the trial court abused its discretion by prohibiting the leave to amend. The Supreme Court of California ruled on the sole question of whether balance billing was allowed. They reversed the judgment of the appeal court and remanded for further consideration.

Conclusion

The co-pays for emergency care are now significant with high-deductible insurance plans. Problems and complaints should be referred to accounting and billing services for resolution at a later point, when they can be more calmly assessed. Thankfully, in the ED we deliver care at the point of need, allowing other members of the hospital professional staff to address reimbursement issues after the care has been delivered.

References

1. 42 C.F.R. §§482.55 – Condition of Participation: Emergency Services, 489.24 – Special Responsibilities of Medicare Hospitals in Emergency Cases.

2. *Gatewood* v. *Washington Healthcare Corporation*, 933 F.2d 1037 (1991).

3. *Correa* v. *Hospital San Francisco*, 69 F.3d 1184 (1995).

4. Norton EC, Staiger DO. How hospital ownership affects access to care for the uninsured. *RAND J Econ.* 1994;25(1):171–185.

5. Davidoff A, Dubay L, Kenney G, Yemane A. The effect of parents' insurance coverage on access to care for low-income children. *Inquiry.* 2003;40(3):254–268. DOI:10.5034/inquiryjrnl_40.3.254.

6. Patient Protection and Affordable Care Act (Public Act 111–148), 42 U.S.C. & 18001 et seq (2010).

7. *Prospect Medical Group* v. *Northridge Emergency Medical Group.* 198 P.3d 86 (2009).

Intoxication

Case

The paramedics described a moderate-speed motor vehicle collision, in which no one seemed to be hurt, but the patient was brought in to the emergency department (ED) for evaluation to be sure. She was a bus driver, driving the bus home at the end of the day right before the shift ended. She had collided with another vehicle while trying to return the bus to the station. She said that she was tired and fell asleep, but she seemed a little shaky and her speech was a little slurred on presentation.

The ED physician decided to complete the standard trauma workup, including imaging of her head, neck, chest, and abdomen, based on their protocol for altered mental status. They sent off the standard blood work, including serum alcohol and urine drug screen. After a couple of hours, the standard radiographic screening was complete and interpreted to be normal. However, the screening for intoxicants found both a low level of serum alcohol (0.04 mg/dL) and a urine drug screen that was positive for opiates.

The department got busy and the physician had to attend to another emergency. The patient's discharge instructions were completed and the nurses were told to make sure that she had safe transport home. Her family arrived and she was discharged with a diagnosis of musculoskeletal trauma to follow up with her primary care physician.

A few months later, the hospital attorney contacted the ED to say that they had received a complaint concerning this patient's evaluation. Apparently, a complaint had been filed with the state medical board and the patient had lost her job as a school bus driver. She had a commercial driver's license (CDL) and, although she had transported all the students for the day, her employment was terminated because the testing had revealed intoxicants in her system. Her attorney alleged that this release of information was not discussed with her. She did not give informed consent to have blood drawn or urine obtained to be evaluated for intoxicants.

The provider stated that the patient had a clinical presentation of altered mental status and in the setting of the trauma evaluation, it was a necessary part of the evaluation to assess the veracity of her exam and history.

Medical Approach

When a patient presents with an altered mental status in a trauma setting, it is a necessary part of the evaluation from a medical perspective to evaluate for intoxicants. This allows one to interpret the veracity of a patient's history and physical exam. In this case the standard is especially high since the patient has a CDL, which requires a high degree of function on her part. The fact she presented with an altered mental status means that she abrogates the right to consent for the assessment of intoxicants, if she has an issue while at work. This is a higher standard than would be necessary for a patient who had been involved in an accident with their personal vehicle, although the requirement would still likely exist in most jurisdictions for most situations.

An estimated 20–25% of patients treated in the ED or as trauma inpatients have been drinking, with a blood alcohol concentration (BAC) of 0.10 g/dL (22 mmol/L) or greater. Many of these patients abuse alcohol, tobacco, and other drugs. Proper management of the trauma patient includes BAC determination, careful history for alcohol abuse, referral for treatment, and assessment for drug abuse.[1] Failure to do so may expose the physician to medicolegal risk if the patient hurts themselves or others.

Despite harsh legislation, driving under the influence of alcohol (DUI) is exceedingly common in motor vehicle collisions. Biffl et al. evaluated 525

Table 58.1 ED high-risk substance abuse profile

1. Males
2. Young
3. Metropolitan center
4. After midnight
5. Weekends
6. Violence
7. Trauma
8. Motor vehicle accident
9. High acuity
10. Psychiatric morbidity

Reference: El-Guebaly et al.[3]

Table 58.2 Medical care of the intoxicated patient

1. Added caution in medical evaluation
2. Heightened confidentiality requirements
3. Prudent discharge diagnosis and instructions
4. Discharge to safe environment with caregivers
5. Societal protection from patient's irresponsible actions

drivers, in which 74% (387) had serum alcohol measured, and 35% (137) had a BAC level greater than 100 mg/dL.[2] There were 113 state residents, of whom 19% (22) were charged with an offense related to the collision. Of these, 54% (12) were charged with DUI, and 83% (10) convicted, with an overall conviction rate of 9%. There was an established recidivism rate, in which 32% (7) of those charged had prior charge or conviction. Screening for alcohol and drug abuse and acute intervention are crucial for effective diagnosis and treatment.

Substance abuse may also be pervasive in certain ED and trauma populations. El-Guebaly et al. reported a substance use prevalence rate of 9–47% based on the population and location tested.[3] They found most common drugs – marijuana, benzodiazepines, and cocaine – followed a pattern similar to alcohol. They advocate the use of screening tools in high-risk populations. This risk group includes males, younger patients, metropolitan centers, after midnight, weekends, violent events, trauma, motor vehicle accidents, high acuity, and individuals with psychiatric morbidity (Table 58.1) Once screening is performed, it should be complemented by intervention, referral, and treatment programs.

Legal Analysis

In *Schmerber* v. *California*, the petitioner was noted to be intoxicated at the scene, was arrested at the ED, and was notified of his Miranda rights to stay silent and be represented by counsel.[4] However, the arresting officer directed the physician to draw a blood sample despite the patient's refusal at the request of counsel. The petitioner was convicted of a criminal offense of DUI, after

chemical analysis and admission as evidence under protest. The trial court convicted and decision was upheld by the appellate court, rejecting all arguments of denial of due process (Ad. V and XIV), right against self-incrimination (Ad. V), right to counsel (Ad. VI), and right to not be subjected to unreasonable search and seizure (Ad. IV and XIV).[5-8] The Supreme Court of the United States held that there is no constitutional prohibition of a compelled blood sample for diagnosis of intoxication, as long as there is probable cause.

In *Scott* v. *Uljanov*, the patient presented to the ED after allegedly ingesting alcohol and benzodiazepines and had a documented BAC of 0.29 g/dL.[9] He subsequently fell from a hospital bed, had a cut treated, and was admitted to the psychiatric unit. He sued the hospital and physician for wrongful detention. He also alleged that he was negligently supervised in his intoxicated state. The Supreme Court of New York dismissed these claims, based on a time claim barred statute of limitations, CPLR 214-a, of two and a half years.[10] The Appellate Division reversed, claiming the allegation resides in negligence, subject to a three-year statute, CPLR 214. The appeal court concluded again that the claims were considered medical malpractice and not simple negligence. Claims against the individual defendant were dismissed because he was not an aggrieved party, and claims against the corporate defendants were dismissed as time barred.

Conclusion

The presence of a patient in an intoxicated state invokes a number of provider obligations. First, the requirement for added caution in any medical evaluation, due to the unreliability of history and physical exam. Second, heightened confidentiality requirements for the patient care encounter. Third, particular precautions relating to discharge diagnosis and instructions. Fourth, the patient's need be discharged to a safe environment, with acceptance of this responsibility ideally by family, if available. Fifth, it is crucial that society at large be protected from an irresponsible individual, which addresses issues of driving, workplace safety, and social responsibility (Table 58.2).

References

1. Waller JA. Management issues for trauma patients with alcohol. *J Trauma*. 1990;30(12):1548–1553.

2. Biffl WL, Schiffman JD, Harrington DT, Sullivan J, Tracy TF, Cioffi WG. Legal prosecution of alcohol-impaired drivers admitted to a level i trauma center in Rhode Island. *J Trauma*. 2004;56(1):24–29.

3. El-Guebaly N, Armstrong SJ, Hodgins DC. Substance abuse and the emergency room: programatic implications. *J Addict Dis*. 1998;17(2):21–40. DOI:10.1300/J069v17n02_03.

4. *Schmerber* v. *California*, 384 U.S. 757 (1966).

5. U.S. Const. Amend V.

6. U.S. Const. Amend XIV.

7. U.S. Const. Amend VI.

8. U.S. Const. Amend IV.

9. *Scott* v. *Uljanov*, 74 N.Y. 2d 673 (1989).

10. New York Civil Practice Law and Rules (CPLR) SS 214. Actions to be commenced within three years: for non-payment of money collected on execution; for penalty created by statute; to recover chattel; for injury to property; for personal injury; for malpractice other than medical, dental or pediatric malpractice; to annul a marriage on the ground of fraud, 1214-a. Action for medical, dental or podiatrist malpractice to be commenced within two years and six months; exceptions.

Laboratory Testing

Case

In the emergency department (ED) the shift was coming to an end. There was a single patient left with a couple of laboratory results that were still pending. The departing physician was ready to go home, and the incoming physician had already arrived. The departing physician told him that, apart from the patient who was waiting for laboratory results and two patients awaiting transportation, all other patients were either discharged or admitted, all the calls had been made, and discharge instructions were done. That patient who was waiting for test results was most likely to be discharged home as well. She was an elderly woman with history of a fall and was on coumadin. They had scanned her head, which was normal, and had sent off the prothrombin time (PT) and international normalized ratio (INR) tests to the laboratory just to ensure that the patient was not over-anticoagulated. The departing physician asked that the oncoming physician check the PT before discharging the patient, and then went home after his busy day.

When he returned for his next shift 3 days later, one of the nurses told him that a patient who had been discharged had returned with an intracranial hemorrhage. After the discussion, the physician remembered the patient, who had a negative CT scan and was waiting for her PT result to go home. The issue was that the PT had actually come back significantly elevated, but the patient had been discharged before the PT result came back. Apparently, at the time no one had noted that it was significantly abnormal. She then came back two days later with an intracranial hemorrhage and was admitted to the intensive care unit (ICU). She was still in the ICU, was doing OK, and didn't require surgery.

Medical Approach

There is a clear precedent suggesting that the person who orders a test needs to follow up on it, even in the ED or in an ambulatory setting. Anyone who orders a laboratory test must make arrangements to follow up on abnormal results of that test, either through the ED, the ambulatory care center, or the primary care physician (PCP) of record.

Most EDs have a laboratory follow-up system, whether it is a de facto evaluation by the charge nurse, a quality assurance nurse, or the oncoming shift physician. There should be a standardized screening process that flags abnormal test results and places decision-making with the physician in charge of follow-up testing. Failure to do so will incur significant medicolegal liability.

The analysis of laboratory error includes evaluation of interpretation issues as well as laboratory procedures and processes.

Bonini et al. found considerable concordance of error distribution throughout the laboratory process.[1] Most errors occur in the pre- or post-analytic phase (68–87%) with the minority (13–32%) occurring in the analytic portion of the laboratory analysis. The preanalytic phase involves ordering, patient identification, and sampling. The analytic phase involves the specimen processing. The post-analytic phase is the clinical period when results are interpreted and discussed with the patient or other providers for follow-up. Substantially more errors were reported using a standardized assessment process compared to those from complaints or near-accident reports.

The obvious concern is the responsibility for laboratory and radiology test ordering, tracking, and follow-up. The premise is that the ED physician is obligated to follow up on any test ordered, even if it is not reported back to them directly.[2] This is most problematic when the test is reported after their shift has ended. Appropriate follow-up mechanisms must be in place to optimize patient care and minimize medicolegal liability. The key is to have a reliable reporting mechanism, so results can be discussed with the patient and their PCP or specialist.

There are numerous approaches to dealing with late-arriving laboratory results in the ED. Greenes et al. developed computerized notification, the Automated Late-Arriving Results Monitoring System system.[3] They analyzed cases over a two-year period and studied three tests prospectively. They found that among late-arriving tests, 75% (3/4) of positive pregnancy tests, 59% (23/39) positive chlamydia cultures, and 33% (6/18) of abnormal lead levels were not adequately reported. Specifically, there was no documented follow-up of abnormal results within one week. They postulate that an automated system would minimize this error rate.

Legal Analysis

In *Mehlman* v. *Powell*, the patient had dyspnea and saw his personal physician, who ordered a battery of tests and a ventilation–perfusion (VQ) lung scan.[4] He worsened at home, was unable to reach his physician, and proceeded to the ED. There were undisputed EKG changes, consistent with heart failure due to a pulmonary embolism (PE), allegedly not appreciated by the ED physician. The patient was discharged with a diagnosis of pneumonitis, and died at home. Suit was brought against the PCP, the ED physician, and the hospital with plaintiff verdict in trial court, and a cross-claim by the hospital against the ED physician for damages. The Court of Appeals of Maryland ruled that the hospital gives an appearance of the ED physicians being hospital employees rather than independent contractors, and are liable for the physician's actions as well. However, they affirmed the trial court ruling that the facility had no independent negligence that contributed to the patient's death. Likewise, they affirmed the trial court properly allowed expert testimony concerning the PCP's compliance with medical care standards.

In *Norman-Bloodsaw* v. *Lawrence Berkeley Laboratory*, the issue on appeal is whether an employee who undergoes a general employee health screening, can without their knowledge, be screened for private and sensitive medical conditions.[5] Here, a group of clerical and administrative workers underwent job preplacement and periodic health examinations, looking for conditions such as syphilis, sickle cell trait, and pregnancy. The aggrieved group asserted the testing violates Title VII of the Civil Rights Act of 1964, the Americans with Disabilities Act (ADA), and the right to privacy guaranteed by the Fourth Amendment of the US Constitution and Article 1, §1 of the California Constitution.[6–9] The district court granted the defendants-appellees' motion for dismissal, judgment on pleadings, and summary judgment on all the plaintiffs-appellants' claims. They concluded the claims were time barred and failed to state a cognizable Title VII claim. The United States Court of Appeals, Ninth District affirmed the ADA claim dismissal, but reversed the Title VII and federal and state privacy claims dismissals. The mere fact that the prospective employee had provided a specimen does not provide notice of testing, the nature of the testing, and the need for that specific testing. This analysis will require examination at trial to decide these issues.

In *Sharpe* v. *St. Luke's Hospital*, the question arises of whether a hospital that collects urine samples for drug testing for an employer owes a greater duty of care to the patient, regardless of their employee status.[10] The employee presented for random drug screening and the hospital forwarded the sample to an outside laboratory for testing. The employee's sample was allegedly positive for illicit substances, resulting in termination of her employment. The ousted employee filed suit, alleging deviations in the standard chain of custody process. The hospital filed a motion for summary judgment, maintaining that the complainant could not establish that a duty was owed, which was awarded by the trial court. The Supreme Court of Pennsylvania held that indeed the appellant was owed a duty of reasonable care regarding specimen handling. The superior court order was reversed and case remanded for further consideration.

Conclusion

Laboratory testing is a particularly problematic area from a medicolegal perspective. There is a defined obligation to follow-up any laboratory test performed in the ED. In terms of patient informed consent, there should be a clear delineation between testing ordered for patient care, and testing ordered by contractual employer obligation or for forensic purposes by law enforcement. Heightened confidentiality is required when reporting on any toxicological testing results.

References

1. Bonini P, Plebani M, Ceriotti F, Rubboli F. Errors in laboratory medicine. *Clin Chem.* 2002;48(5):691–698.

2. Moore GP. Liability of emergency physicians for studies ordered in the emergency department: court cases and legal defenses. *J Emerg Med.* 2011;40(2):225–8. DOI:10.1016/j.emergmed.2009.08.047.

3. Greenes DS, Fleisher GR, Kohane I. Potential impact of a computerized system to report late-arriving laboratory results in the emergency department. *Pediatr Emerg Care.* 2000;16(5):313–315.

4. *Mehlman* v. *Powell*, 378 A.2d 1121 (1977).

5. *Norman-Bloodsaw* v. *Lawrence Berkley Laboratory*, 135 F.3d 1260 (1998).

6. Title VII, Civil Rights Act of 1964, 42 U.S.C. §2000 et seq (1964).

7. Americans with Disabilities Act of 1990, 42 U.S.C. §12102.

8. U.S. Const. Amend IV.

9. California Constitution. Article 1, Section 1: Right To Privacy.

10. *Sharpe* v. *St Luke's Hospital*, 821 A.2d 1215 (2003).

Left without Being Seen, Left without Treatment, and Elopement

Case

It was a very busy day in the emergency department (ED). The waiting room was packed and every bed was full. The winter flu season was raging, and the department was at a standstill as it was clear that patients were not being admitted upstairs. The backup physician was called in from home to begin to treat patients in the ED waiting room. The nursing supervisor came down to the ED to help, and the hospital medical director came in from home to evaluate the discharge and floor transition process.

Luckily, there were no acute patient emergencies although the sheer number of patients was overwhelming for the department. Eventually, by that evening the patient admissions were moved into the system. By the next morning the department had returned to normal and all patients had been transferred to their floor beds.

Next day there was a call from the patient advocate, as concerns had been raised by patients and families. Some patients had left the waiting room and others who had been given bed spaces and waited for additional care had also left the department due to the prolonged waits.

An explanation was offered describing the triage process, and the extra medical and nursing resources that were brought in to care for patients. It was suggested that the ED should implement a staging system program for non-urgent complaints that could be dealt with in a clinic setting, to allow the ED to continue to operate in times of stress.

Medical Approach

In times of ED stress patients can often leave in an unpredictable fashion when the wait becomes too long. Many hospitals have instituted a contingency plan to deal with this extra flow, but with heavy patient numbers this may sometimes not be successful even with the best advance planning.

From a quality assurance perspective, we define patients that leave without being seen (LWBS) as patients who have presented to an ED, completed the registration process, but leave before they undergo the medical screening exam (MSE), typically performed by the physician (Table 60.1). Those who have received an MSE by the physician, but then leave prior to complete evaluation by the physician, are defined as left without treatment (LWOT) or left before treatment complete (LBTC). Patients who are evaluated by the physician and leave before the diagnosis and treatment plan can be completely implemented are defined as leaving against medical advice (AMA). There is usually a physician discussion of repercussions and documentation confirming the discrepancy of opinion, that may or may not be signed. Lastly, the term 'elopement' is typically used to describe the unannounced departure of a patient, who may be described as impaired, at any stage of the care process prior to official discharge, without the physician's knowledge.

The Emergency Department Performance Measures and Benchmarking Summary: Consensus Statement defined three performance measures referencing the MSE.[1] These are: (1) patients leaving before the MSE; (2) patients leaving after the MSE, but before provider documented treatment complete; (3) patients who leave AMA, where the patient is recognized by the institution, interacts with ED staff, but leaves before the encounter is complete (Table 60.2). However, there is accompanying documentation of patient competence, discussion of risks and benefits, and completion or refusal to complete document confirming intent to leave against medical staff recommendations (Table 60.3).

The analysis of the problem of patients leaving before their ED evaluation is complete has been

Table 60.1 Premature departure: quality markers

	Status	Parameters
1.	Left without being seen (LWBS)	After registration, before MSE
2.	Left without treatment (LWOT)	After MSE, before disposition
3.	Against medical advice (AMA)	Plan implementation discrepancy
4.	Elopement	Departs unannounced

Table 60.2 ED performance measures and benchmarking summary

Status. Parameters
1. Leaving before medical screening exam (PLBM). Before MSE
2. Leaving after medical screening exam (PLAM). Before provider complete
3. Leave against medical advice (LAMA) Before complete with discussion

Reference: AHRQ Consensus Statement[1]

Table 60.3 Against medical advice: criteria

1. Documented patient competence
2. Discussion of risks and benefits
3. Completion or refusal to sign
4. Intent to leave against staff recommendations

Reference: AHRQ Consensus Statement[1]

Table 60.4 LWBS survey of 262 hospitals and 9.2 million visits

Incidence	
Overall 2.6%	Range 0–20.3%
Multivariate analysis	
Increase 1.15	10% increase poorly insured
Decrease 0.86	$10,000 increase in income
Early departure demographic	**OR**
Teaching program	2.14
County ownership	2.09
Trauma center	1.62

Reference: Hsia et al.[2]

studied extensively. It is important to note that the data is specific to site, region, and circumstance. Hsia et al. reported on a large study sample of 9.2 million ED visits evaluated in 262 hospitals, in which the median LWBS rate was 2.6% with a range of 0–20.3%.[2] Multivariate analysis finds that the LWBS rate increases by a factor of 1.15 for every 10% point increase in poorly insured patients, and decreased by a factor of 0.86 for each $10,000 increase in income. Hospital demographic descriptors such as teaching program affiliation (OR 2.14), county ownership (OR 2.09), and trauma center designation (OR 1.62) increase the likelihood of the patient leaving. Facilities that have a large proportion of low-income and poorly insured patients are at greatest risk for those leaving the department without proper care (Table 60.4).

A study by Pham et al. evaluating the National Hospital Ambulatory Medical Care Survey (NHAMCS) from 1998 to 2006 reported an LWBS rate of 1.7 (95% CI 1.6–1.9) patients per 100 ED visits annually.[3] These were patients who were triaged but not evaluated by a physician. Multivariate analysis of demographic correlates finds that patients at age extremes (<18 years, >65 years) and nursing home residents were associated with lower LWBS rates. (Table 60.5). Those who were non-white or Hispanic, on Medicaid, self-pay, or other insurance status had higher LWBS rates.

Visit characteristics more likely correlated to higher LWBS rates include visits for musculoskeletal complaints or injury/poisoning/adverse events and are higher for miscellaneous complaints. Those with lower acuity visits were more likely to leave, and those with work-related injury more likely to remain. Institutional characteristics associated with patients who LWBS were those in metropolitan areas and teaching institutions. To be most effective, prediction and benchmarking of LWBS rates should control for visit and facility characteristic rates.

Rowe et al. reported on a cohort of 4.5% (711) of 15,660 registered ED patients who were LWBS cases.[4] Of the 498 patients who responded, who waited an average of 87 minutes prior to seeing the physician, 49% said they were "fed up with waiting." Overall 60% (299) of the LWBS cases sought medical attention within one week, with 4.6% (14) hospitalized and with one requiring urgent surgery (Table 60.6). Triage level was not associated with the likelihood of seeking medical attention. Of those 39% (198) of patients who did not seek attention, 26% (50) were triaged as

Table 60.5 National Hospital Ambulatory Medical Care Survey (NHAMCS), 1998–2006

		LWBS rates 1.7 (95% CI 1.6–1.9)	Lower OR (95% CI)	Higher OR (95% CI)
Status				
Age	(<18 years)		0.80 (0.66–0.96)	
	(>65 years)		0.46 (0.32–0.64)	
	Nursing home		0.29 (0.08–1.00)	
Demographics				
Race	Non-white			1.41 (1.22–1.63)
	Hispanic			1.25 (1.04–1.49)
Insurance	Medicaid			1.47 (1.27–1.70)
	Self-pay			1.96 (1.65–2.32)
	Other insurance			2.09 (1.74–2.52)
Diagnosis	Musculoskeletal		0.70 (0.57–0.85)	
	Injury/poisoning/adverse		0.65 (0.53–0.80)	
	Miscellaneous			1.56 (1.19–2.05)
Classification	Low triage acuity			3.59 (2.81–4.58)
	Work-related		0.19 (0.12–0.29)	
Facility	Metropolitan			2.11 (1.66–2.70)
	Teaching institution			1.33 (1.06–1.67)

Reference: Pham et al.[3]

Table 60.6 LWBS patient opinion survey

	LWBS rate	4.5% (15 660)
	Average wait	87 minutes
	Questionnaire response	411
Profile		**Incidence (%)**
Rationale	"Fed up waiting"	49
Follow-up	Sought attention within 1 week	60
	Hospitalized	4.6
	Surgery	0.2
Status	Did not seek attention	39
	Triage urgent	26

Reference: Rowe et al.[4]

urgent. Overall, most patients leave at the peak, busy times. Complications are rare, but can be significant.

Fernandes et al. reported a similar experience with 1.4% (423/23,933) patients who were LWBS cases with follow-up in 39% (165).[5] The most common reasons for leaving included prolonged wait times (60%, 99/165); perceived difficulties with hospital staff (28%, 46/165); and pressing commitments elsewhere (27%,

45/165). The vast majority (92%, 152/165) of patients believe they should be evaluated by a physician within one hour. The majority of people who left (67%, 284/423) had low acuity ratings, and 65% left between 30 minutes and 2 hours after registration on average (Table 60.7). Roughly half of the patients (48%, 80/165) sought medical attention within 24 hours with their personal physician (39%, 65/165) and other EDs (18%, 29/165). The majority of patients who left had low acuity, left because of prolonged waiting times, and sought additional care.

Monzon et al. reported a cohort of 3.57% (386/10,808) patients who were LWBS cases.[6] One-third of the patients had no fixed address or telephone, and only 23.8% (92/386) consented to a phone interview (Table 60.8). One-third (36.7%) cited excessive wait time as their reason for leaving. Interestingly, they were no more likely than the control (70%) group to seek care after departure. The LWBS group often lacked a regular physician (39.1% vs. 21.7%, P = 0.01) and were more likely to present to an ED or clinic (34.8% vs. 12.0%, P < 0.001). The control group was more likely to follow up with a family physician (37.0% vs. 23.9%,

Table 60.7 LWBS survey

Patients	23 933	
LWBS	1.4% (423)	
	Outcome	**Incidence (%)**
Follow-up		39
Rationale		
1.	Prolonged wait times	60
2.	Perceived difficulty with staff	28
3.	Pressing commitments	27
Perception		
4.	Evaluated by physician within 1 hour	92
Departure demographic		
Low acuity		67
Timing post registration		30–120 min
Follow-up within 24 hours		
	PCP	39
	ED	18

Reference: Fernandes et al.[5]

Table 60.8 LWBS cohort characteristics

Patients	10,808
LWBS	3.57% (386)
Factors	**Incidence (%)**
No address or phone	33.3
Phone interview	23.8
Rationale	
Excessive wait times	36.7
Post-departure care	70
Cohort	**Comparison (%)**
LWBS	
Lacked regular physician	39.1 vs. 21.7, $P = 0.01$
Present to ED or clinic	34.8 vs. 12.0, $P < 0.001$
Control	
Present to PCP	37.0 vs. 23.9, $P = 0.06$

Reference: Monzon et al.[6]

Table 60.9 Parent–pediatric LWBS

Patients	11,087	
LWBS	3% (289)	
Profile		**Incidence (%)**
1.	Urgent triage	15
2.	Taken elsewhere	63
Rationale		
3.	Waited too long	58
4.	Symptoms resolved	37
Multivariate analysis		**OR (95% CI)**
5.	Lower acuity	4.0 (2.2–7.2)
6.	Midnight–4 a.m.	5.9 (2.8–12.5)
7.	Seek care elsewhere	4.3 (2.9–6.4)

Reference: Goldman et al.[7]

$P = 0.06$). Interestingly, the groups did not differ in health status, nor in subsequent hospital revaluation.

Goldman et al. reported on the pediatric experience in which 3% (289/11 087) LWBS.[7] This group consisted of 15% (24/158) of children triaged as urgent, with 63% (99) taken elsewhere for care. Parents suggested that waiting too long (58%, 92) and resolution of symptoms (37%, 58) were the reasons for leaving. Multivariate analysis revealed that children who left had a lower acuity (OR 4.0, 95% CI 2.2–7.2), were more likely to register between midnight and 4 a.m. (OR 5.9, 95% CI 2.8–12.5), and more likely to be taken somewhere else for follow-up care (OR 4.3, 95% CI 2.9–6.4) (Table 60.9).

McMullan and Veser compared the LWOT incidence to the ED volume, reporting a rate of 3.4% (629/18 664).[8] They found that when shift volume exceeded 25 patients per 12-hour shift, or 2.1 patients per hour for a single physician site, significantly more patients were LWOT (Table 60.10). They also found the same result if there were more than five high-acuity patients per shift. Evaluation of this cohort found at least one of these maxima was exceeded in over half the cases. They suggested a predictive model based on these parameters to assist in staffing models. Overall, the LWBS rate extrapolated from this study group was 2.88% with a range of 1.4–4.5% (Table 60.11).[2–8]

Legal Analysis

One area of caselaw focus is on elopement of patients admitted with a psychiatric diagnosis.

Table 60.10 LWOT compared to volume

Patients	18,664	
LWBS	3.4% (629)	
Factors in solo-staffed department		
1.	Shift (12-hour) volume	> 25 patients
2.	Patients per hour	> 2.1
3.	High-acuity patients	> 5 per shift

Reference: McMullan and Veser[8]

Table 60.11 LWBS overview

Incidence (%)		Study	Patients	Reference
Overall	**Range**			
2.88	1.4–4.5			
2.6		Hsia	9.2 million	2
1.7		Pham	136 million	3
4.5		Rowe	15,660	4
1.4		Fernandes	23,937	5
3.5		Manzon	10,508	6
3.0		Goldman	11,087	7
3.4		McMullan	18,664	8

In *Burchfield* v. *United States of America*, the patient presented to the ED, and was transferred to an open ward of the psychiatric facility.[9] He eloped from the facility, as noted during a bed check, broke into a local residence and assaulted the inhabitant, and was charged and convicted of this crime. The householder sued the facility, alleging the elopement was due to a failure to follow their policies and procedures, pursuant to the Federal Tort Claims Act.[10] The facility defended the elopement by stating they could encourage but not force a voluntary patient to stay. They testified he had not been a problem previously, but was restrained once previously. The district court held that since this patient was admitted with voluntary status and the plaintiff was a random subject of attack, no duty was owed, so there was no breach of that duty.

In *Gonzalez* v. *Paradise Valley Hospital*, a patient with a long-standing psychiatric history allegedly attacked a family member and was taken to the ED by police, who requested a 72-hour patient hold.[11] The patient was found to be agitated and "clearly psychotic." He ran out of the door, but was returned to the ED by law enforcement, placed in restraints, and medicated. He was admitted to a locked psychiatric facility as he was felt to be a danger to others, but escaped the next afternoon, broke into a local apartment and cut himself, resulting in his death. The Welfare and Institutions Code §5150 provides for a 72-hour involuntary commitment, while Section 5278 immunizes defendants from breaches of the applicable standard of care during the detention.[12] The trial court granted summary judgment motion for the physician and the hospital, citing the opinion in *Heater* v. *Southwood Psychiatric Center* (1996).[13] The appeal court reversed the trial court judgment for the defendant, holding there was no statutory immunity for negligence during the 72-hour hold, citing a later decision in *Jacobs* v. *Gross* (2003).[14]

Administrative disability hearings often have ED visits as a significant focus of the analysis. In *Emery* v. *Astrue*, the plaintiff brought an action pursuant to 42 U.S.C. §405 (g) and 1383 (c) (3) for final review of the final determination of the Commissioner of Social Security denying her application for Disability Insurance Benefits (DIB) and Supplemental Security Income (SSI) under Titles II: Federal Old Age, Survivors and Disability Insurance Benefits (§§401–434) and XVI: Supplemental Security Income For

Table 60.12 Social security five-step disability analysis

1. Engaged in substantial gainful activity
2. Severe impairment
3. Meet special impairment criteria
4. Capable of performing past work
5. Residual functional capacity to perform

Reference: C.F.R.[21]

Aged, Blind And Disabled (§§1381–1385) of the Social Security Act, 42 U.S.C. Chapter 7.[15–18] The patient complained of numerous and various pain syndromes, had seen multiple providers, and had numerous ED presentations accompanied by elopement if specific pain medication requests were not accommodated.

Under the Social Security Act, an individual is considered disabled when they are:

unable to engage in any substantial gainful activity by reason of any medically determinable physical or mental impairment which can be expected to result in death or has lasted or can be expected to last for a continuous period of not less than 12 months.

The plaintiff alleged that the proper decision requires consideration of the opinion of the treating physician, and the patient's subjective complaints. The district court held that the administrative-law judge failed to properly consider the patient's treating physician, and the case was remanded for reconsideration.

In *Holden* v. *Astrue*, the plaintiff sought judicial review for final decision of the Commissioner denying application for SSI pursuant to Title XVI of the Social Security Act.[19,20] The patient had presented to the ED on multiple occasions, with various complaints, requiring analgesics and muscle relaxants. After numerous visits, the patient was informed there would be prescription restrictions, as no findings were identified other than degeneration. She then made a rapid departure from the ED. The district court affirmed the administrative-law judge's decision as being supported by substantial evidence and based on proper legal standards. The Commissioner promulgated the five-step sequential process for analyzing alleged disability:[20–22] Step 1: Is claimant engaging in substantial gainful activity? Step 2: Does the claimant have a severe impairment? Step 3: Does a specified disability exist? Step 4: Is claimant capable of doing past work? Step 5: Does the claimant have the residual functional capacity to perform other work? (Table 60.12).

In *Picklesimer* v. *Colvin*, action was again filed pursuant to 42 U.S.C. §405 (g) to obtain judicial review of the Commissioner's final decision denying the plaintiff's claim for DIB and SSI.[23,24] The administrative-law judge's record included reference to numerous ED visits for various different pain complaints, for which specific analgesics were sought, accompanied by a large number of elopements without formal discharge. The district court reviewed the administrative record as a whole, and concluded the plaintiff was not disabled as the decision was supported by ample evidence.

It is crucial to recognize that the ED records are often reviewed focusing on elopement prior to official discharge, as well as the incidence of patients leaving AMA or LWOT.

In *IASIS Healthcare* v. *Apollo Physicians of Texas*, the health-care organization appealed a jury decision awarding an EM physician group damages concerning a contract dispute.[25] The Court of Appeals of Texas, Thirteenth District eventually reversed and remanded this decision. There were no grounds for tortious interference, the facility acted in good faith, the lost profit evidence is not sufficient, no viable tort theory was offered, and prejudicial evidence was admitted. However, a contract stipulation benchmarking performance quality standards for the ED group included an AMA and LWOT rate of 1% of the patient population, among other parameters. These parameters were not met. The physician group felt these were worthy benchmarks, but largely beyond their control. They alleged, but did not prove, the administration tried to supplant the decision-making of licensed medical professionals.

Conclusion

These quality markers should be tracked with nursing and physician staff and gauged appropriately to patient flow. Hospital-based rapid processing and discharge programs should also be instituted to increase discharge efficiency in times of stress. Studies show that reducing overall length of stay in the ED demonstrates corresponding decreases in the proportion of patients who leave the ED before their evaluations are complete.[26]

References

1. AHRQ Emergency Department Performance Measures and Benchmarking Summit: The Consensus Statement.2006 www.qualityindicators.ahrq/gov. Accessed May 20, 2016.

2. Hsia RY, Arch SM, Weiss RE, Zingmond D, Liang LJ, Han W, et al. Hospital determinants of emergency department left without being seen rates. *Ann Emerg Med.* 2011;58(1):24–32.

3. Pham JC, Ho GK, Hill PM, McCarthy ML, Pronovost PJ. National study of patient, visit and hospital characteristics associated with leaving an emergency department without being seen: predicting LWBS. *Acad Emerg Med.* 2009;16(10):949–955. DOI:10.1111/j.1553–2712.2009.00515.x.

4. Rowe BH, Channan P, Bullard M, Blitz S, Saunders LD, Rosychuk RJ, et al. Characteristics of patients who leave emergency departments without being seen. *Acad. Emerg Med.* 2006;13(8):848–852. DOI:10.1197/j.aem.2006.01.028.

5. Fernandes CM, Daya MR, Barry S, Palmer N. Emergency department patients who leave without seeing a physician: the Toronto Hospital experience. *Ann Emerg Med.* 1994;24(6):1092–1096.

6. Monzon J, Friedman SM, Clarke C, Arenovich T. Patients who leave the emergency department without being seen by a physician: a case-matched study. *CJEM.* 2005;7(2):107–113.

7. Goldman RD, Macpherson A, Schuh S, Mulligan C, Pirie J. Patients who leave the pediatric emergency department without being seen: a case-control study. *CMAJ.* 2005;172(1):39–43. DOI:10.1503/cmaj.1031817.

8. McMullan JT, Veser FH. Emergency department volume and acuity as factors in patients leaving without treatment. *South Med J.* 2004;97(8):729–33.

9. *Burchfield* v. *United States of America*, 750 F. Supp. 1312 (1990).

10. Federal Tort Claims Act, 28 U.S.C. §§1346 (b), 2671–2680.

11. *Gonzalez* v. *Paradise Valley Hospital*, 111 Cal. App.4th 735 (2003).

12. California Welfare and Institutions Code §5150: Involuntary Psychiatric Hold (1967).

13. *Heater* v. *Southwood Psychiatric Center*, 49 Cal. Rptr.2d 9 (1996).

14. *Jacobs* v. *Grossmont Hospital*, 133 Cal. Rptr.2d 9 (2003).

15. *Emery* v. *Astrue*, No. 2:08cv551, September 17, 2009.

16. 42 U.S.C. §405–Evidence, Procedure and Certification For Payments (2006).

17. 42 U.S.C. §1383 (c) (3): Procedure for Payment of Benefits.

18. Social Security Act 42, U.S.C Chapter 7, Pub.L.74–271, 49 Stat.620 (1935).

19. *Holden* v. *Astrue*, Case No. 1:11-cv-00716-SMS. November 28, 2012.

20. Social Security Act, Title XVI, 42 U.S.C. §301 et seq.

21. 20 C.F.R. §§404.1520 (a)–(f):Evaluation of Disability in General, 416.920 (a)–(f):Evaluation of Disability of Adults, in General.

22. *Lester* v. *Chater*, 81 F.3d 821 (1995).

23. *Picklesimer* v. *Colvin*, No. 3:13–1457, October 13, 2015.

24. 42 U.S.C. §405 (g): Evidence, Procedure and Certification For Payments.

25. *IASIS Healthcare* v. *Apollo Physicians*, Case No.13-10-00173-CV (TX. Court of App. 13, October 20, 2011).

26. Sharieff GQ, Burnell L, Cantonis M, Norton V, Tovar J, Roberts K, et al. Improving emergency department time to provider, left-without-treatment rates, and average length of stay. *J Emerg Med.* 2013;45(3):426–432. DOI:10.1016/j.emergmed.2013.93.014.

Chapter 61

Malpractice Claims

Case

At a medical executive committee meeting, the emergency department (ED) medical director was asked about a medical malpractice case affecting the ED. A visiting board member had asked a question concerning the likelihood of ED medical malpractice. He said that he thought lawsuits were probably more common in emergency medicine than in other medical specialties. The ED director suggested there are reasons why litigation may be more common in emergency medicine. These issues are related to the patient population, including high-acuity conditions, some patient non-compliance, and lack of established physician–patient relationship. But it was by no means the specialty most associated with lawsuits, as the ED has many programs and protocols in place to address patients who present in an irregular and uncertain fashion.

The director invited the board member to visit and tour the ED, and to interact with the physicians, nurses, and other providers who care for this difficult patient population.

Medical Approach

There is often a misconception that emergency medicine is especially prone to litigation. The reasons why relate to the high-acuity patient population, repeat visits, irregularity of presentation, poor patient compliance, and lack of established relationship for post-discharge follow-up. In fact, emergency medicine pales in comparison to other practice specialties including neurosurgery, cardiothoracic surgery, general surgery, as well as internal medicine and its specialties, which all have higher rates of malpractice incidence.

Macroanalysis typically focuses on adverse events and patient outcome. There is thought to be an association between adverse events and medical malpractice,

but Brennan et al. evaluated the relationship between negligent adverse events and subsequent medical malpractice litigation in 46 closed claims.[1] The found that 41.6% (10/24) of cases with no adverse event identified settled for a mean plaintiff award of $28,760; 46.1% (6/13) of cases with adverse events, but no negligence, with mean payment of $66,944; 55.5% (5/9) cases with adverse events due to negligence with a mean payment of $66,944; 87.5% (7/8) of cases with associated permanent disability settled for $201,250 on average. Multivariate analysis revealed the only significant predictor of payment was disability ($P = 0.03$), and not related adverse events or negligence.

Studdert et al. evaluated a group of 1452 closed malpractice claims and found that in 3% there was no verifiable medical injury, and 37% did not involve medical errors at all.[2] The majority of claims were not associated with error (72%, 370/515) or injury (84%, 31/37) and did not result in payment. However, most that involved error or injury (73%, 653/889) did involve compensation. The average payment was higher for incidents involving error than not ($313,205 vs. $521,560, $P = 0.004$)

Information from the Physician Insurers Association of America database was analyzed to reveal 11,529 claims accounting for $664 million in liability over a 23-year period.[3] The most common error encountered was that in diagnosis (37%), followed by procedural errors in 17%, and in 18% no error was identified at all. The majority (70%) of the claims closed without payment, 29% were settled for payment. Only 7% of claims were resolved by verdict, and the majority (85%) were resolved in favor of the clinician.

There are diverse factors that would cause a patient to file a lawsuit. Hickson et al. asked 508 families of pediatric patients their reasons for filing.[4] They stated they were advised by knowledgeable

Table 61.1 Factors that prompted families to file malpractice claims

	Reason	Incidence (%)
1.	Advised by knowledgeable acquaintances	33
2.	Recognized "cover-up"	24
3.	Needed money	24
4.	Recognized child would have "no future"	23
5.	Needed information	20
6.	Seeking "revenge," or protecting others from "harm"	19

Reference: Hickson et al.[4]

acquaintances (33%), recognized a "cover-up" (24%), needed money (24%), recognized "limited future" for child (23%), needed information (20%), and decided to seek "revenge" or protect others from harm (19%) (Table 61.1). A pervasive theme was dissatisfaction with physician communication, and this should be noted and addressed.

Legal Analysis

The caselaw focuses on procedural issues as often as on case merit. Statute of limitations issues are often invoked. In *Borgia* v. *City of New York*, the infant and father took judgment against New York City for alleged medical malpractice at a city hospital.[5] The appellate court reversed and dismissed based on a time-barred statute, in which the notice of claim needed to be filed within 90 days.[6] The remaining legal question was whether the claim accrued on the date of the alleged negligent act, or at the end of a continuous course of treatment.

The statute of limitations bar to action also figured prominently in *Scott* v. *Uljanov*,[7] in which the action was dismissed under the 2.5-year medical malpractice statute.[8] However, the plaintiff refiled under a simple negligence theory with a 3-year statute of limitations, which was allowed. The appeal court noted the absence of a line between negligence and a specialized medical malpractice action. The patient was 15 months old, suffered severe second- and third-degree burns from a coffee spill, was admitted to a ward setting, and suffered shock and an anoxic brain injury the next day. The Court of Appeals of the State of New York reversed the

appellate court, reinstating the trial court decision. They held that, "when the course of treatment, that includes the wrongful act or omissions, has run continuously, is related to the original condition or complaint, the accrual comes only at the end of the treatment period."

The standard of proof for negligence is often the point of controversy in a medical malpractice action. In *Gooding* v. *University Hospital Building*, the patient presented to the ED suffering from lower abdominal pain, and had a syncopal episode.[9] There was allegedly a delay in evaluation while waiting for the patient's gastroenterologist to arrive, and the patient succumbed allegedly to a ruptured abdominal aortic aneurysm. The family filed suit, alleging the proper history, exam, and testing was not performed to diagnose his condition before the cardiopulmonary arrest. The trial court instructed the jury that they could find for the plaintiff if the hospital "destroyed" his chance to survive. The Supreme Court of Florida addressed the question of whether, in a wrongful-death action, they must prove that more likely than not the death was caused by the defendant's negligence, and affirmed that this was indeed the case. However, they evaluated negligence standards from other jurisdictions.

The negligence standards have included a loss of chance to survive, even when a patient was less than likely or equally likely to survive or not. In *Hernandez* v. *Clinica Pasteur*, there was an alleged failure to treat a heart condition.[10] The defined proximate cause standard was, a "better chance to survive" if the patient had received prompt medical attention. This standard is sufficient to form the basis for submission to a jury. In *Dawson* v. *Weems*, a patient was given banked rather than fresh blood depriving him of the "best chance" to survive.[11]

The "loss of a chance" to survive rationale is best stated in *Hicks* v. *United States*; if there is any "substantial possibility" of survival and the defendant has destroyed it, they are answerable.[12] However, the "more likely than not" survival test was met as testified by the expert that the patient "would have survived." In *Cooper* v. *Sisters of Charity of Cincinnati*, the providers were sued over an ED care event in which the expert testified to a 50% chance of survival.[13] The *Gooding* court held there was no reason to relax the "more likely than not" negligence standard. They agreed with the *Cooper* standard, that more than a decreased chance of survival must be shown because of the defendant's conduct. To establish a jury question on proximate cause, the plaintiff must show that the injury "more likely than not" resulted from defendant's negligence. The district court properly ruled that the trial court should have granted the hospital motion for directed verdict.

Another debate in the medical malpractice arena is whether the proper standard of care has a local, regional, or national standard of care. In *Shilkret v. Annapolis Emergency Hospital Association*, the question raised was whether the "strict locality" negligence standard would be applied to a medical malpractice case.[14] The medical expert testified that facilities belonging to the American Hospital Association, one of several members of the accrediting body, the Joint Commission, should meet the national standard of care. The trial judge held that the "strict locality" rule practiced in that area was the standard, rather than the "national standard," not tied to a particular area, or the "similar locality" standard observed by physicians of ordinary skill and care in the defendant physician's locality or in a similar community. The trial court held that the plaintiffs failed to establish a sufficient standard for the jury, and this was affirmed by the Court of Special Appeals. The Court of Appeals of Maryland reversed and remanded for a new trial. They held that:

> a hospital is required to use that degree of care and skill which is expected of a reasonably competent hospital in the same or similar circumstances. As in cases brought against physicians, advances in the profession, availability of special facilities and specialists, together with all of the relevant considerations are to be taken into account.

The "loss of chance" doctrine was reviewed in *McKellips* v. *St Francis Hospital*, in which the patient with risk factors presented to the ED allegedly with chest pain, was discharged with gastritis, and returned in cardiac arrest.[15] The district court concluded the appellant's evidence was not sufficient. The proximate cause analysis consists of two elements: cause in fact, the "but for analysis" concerning this case; and legal causation, that determines whether legal liability is imposed if the defendant's conduct is causative. The loss of a less than even chance of recovery or survival, related to the defendant's conduct, becomes a question of proximate cause for the jury. If the defendant's negligence is felt to be the proximate cause of injury, there is only liability for injuries which aggravate a pre-existing condition.

Conclusion

Greater awareness of proper risk management practice is likely to mitigate subsequent malpractice experience. Providers should be familiar with current standards of care, risk avoidance and mitigation strategies, and local, state, and federal guidelines.

References

1. Brennan TA, Sox CM, Burstin HR. Relation between negligent adverse events and the outcomes of medical-malpractice litigation. *N Engl J Med*. 1996;335(26):1963–1967. DOI:10.1056/nejm199612263352606.

2. Studdert DM, Mello MM, Gawande AA, Gandi TK, Kachalia A, Yoon C, et al. Claims, errors and compensation payments in medical malpractice litigation. *N Engl J Med*. 2006;354(19):2024–2033. DOI:10:1056/nejmsa054479.

3. Brown TW, McCarthy ML, Kelen GD, Levy F. An epidemiologic study of closed emergency department malpractice claims in a national database of physician malpractice insurers. *Acad Emerg Med*. 2010;17(5):553–560. DOI:10.1111/j.1553–2712.2010.00729.x.

4. Hickson GB, Clayton EW, Githens PB, Sloan FA. Factors that prompted families to file medical malpractice claims following perinatal injuries. *JAMA*. 1992;267 (10):1359–1363. DOI:10.1001/jama.1992.03480100065032.

5. *Borgia* v. *City of New York*, 12 N.Y.2d 151 (1962).

6. Administrative Code of City of New York, §394a-1.0.

7. *Scott* v. *Uljanov*, 74 N.Y.2d 673 (1989).

8. New York Civil Practice Law and Rules §214-a. Action for Medical, Dental or Podiatric Malpractice to Be Commenced Within Two Years and Six Months; Exceptions.

9. *Gooding* v. *University Hospital Building*, 445 So. 2d 1015 (1984).

10. *Hernandez* v. *Clinica Pasteur, Inc.*, 293 So. 2d 747 (1974).

11. *Dawson* v. *Weems*, 352 So. 2d 1200 (1977).

12. *Hicks* v. *United States*, 368 F.2d 626 (1966).

13. *Cooper* v. *Sisters of Charity of Cincinnati*, 272 N.E.2d 97 (1971).

14. *Shilkret* v. *Annapolis Emergency Hospital Association*, 349 A.2d 245 (1975).

15. *McKellips* v. *Saint Francis Hospital*, 741 P.2d 467 (1987).

Mandatory Care

Case

The patient presented to the emergency department (ED) with a myriad of complaints and a varied symptom complex that included nausea, vomiting, muscle aches, a lump that had been present for 6 months, and a skin rash. The workup showed a symptom complex of tracheobronchitis as there was no fever, no elevation of the white blood cell count, and a minimally productive cough that had been present for a week. The decision was made to start the patient on outpatient antibiotics, as well as topical cream for the rash. He was able to eat and drink in the ED and had showed no objective evidence of dehydration.

At the conclusion of the visit, he was discharged home with a family member coming to pick him up. When the family member arrived they requested the patient be admitted, although he wanted to go home and did not have a diagnosis. The presentation was consistent with an outpatient management plan. The patient's primary care physician (PCP) was consulted and he concurred as well.

The family member on the other hand again asked that he should be admitted because he believed that was supposed to happen if the family wanted it. Social service was consulted and additional outpatient resources were arranged for the patient. Additional family members came and stated they were happy with the outpatient treatment plan and with the additional visiting nurse appointments for the coming week. The patient was discharged home uneventfully.

Medical Approach

There are some obvious misconceptions about what a hospital is required to do when the patient presents to the ED. Typically a comprehensive history is taken and a physical exam is performed. There is a diagnostic evaluation and a treatment plan is designed. The appropriate medical diagnosis is made, therapeutics

offered, and follow-up arranged for a patient discharge. For an inpatient admission, additional psychosocial support may often be offered.

Accessibility to emergency medical care is often discussed when there is an issue of care availability. Legal issues begin with an analysis of ambulance diversion policies and protocols.[1] Second, the duty of care is defined by proximity, foreseeability, and reliance by the patient to establish that duty. Patients and family have a general expectation that patient care is universally available in an ED setting. Third, availability of care is often dictated by moral and ethical considerations. Fourth, there is felt to be a clearer pathway if there is a pre-existing relationship between the patient and a physician or hospital. Fifth, this area is often a matter of public policy debate and significant legislative activity. Sixth, the duty to treat has a significant resource and financial impact on physicians and hospitals (Table 62.1).

The issues with care availability are often manifest in ambulance diversion policies. The New York State Emergency Medical Services Council offers the Emergency Patient Destination and Hospital Diversion Policy Statement.[2] These and similar guidelines suggest that first, all ambulance patients should be informed of the need to be taken to a facility capable of providing the needed care; second, the triage and transport of out-of-hospital patients must be based on principles of emergency medical services (EMS) practice and pre-established regional and state medical protocols; third, patients who meet specialty criteria are transported to facilities that specialize in trauma or stroke care; fourth, a diversion request may be honored if a facility's capacity to treat additional patients promptly is exceeded (this is not a literal interpretation and the facility does not need to be physically at bed space capacity); fifth, the hospital cannot, however, refuse to treat a patient if they present for care to the facility (Table 62.2).

Table 62.1 Duty to provide emergency care

1.	Ambulance diversion policies
2.	Duty of care
3.	Proximity, foreseeability, and reliance
4.	Ethical considerations
5.	Pre-existing patient relationship
6.	Public policy
7.	Legislation
8.	Impact of duty

Reference: Walker[1]

Table 62.2 New York emergency patient destination and hospital diversion policy

1.	Inform all patients of diversion to capable facility
2.	Triage and transport based on existing regional or state protocols
3.	Disease specifics mandate transfer to specialty facility
4.	Diversion request if facility capacity exceeded
5.	Hospital cannot refuse treatment after patient's arrival

Reference: New York Bureau of Emergency Medical Services[2]

Table 62.3 Patient Protection and Affordable Care Act and grandfathered health insurance plans

Job-based grandfathered plans:	
1.	Have not cut benefits or increased costs
2.	Notify insured of grandfathered plan
3.	Have continuously covered one person since March 23, 2010
All health plans must:	
1.	End lifetime limits
2.	End arbitrary cancelations
3.	Cover adult children to age 26
4.	Provide summary of benefits and coverage (SBC)
5.	Spend majority of premiums on health care, not costs or bonuses
Protections that don't apply to grandfathered plan:	
1.	Provision of free preventive care
2.	Guaranteed right to appeal
3.	Protected doctor choice and emergency care access
Protections that don't apply to individual grandfathered plans:	
1.	Ending yearly limits on coverage
2.	Covering a pre-existing health condition
Doctor choice and ED access	
1.	Choose your own doctor
2.	No referrals for ob-gyn services
3.	Access to out-of-network ED service
	Can't require higher co-payment or co-insurance
	Can't require prior approval for ED service

Reference: www.healthcare.gov[5]

There are state guidelines which may augment federal patient care mandates. The State of Illinois offers emergency medical care coverage guidelines.[3] They specify that care is provided for an emergency medical condition (EMC) when it occurs suddenly and unexpectedly, is caused by illness or injury, and requires immediate attention to prevent serious jeopardy to patient's health or serious impairment to bodily functions or parts. Chronic conditions, terminal illness, and long-term care do not necessarily meet the criteria for emergency care. End-stage renal disease is an emergency condition, extending to noncitizens as well, but coverage is limited to dialysis services only.

There has been less discussion on this topic since the adoption of the Patient Protection and Affordable Care Act.[4] Most accept a mandatory care obligation in the world of emergency medicine. However, it is complex and nuanced in the case of grandfathered health insurance plans that after March 23, 2010 may enroll patients in plans that (1) have not substantially cut benefits or increased costs, (2) have notified the insured they have a grandfathered plan, and (3) have continuously covered one person since March 23, 2010 (Table 62.3).[5]

All health-care plans must: (1) end lifetime limits; (2) end arbitrary cancelations; (3) cover adult children up to the age of 26 years; (4) provide an easily understandable summary of benefits and coverage; (5) spend the majority of premiums on health care, not administrative costs and bonuses.

Protections that do not apply to grandfathered plans include: (1) coverage of free preventive care; (2) guaranteed right to appeal a coverage decision; (3) choice of doctors and access to emergency care. In addition, individual grandfathered plans do not have to end yearly limits on coverage or cover preexisting health conditions.

Access to out-of-network ED services is mandatory except in qualified grandfathered plans that may have additional requirements. Normally, insurance plans cannot require higher co-payment or co-insurance for out-of-network ED care. Nor can they require prior approval for out-of-network ED care.

Legal Analysis

In *Miller* v. *Medical Center of Southwest Louisiana*, the patient presented to the ED after an automobile accident.[6] The physician thought the patient would benefit from transfer to a facility with orthopedic and surgical capability. He contacted for transfer, the patient was accepted, but the original facility was allegedly notified by the receiving hospital administrator not to send the patient due to lack of insurance. The family filed suit citing an Emergency Medical Treatment and Labor Act (EMTALA) claim.[7] The district court held that the patient never "came to" the receiving hospital proper within the meaning of the statute, granting the defendant motion to dismiss for failure to state a claim.[8] The plaintiff appealed and the United States Court of Appeals (USCA), Fifth Circuit affirmed that the receiving hospital was not obliged to provide care as the patient did not truly present for care. They cited *Johnson* v. *University of Chicago Hosp*, in which a centralized telemetry-based paramedic control center directed hospital transports.[9] The paramedics were notified of a pediatric patient who stopped breathing, and the telemetry operator directed them to transport past a closer facility. The family sued, the trial court dismissed, and the USCA, Seventh Circuit upheld the claim dismissal. Again, they held that the baby "never came to" the hospital and never crossed the threshold of EMTALA liability.

In *Collins* v. *DePaul Hospital*, the patient presented to the ED after a severe accident. Most of his injuries were addressed, except for a hip fracture that was not radiographed.[10] He presented in an unconscious condition and was poorly communicative for a large proportion of his stay. He was discharged that month, and allegedly told to follow up with another physician on an outpatient basis. The patient filed suit, alleging "lost opportunity" for correction of hip fracture, and the district court granted the hospital's summary

judgment motion. The USCA, Tenth Circuit affirmed the trial court decision, holding that EMTALA addressed the screening process.[7] The patient was not just "sent home," but was treated for almost a month. The missed injury was not due to lack of screening, however, and the claimant has a right to assert a medical malpractice action.

Conclusion

To be clear, hospitals try to accommodate family requests and wishes almost all the time. However, they are not mandated to admit a patient simply because the family requests it. It is important to note that family opinion about a patient recovery's is important. They obviously know their family member better than the health-care professionals involved, but this is just one factor in the decision-making that is done by a comprehensive multidisciplinary team.

References

1. Walker AF. The legal duty of physicians and hospitals to provide emergency care. *CMAJ*. 2002;166 (4):465–469.

2. New York Bureau of Emergency Medical Services. Emergency Patient Destinations and Hospital Diversion. Policy Statement 06-0. January 11, 2006.

3. Illinois Department of Human Services. Emergency Medicine Coverage for Non-citizens. March 21, 2003.

4. Patient Protection and Affordable Care Act (Public Act 111–148), 42 U.S.C. & 18001 et seq. (2010).

5. Grandfathered Health Insurance Plans. www .healthcare.gov. Accessed May 30, 2016.

6. *Miller* v. *Medical Center of Southwest Louisiana*, 22 F.3d 626 (1994).

7. EMTALA, U.S.C. §1395dd (a).

8. Federal Rules of Civil Procedure Rule 12 (b) (6): Motion for Failure to State a Claim.

9. *Johnson* v. *University of Chicago Hosp.*, 982. F.2d 230 (1992).

10. *Collins* v. *DePaul Hospital*, 963 F.2d 303 (1992).

Mandatory Reporting

Case

When the patient present to the emergency department (ED) he looked dehydrated, with nausea and vomiting for days. He had a slight fever at home but was otherwise healthy. There was no travel history, no other health conditions, but he felt sick for a day or two and then had profuse diarrhea, too many events to count. He worked in the food industry, and was a back-line cook in a restaurant.

The standard laboratory screening tests showed an elevated white blood cell count, normal urinalysis, and no laboratory evidence of dehydration. He was given fluids and anti-nausea medication, and stool cultures were performed. He was discharged home with a work excuse until symptoms resolved completely, and oral rehydration instructions. Two days later his stool culture was found positive for shigella, an antibiotic prescription was called in, and the appropriate notification was made to the county health agency, as this was a mandatory disease reporting requirement.

Two weeks later, the risk manager called the ED, telling them that the patient had requested compensation for his time off work. He also asserted the hospital had violated his confidentiality by reporting this infectious diarrhea to his workplace. He was forced to stay off work for a week and wanted to be paid for the lost time. The ED physician informed the risk management department this was a reportable infectious disease and they were obliged to file a report with the county health department. It was the physician who had contacted his workplace as this was a local statutory requirement. The hospital only informed the patient of his culture results.

Medical Approach

It is important to realize there are mandatory reporting requirements for numerous communicable disease conditions. Requirements vary by state, county,

or local jurisdiction and every practitioner should know the requirements in their area. A formalized approach involving the laboratory follow-up process should be used to notify the patient, and if there is a requirement to report to government agencies the report should be formally documented.

Mandatory reporting statutes require designated individuals to report certain illnesses, injuries, or cases of neglect to regulatory or law enforcement agencies, usually with the assistance of social services. There are statutory obligations to report cases of child abuse, elderly abuse, sexual assault, domestic violence, gunshot wounds, and vulnerable adults at risk for harm.[1] The mandatory reporting statutes require and empower the ED physician to notify a monitoring agency of a tracked event or action.

The communicable disease reporting requirements are probably most widely known by practitioners. The New York State Sanitary Code imposes these requirements on the physicians primarily to report specified diseases to the local health department within 24 hours of diagnosis.[2] The New Jersey Administrative Code requires reporting for communicable diseases and work-related conditions.[3] Here, based on the pathogen concerned, reporting for confirmed or suspected cases is required either immediately or within 24 hours of diagnosis, some to the local health department and some to the state department of health. As well, the state has a provision for occupational exposure, environmental disease, injuries, and poisonings.

Surveillance is a key component of the public health overall assessment process. Roush et. al. performed an analysis of 58 diseases and conditions recommended for national reporting.[4] They found 33% (19) of the diseases were reportable in all states, 60% (35) were reportable in 90% of states, 26% (15) in 75–90% of states, and 14% (8) in less than 75% of states. There is significant variability in reporting requirements, so it is essential for providers to know their local requirements.

The laboratory system is an integral part of the surveillance process. The Vermont Department of Health reviewed 2035 reports of selected notifiable diseases, in which 80.3% were confirmed cases.[5] The laboratory provided 71% (1160) of the referred cases. Physicians indicated that 18% always reported notifiable cases. The most frequently cited reason for physicians not to report was that was the laboratory would do the reporting.

Tan evaluated a cohort of 1250 clinics with 1093 private physicians, in which 37.2% (406) of physicians reported a communicable disease at some point.[6] They cited various reasons not to report including privacy violation, troublesome procedure, and not sure whether it was reportable. The largest proportion (62.5%) of non-reporting physicians suggested a simplified reporting approach would help.

Legal Analysis

One of the most difficult areas of mandatory reporting involves employment-related issues. In *Leckelt v. Board of Commissioners of Hospital District No.1*, the employee, a licensed practical nurse, appealed his dismissal from a local county hospital.[7] He functioned as a nurse in the ED and intensive care unit (ICU) wearing gloves for sterile procedures, but not for intravenous starts and dressing changes. The facility in which he worked required he submit to testing for infectious diseases and refused to permit him to work until he submitted the results, which he declined to do. Following a bench trial, the court concluded that:

> the hospital has the right to require such testing, of an employee who has a high risk of infectious disease in order to fulfill their obligation to its employees and the public concerning infection control and health and safety in general, and termination is justified for refusal.

On appeal the claimant alleged violations of the Federal Rehabilitation Act of 1973, the Louisiana Civil Rights For Handicapped Persons Act, the Equal Protection Clause of the Fourteenth Amendment and Right to Privacy under the Fourth and Fourteenth Amendments.[8-12] The appeal court held that the facility's strong interest in maintaining a safe workplace through infection control outweighed the limited intrusion on any privacy interest of the employee in the test results.

Table 63.1 Persons required to report suspected child abuse

1.	Licensed physician
2.	Osteopath
3.	Medical examiner
4.	Coroner
5.	Funeral director
6.	Dentist
7.	Optometrist
8.	Chiropractor
9.	Podiatrist
10.	Intern
11.	Registered nurse
12.	Licensed practical nurse
13.	Hospital personnel engaged in admission, examination, care, or treatment
14.	Christian Science practitioner
15.	School administrator
16.	Schoolteacher
17.	School nurse
18.	Social services worker
19.	Daycare center worker
20.	Childcare worker
21.	Foster care worker
22.	Mental health professional
23.	Peace officer
24.	Law enforcement official

Reference: Pennsylvania Consolidated Statutes.[14]

In *Heinrich* v. *Conemaugh Valley Memorial Hospital*, a pediatric patient had a fall from a walker at home, and 2 days later was taken to the family's pediatrician for an ear infection.[13] The child was taken to the ED after the mother noticed posterior auricular swelling. A number of interventions were performed by the ED staff in consult with the pediatrician, and concerns over suspected child abuse were discussed with the family. These concerns were reported to the proper authorities, and the family filed suit alleging corporate negligence, defamation, and intentional infliction of emotional distress. The trial court granted preliminary objections, in the nature of a demurrer from the hospital appellees, which was affirmed by the Superior Court of Pennsylvania. They held there was no dispute, in that there was both a mandatory reporting obligation and immunity. The general rule is that if anyone has "reasonable cause to suspect" that a child coming before them in the course of their employment or profession is a victim of abuse, they must report it, and that report is privileged.[14] Persons required to report (but are not limited to) are listed in Table 63.1. A person or institution participating in good faith in a report or investigation of suspected child abuse is immune from any liability that may result from these actions.[14]

Conclusion

It can be difficult for patients to understand a mandatory reporting strategy, as they hear so much about patient confidentiality and privacy. When assessing for diseases or conditions that have a mandatory reporting requirement it is helpful to explain this at the start.

References

1. Mindlin J, Brandl B. Respecting elders, protecting elders: untangling the mystery of what sexual assault advocates need to know about the mandatory reporting of elder abuse. *National Clearinghouse on Abuse in Later Life (NCALL)*, 2011.

2. Communicable Disease Reporting Requirements (10 NYCRR 2.10.2.14). New York State Department of Health. DOH-389. February 2011.

3. New Jersey Administrative Code Title 8, Chapters 57, 58. July 2013.

4. Roush S, Birkhead G, Koo D, Cobb A, Fleming D. Mandatory reporting of diseases and conditions by health care professionals and laboratories. *JAMA*. 1999;282(2):164–170. DOI:10.1001/jama.282.2.164.

5. Schramm MM, Vogt RL, Mamolen M. The surveillance of communicable disease in Vermont: who reports? *Pub Health Rep*. 1991;106(1):95–97.

6. Tan HF, Yeh CY, Chang HW, Chang CK, Tseng HF. Private doctors' practices, knowledge, and attitude to reporting of communicable diseases: a national survey in Taiwan. *BMC Infect Dis*. 2009;9(11):1–8. DOI:10.1186/1471-2334-9-11.

7. *Leckelt v. Board of Commissioners of Hospital District No. 1*, 909 F.2d 820 (1990).

8. Louisiana Laws Revised Statutes. Civil Rights for Handicapped Persons Act: RS 46:2251 (2013).

9. Federal Rehabilitation Act of 1973, 29 U.S.C. §701 et seq.

10. Louisiana Civil Rights for Handicapped Persons Act, R.S. 46:2251 et seq.

11. U.S. Const. Amend. IV.

12. U.S. Const. Amend. V.

13. *Heinrich* v. *Conemaugh Memorial Hospital*, 648 A.2d 53 (1994).

14. Pennsylvania Consolidated Statutes 23 Pa.C.S. §6311 Domestic Relations, §6318 Immunity From Liability.

Medical Education

Case

The resident physician completed her second year of residency, and performed quite admirably. She was a good clinician, with good communication skills and a good interface with the patients. She was considering fellowship training and she filled out an additional application at her institution. The application had a long list of questions concerning out-of-hospital behaviors. She answered "no" to all the above questions, although thinking hard about one of them.

The rotation was busy, and the resident physician had not heard much about her fellowship application. However, a month later she was summoned by the residency director for a meeting. It appears there had been an issue when she was a minor that resulted in her arrest, and she had neglected to mention this on the application. In addition to concerns about her fellowship application, the director looked retrospectively at the residency application and was concerned that the same answers were listed there. The residency committee was convened to discuss the issue, questioning the physician's honesty and integrity.

She stated that she thought this issue was unrelated, as she was told the charges had been dismissed. However, a criminal background check did not corroborate this information, and the charges still appeared to be active. The physician was placed on probation from the residency and transferred to another program in a different city.

Medical Approach

Numerous issues may arise in a residency training program, relating to education, performance, regulatory issues, or public awareness. However, it is important to realize there are various levels of scrutiny and concern regarding honesty and integrity issues in training programs, as well as medical licensure in general.

The key is heightened awareness at times of stress and transition. Yao and Wright performed a national survey of internal medicine residency program directors to define the characteristics of "problem residents."[1] The "problem resident" was defined as "a trainee who demonstrates a significant enough problem that requires intervention by someone of authority." They solicited 404 programs with a 74% (298) response rate. The mean point prevalence of problem residents was 6.9% (SD 5.7%) with a range of 0–39% (Table 64.1). However, 94% of programs acknowledged having a problem resident at some point. The most frequently reported difficulties included

Table 64.1 Survey of "problem residents" in internal medicine training programs

Programs (404)	94% issue at some point	
Prevalence	6.9% (0–39%)	
Issues		**Incidence (%)**
Difficulties		
1. Insufficient medical knowledge		48
2. Poor clinical judgment		44
3. Inefficient time use		44
Problems		
4. Stressors		42
5. Depression		24
Identifier		
6. Chief resident		84
7. Attending physician		76
8. Resident self-report		2
Intervention		
9. Feedback sessions		65
10. Structured supervision		53

Reference: Yao and Wright.[1]

Table 64.2 Emergency medicine residency application inaccuracies

Inaccuracy	Significance % (95% CI)
1. Misrepresentation	
N = 173	
Single	13.3 (8.8–19.5)
Multiple	4.0 (1.8–8.5)
2. Authorship	
N = 47 (27.2%)	
Single	21.3 (11.2–36.1)
Multiple	12.8 (5.3–26.4)
3. AOA membership	
N = 14 (8.1%)	35.7 (14.0–64.4)
4. Advanced degree	
N = 15 (8.7%)	26.7 (8.9–55.2)

Reference: Roellig and Katz.[2]

Table 64.3 Residency interview: potentially discriminatory questions

Interview question	Incidence (%)
1. Marital status	86
2. Where born	54
3. About children	31
4. Religious or ethical beliefs	24
5. National origin	15
6. Plans for pregnancy	10

Reference: Santen et al.[3]

insufficient medical knowledge (48%), poor clinical judgment (44%), and inefficient use of time (44%). Accompanying problems identified included stressors (42%) and depression (24%). Issues were most frequently identified by the chief resident (84%) or the attending physician (76%), but rarely by the residents themselves (2%). They stressed that frequent feedback sessions (65%) and structured supervision (53%) were the most helpful interventions.

Honesty and integrity are important cornerstones of the medical profession. Roellig and Katz studied inaccuracies in emergency medicine residency training applications.[2] They screened 194 (58.3%) applications and 173 (89.1%) were enrolled in the study. There was a single misrepresentation in 13.3% (23) and multiple misrepresentations in 4.0% (7) (Table 64.2). Authorship of at least one peer-reviewed article was improperly claimed by 27.2% (47), with 21.3% (10) having one inaccuracy and 12.8% (6) having two or more. American Osteopathic Association (AOA) membership was claimed by 8.1% (14), but 35.7% (5) were inaccurate. Advanced degrees were claimed by 8.7% (15) and 26.7% (4) were in error. It is essential to verify application claims.

Conversely, incoming residents may raise concerns about the programs. Santen et al. surveyed fourth-year medical students from a single institution, in which 90% of the 63 respondents felt they were asked a discriminatory question (Table 64.3).[3] They were asked about marital status (86%), where they were born (54%) and/or their national origin (15%), whether they had children (31%), their religious or ethical beliefs (24%), and any plans for pregnancy (10%). Most felt they were asked at least one discriminatory question, but this typically did not affect their program ranking.

Although litigation seems more pervasive in medical education, there has always been a general undercurrent at all stages of the health-care continuum. Helms and Helms analyzed 40 years of resident training litigation.[4] They identified 174 legal decisions, in which 22% (38) involved disputes over general programmatic issues. The majority addressed administrative decision-making, especially relating to the dismissal of residents from a program. The programs were more likely to prevail than the resident claimant. Helms and Helms recommend attempts at accommodation, although they found it unlikely to decrease the incidence of litigation.

Minicucci and Lewis analyzed medical education litigation.[5] They found the majority of claims filed against institutions by medical education participants concern termination of residents from their respective institution. The claimant most often cited discrimination or failure to provide adequate due-process protections. They recommend documenting all residency-relevant events, both positive and negative, and ensuring there are proper policies and protocols to deal with this issue.

The advent of the Rehabilitation Act of 1973 Section 504 and the Americans with Disabilities Act

Table 64.4 Medical education and disability interface

1. Qualified physicians with disabilities
2. Essential tasks to be performed
3. Reasonable accommodations
4. Communication: student, faculty, administrator

Reference: Helms and Helms[4]

(ADA) of 1990 are at the forefront of litigation involving some students with disabilities and health-care programs.[6,7] The courts and medical educators will help to refine policies to help identify people with disabilities and assist in avoiding the issue.[8] Important criteria include: (1) when physicians with disabilities are otherwise qualified; (2) what are the essential tasks performed by the physician; (3) what are reasonable accommodations; (4) how communication concerning disability should be accomplished involving administrators, faculty, and students (Table 64.4).

Legal Analysis

In *Buchwald* v. *University of New Mexico School of Medicine (UNMSM)*, the medical school had a stated policy that, all things being equal, they would favor long-term over short-term state residents in the admission process.[9] The district court found this preference to violate "clearly established" law concerning the fundamental right to travel and ruled that admissions officials were not entitled to qualified immunity. The court issued an injunction prohibiting the use of length of residency in admission decisions and the interlocutory appeal followed. The United States Courts of Appeal (USCA), Tenth Circuit held that the plaintiff did not have standing to bring the suit and vacated the injunction. Likewise, the institutional defendants are immune from suit based on the Eleventh Amendment, "the judicial power of the United States shall not be construed to extend to any suit in law or equity, commenced or prosecuted against one of the United States by citizens of another state, or by citizens or subjects of any foreign state."[10] The district court was reversed where it allowed the suit to proceed against the UNMSM Board of Regents or Admissions Committee, and the denial of defendant's summary judgment motion to dismiss. However, the appeal court affirmed the district court decision that permitted the plaintiff to seek injunctive relief to immediately place her in the entering class under

the *Ex parte Young* exception and remanded for further consideration. The *Ex parte Young* case allowed the suit to proceed as the state official was not acting on behalf of the state when he sought to enforce an unconstitutional law.[11]

In *Doe* v. *National Board of Medical Examiners*, the medical student took the US Medical Licensing Examination Steps 1 and 2 with accommodations under Title III of the ADA.[12,13] The accommodation allowed extra testing time, and this was noted on the final testing result. He applied for residency and sought a motion for an injunction to prohibit the National Board of Medical Examiners from annotating his scores, as in his opinion he would be irreversibly harmed by this. The district court granted his motion, in that he had standing to sue and reasonable likelihood of success on his claim of taint and the irreparable harm that could occur. The USCA, Third Circuit held that the plaintiff failed to meet his burden under Section 309 of the ADA, proving his scores were comparable to the non-accommodated scores in terms of proving future success. As well, they felt the proper filing was under Section 309 specifically covering examinations, not Section 302 governing public accommodations. They vacated the order granting the preliminary injunction.

In *Roth* v. *Lutheran General Hospital*, the claimant applied to medical school acknowledging a problem with his vision, "that no longer confronts him."[14] He had difficulty early in his medical training with visual fine detail work, saw an ophthalmologist, was diagnosed with fatigue-induced visual impairment, and requested accommodation. The school offered a modified schedule featuring no night call, lighter rotation schedules, and no requirement to perform surgical procedures. He filed a complaint with the US Department of Education due to a low clerkship grade. They concluded he was an individual with disabilities under both the ADA and the Rehabilitation Act (RA), and both Acts were violated. He completed his medical school curriculum in the top 25% of his class, and the grade was reevaluated.[6,7] He filed additional complaints concerning an honor society application and other clerkship grades, which were not found to be consistent with discrimination. He then applied to residency, had numerous discussions with faculty advisers, with some discussion of his visual issues and disagreement on his ranking and did not match for a residency position at that site. Although he attempted to solicit a residency position before the match, he did not contact the residency program for an unmatched open training spot afterward. He reapplied the next year, did not match, and did not seek an additional open spot after the match. He alleged retaliation for his disability and filed for injunctive relief to compel admission, which was denied. The USCA, Seventh Circuit affirmed the trial court denial. They held that the legislative intent of the ADA and RA are to integrate people with a disability into the economic and social mainstream, and to ensure they will not be stereotyped for any impairment. However, there is a clear line of demarcation between extending the statutory protection to a person with a disability and allowing an individual with marginal impairment to use the disability laws as bargaining chips to obtain an unfair advantage.[15]

In *Jakubowski* v. *Christ Hospital*, the resident obtained his program portion after a failure to match, allegedly had difficulties, had a remediation period, and had his contract not renewed after his internship year.[16] He filed suit against his residency program and director for lack of accommodation, alleging violations of the RA (29 U.S.C. §794),[6] the ADA (42 U.S.C. §12112),[7] and the Ohio Revised Code (§4112.02).[17] The defendants moved for summary judgment, which the district court granted. The USCA, Sixth Circuit affirmed, noting that for the accommodation to be successfully applied, the claimant must prove a baseline competence and the chance of success may not be too attenuated.

In *Hernandez* v. *State Board of Registration for the Healing Arts*, the plaintiff applied for a license to practice in that state, and that inquiry requested additional information about his residency training.[18] He did not complete the residency program, allegedly at the program's request. After three requests, a non-supportive reference was offered. He moved to another state seeking a new residency program. He was offered an administrative forum to discuss the matter, which he participated in. However, they voted to deny the licensure application, as they cited moral character concerns over an alleged misrepresentation on his application, in which he answered no to a question concerning probation or withdrawal based on a provision of Chapter 324 RSMo 1995.[19] The claimant appealed the denial of license to practice medicine, the circuit court reversed the decision of the Administrative Hearing Commission of the State Board of Registration for the Healing Arts, and the claimant sought compensation for legal fees. The Missouri Court of Appeals reversed the trial court's overturning of the board's decision, and declined the payment of attorney's fees. They held that the declination decision was justified, and the license request could have been denied without offering the administrative forum.

Conclusion

The key is honesty and sincerity when there appears to be a conflict that may be related to integrity. It is best to discuss the issue as early as possible in the process, often bringing it to the applicant's attention before it becomes public, so that a proper remedy may be addressed. Legal advice is always helpful in complicated situations.

References

1. Yao DC, Wright S. National survey of internal medicine residency program directors regarding problem residents. *JAMA*. 2000;284(9):1099–1104. DOI:10.1001/jama.284.9.1099.

2. Roellig MS, Katz ED. Inaccuracies on applications for emergency medicine residency training. *Acad Emerg Med*. 2004;11(9):992–994. DOI:10.1197/j.aem.2004.04.010.

3. Santen SA, Davis KR, Brady DW, Hemphill RR. Potentially discriminatory questions during residency interviews: frequency and effects on residents' ranking of programs in the National Resident Matching Program. *J Grad Med Educ*. 2010;(3):336–340. DOI:10.4300/JGME-D-10-00041.1.

4. Helms LB, Helms CM. Forty years of litigation involving residents and their training: I. General programatic issues. *Acad Med*. 1991;66(11):649–655.

5. Minicucci RF, Lewis BF. Trouble in academia: ten years of litigation in medical education. *Acad Med*. 2003;78(10):S13–S15.

6. Rehabilitation Act of 1973 §504.

7. Americans with Disabilities Act of 1990, 42 U.S.C §12101.

8. Helms LB, Helms CM. Medical education and disability discrimination: the law and future implications. *Acad Med*. 1994;69(7):535–543.

9. *Buchwald* v. *University of New Mexico School of Medicine*, 159 F.3d 487 (1998).

10. U.S. Const. Amend. XI.

11. Ex parte Edward T. Young, Petitioner, 209 U.S. 123 (1908).

12. *Doe* v. *National Board of Medical Examiners*, 199 F.3d 146 (1999).

13. Americans with Disabilities Act (ADA), 42 U.S.C §1281 et seq. Title III, 322, 543.

14. *Roth* v. *Lutheran General Hospital*, 57 F.3d 1446 (1995).

15. *McWright* v. *Alexander*, 982 F.2d 222 (7th Cir. 1992).

16. *Jakubowski* v. *Christ Hospital, Inc.*, 627 F.3d 195 (2010).

17. Ohio Revised Code §4112.02: Unlawful Discriminatory Practices.

18. *Hernandez* v. *State Board of Registration for the Healing Arts*, WD 52275, January 21, 1997.

19. Revised Statutes Missouri Chapter 334 (1995).

Chapter 65

Medical Errors

Case

An external consulting group suggested to hospital administration that medical errors should be tracked as a way to minimize medical malpractice. The medical errors were already being tracked and there was a departmental morbidity and mortality conference to document, address, and develop a remediation program to avoid these errors. The consultants suggested that this was indeed a good idea, but that "near-miss" events should be tracked as well to improve quality and minimize medical malpractice risk. The medical director established a reporting mechanism for near-miss events and went through the same planning process to address issues in the future and avoid litigation.

At the next interdepartmental meeting, one of the staff physicians said she understood the first part of the process, but asked about the evidence for the correlation of near misses with litigation. Her reading on this matter indicated that the correlation between either adverse medical events or near-miss events and subsequent medical malpractice litigation is tenuous at best. The director asked the physician to comply with the departmental request. The research on the issue could be re-presented at the next faculty staff meeting, but in the interim patient care was always paramount and the hospital should do as much as possible to minimize risk and improve care for patients.

Medical Approach

The literature is replete with papers associating adverse medical events with subsequent detrimental impact on patient care, as well as some increase in medical malpractice. Other research has correlated medical malpractice litigation with factors other than adverse events, and in fact some papers have suggested the adverse event itself has no correlation whatsoever with subsequent medical malpractice.

Medical error is a patient outcome that is unexpected, or otherwise not predictable based on the patient and provider circumstances, in which the conventional standards of care are applied. The medicolegal focus is on failure to diagnose, failure to treat, procedural error, failure to consult, or failure to refer, among other possibilities.

The Harvard Medical Practice Study was one of the first to evaluate the relationship between adverse events due to negligence and subsequent malpractice claims.[1] There were 47 malpractice claims among the 30,195 initial emergency department (ED) visits. The overall rate of claims was 0.13% (95% CI 0.076–0.18%). The cohort of patients (8/280) who had an adverse event occur was 1.53% (95% CI 0–3.2%). They estimated the statewide ratio of negligent adverse events (27,179) to malpractice claims (3570) as 7.6 to 1. Therefore, they concluded that the relationship between adverse events and malpractice is more attenuated than is often assumed.

Our understanding is facilitated by appreciating the perception of medical errors by physicians and the public. Blendon et al. evaluated surveys returned by 831 practicing physicians and 1207 members of the public.[2] At that time, 42% of the public and 35% of the physicians reported errors in their own, or a family member's care. Neither group felt this had particular impact on the health care provided. Education is clearly useful in helping the patient, and their family members, understand the significance of the adverse event and its impact on patient care, not just the effect on malpractice.

Another area of focus is patients' and physicians' attitudes regarding disclosure of medical error. Gallagher et al. evaluated focus groups consisting of 52 patients and 46 physicians for their opinions on disclosure of medical errors.[3] The patients wanted full event disclosure: what happened, why the error happened, how the consequences would be mitigated, and plans for prevention of recurrence. Most importantly, they wanted emotional support from the physician if an error occurred, including an apology. The physicians were reticent, however, thinking an apology would create legal liability. As well, the physicians were upset when an error occurred, but were uncertain where they should seek support.

In fact, a work-related error can compound any job-related stress physicians experience. Waterman et al. surveyed an eligible group of 64% (3171/4990) of physicians, examining the effect of error on work and life domains.[4] Physicians involved in a major error experienced anxiety concerning future errors (61%), loss of confidence (44%), sleeping difficulties (42%), reduced job satisfaction (42%), and harm to reputation (13%) (Table 65.1). However, one-third of physicians felt near-miss events also increased their stress. They were more likely to be distressed after serious errors, when they were dissatisfied with error disclosure process, perceived a greater risk of being sued, spent more than 75% of their time in clinical practice, or were female (Table 65.2). Most importantly, only 10% of physicians felt they were adequately supported by the health-care system, a crucial consideration to note.

An important consideration from the patient perspective is to examine the relationship between poor service quality, adverse events, and medical error. Taylor et al. reported on a cohort of patients of whom 80.2% (183/228) reported a perceived quality deficiency in their care.[5] Interestingly, appraisal of objective criteria by chart review found a 28.4% (52/183) incidence of actual adverse events. These were categorized as adverse events (65.3%, 34), close calls (21.1%, 11), and low-risk errors (13.4%, 7). The presence of any service quality deficiency more than doubles the odds of any adverse event, close call, or low-risk error (OR 2.5, 95% CI 1.2–5.4) Specifically, service quality deficiencies involving poor quality of care (OR 4.4, 95% CI 1.4–14.0) were associated with the occurrence of adverse events and medical errors. It is important to recognize that patients' subjective impressions of their care can be helpful to improve system quality.

A significant amount of research has been directed at early medical error disclosure programs. Kachalia et al. described an early disclosure program with offer of compensation, in which the monthly rate of new claims decreased significantly from 7.03 to 4.52 per 100,000 patient encounters (RR 0.64, CI 0.44–0.95); the monthly rate of lawsuits decreased from 2.13 to 0.75 (RR 0.35, CI 0.22–0.58).[6] The median time to claim resolution decreased from 1.36 to 0.95 years. There were financial benefits as well, with the average monthly cost rates decreased for total liability (RR 0.41, CI 0.26–0.66), patient compensation (RR 0.41, CI 0.26–0.67), and legal costs (RR 0.39. CI 0.22–0.67) Early disclosure programs such as this one should be considered in the medicolegal setting.

Legal Analysis

In *Evitt* v. *University Heights Hospital*, the patient presented to the emergency department (ED) with severe chest pain that worsened with inspiration and movement.[7] The patient arrived at 2:30 a.m. and was allegedly discharged in 35 minutes, with instructions to apply heat and contact her primary care physician (PCP) in the morning. The discharge noted her to be non-urgent and stable on discharge. She returned almost 12 hours later and was admitted with a critical cardiac condition. The plaintiff filed suit alleging the Emergency Medical Treatment and Labor Act (EMTALA) failure to screen (§42 U.S.C.1395a) and in the alternative failure to stabilize (§1395b) or to transfer (§1395c).[8] The district court heard the federal

Table 65.1 Physician job-related stress due to medical error

	Issue (%)	Incidence (%)
1.	Anxiety about future error	61
2.	Loss of confidence	44
3.	Sleeping difficulties	42
4.	Reduced job satisfaction	42
5.	Harm to reputation	13

Reference: Waterman et al.[4]

Table 65.2 Physician distress related to serious error

	Issue	Analysis OR (CI)
1.	Dissatisfied with error disclosure	3.86 (1.66, 9.00)
2.	Perceived greater lawsuit likelihood	0.28 (1.50, 3.48)
3.	Clinical practice time (>75%)	2.20 (1.60, 3.01)
4.	Female	1.91 (1.21, 3.02)

Reference: Waterman et al.[4]

case and entered summary judgment in favor of the defendant, without prejudice to the state court action. It was undisputed that the hospital had sufficient staff and equipment to perform the appropriate medical screening exam, and that she received that exam deemed appropriate by the physician. No evidence was offered that she was turned away from the hospital for economic reasons.

In *Molzof* v. *United States*, the patient underwent lung surgery at a Veterans Administration (VA) Hospital, and in the postoperative period there was a ventilator and alarm disconnection, allegedly due to employee negligence, resulting in an anoxic injury.[9] The guardian ad litem filed suit invoking the Federal Tort Claims Act (FTCA) seeking damages for supplemental medical care, future medical care, and loss of enjoyment.[10] The Government admitted liability. The district court awarded continuing free care at the VA, as well as a supplemental care stipend for additional services. However, they did not award damages for duplicative care or for loss of enjoyment. The United States Court of Appeals, Seventh Circuit affirmed any future award of care would be punitive and it was uncertain whether a patient who is in a coma could sustain loss of enjoyment. The Supreme Court of the United States granted certiorari and held that the FTCA provides: "The United States shall be liable, respecting the provisions of this title relating to tort claims, in the same manner and to the same extent as a private individual under like circumstances, but shall not be liable for interest prior to judgment or for punitive damages." 28 U.S.C. §2674.[11] The Supreme Court reversed the appeal court decision and remanded, holding the true intent of recovery in this case was not "punitive" damages sought by the plaintiff. Their recoverability does not depend on proof the defendant has engaged in egregious misconduct, and the sought damages were not meant to punish in the common-law punitive sense.

In *Kramer* v. *Lewisville Memorial Hospital*, the patient had multiple visits to two separate gynecologists for discharge and bleeding, with negative Pap smears reviewed by multiple cytopathology technicians.[12] After continued bleeding, cancer was diagnosed, she was admitted to the hospital, had subsequent ED visits for bleeding, and eventually succumbed to the cancer. Her representative filed suit under the Texas Wrongful Death Act and the Texas Survivorship Statute.[13,14] Before trial the complaint was amended to include the common law premise of "lost chance of survival or cure," stating the patient's chance of survival was significantly worsened by the alleged delay in diagnosis. The trial court rendered a "take-nothing" judgment in favor of the hospital and the appeal court affirmed. The Supreme Court of Texas affirmed the judgment as well. They held that liability for negligent treatment that decreases a patient's chance of avoiding death and other medical conditions, in cases where the adverse result probably would have occurred anyway, is not offered in the pled statutes.

In *Morlino* v. *Medical Center of Ocean County*, the patient, who was 8.5 months pregnant, presented to the ED with a sore throat and was treated with ciprofloxacin.[15] The next day an ultrasound scan revealed the fetus was deceased. The patient filed suit, and a trial court jury gave a unanimous verdict for the defense. There were two issues on appeal: first, the submission of the *Physicians' Desk Reference* (PDR) package insert as evidence of physician standard of care; second, jury instruction in line with the Model Jury Charge 5.36 (A): Exercise of Judgment, that a physician is not liable for diagnosis or treatment resulting from the exercise of the physician's judgment.[16] The appeal court held that a PDR warning is admissible in conjunction with expert testimony, and admissible as a standard of care, but not as prima facie evidence of negligence. As well, they upheld the "exercise of judgment" instruction. The Supreme Court of New Jersey affirmed the judgment of the appeal court. No new trial was ordered.

Conclusion

There is a suggestion that adverse medical events have been associated with worsened patient care outcomes. The correlation is certainly strong enough that we should continue on this path, tracking for near misses and adverse events to improve the quality of care, while still recognizing that the association with medical malpractice litigation may be less clear.

References

1. Localio AR, Lawthers AG, Brennan TA, Laird NM, Hebert LE, Peterson LM, et al. Relation between malpractice claims and adverse events due to negligence – results of the Harvard Medical

Practice Study. *N Engl J Med.* 1981;325(4):245–251. DOI:10.1056/nejm199107253259405.

2. Blendon RJ, DesRoches CM, Brodie M, Benson JM, Rosen AB, Schneider E, et al. Views of practicing physicians and the public on medical error. *N Engl J Med.* 2002;347(24):1933–1940. DOI:10.1056/nejmsa022151.

3. Gallagher TH, Waterman AD, Ebers AG, Fraser VJ, Levinson W. Patients' and physicians' attitudes regarding the disclosure of medical errors. *JAMA.* 2003;289(8):1001–1007. DOI:10.1001/jama 289.8.1001.

4. Waterman AD, Garbutt J, Hazel E, Dunagan WC, Levinson W, Fraser VJ, Gallagher TH. The emotional impact of medical errors on practicing physicians in the United States and Canada. *Joint Comm J Qual Pat Safe.* 2007;33(8):467–476.

5. Taylor B, Marcantonio ER, Pagovich O, Carbo A, Bergmann M, Davis RB, et al. Do medical inpatients who report poor service quality experience more adverse events and medical errors? *Med Care.* 2008;46(2):224–228. DOI:10.1079/MLR.0b013e3181589ba4.

6. Kachalia A, Kaufman SR, Boothman R, Anderson S, Welch K, Saint S, Rogers MAM. Liability claims before and after implementation of a medical error disclosure program. *Ann Intern Med.* 2010;153(4):213–221. DOI:10.7326/0003-4819-153-4-201008170-00002.

7. *Evitt* v. *University Heights Hospital,* 727 F. Supp. 495 (1989).

8. EMTALA 42 U.S.C. §1395 (a–c).

9. *Molzof* v. *United States,* 502 U.S. 301 (1992).

10. Federal Tort Claims Act (FTCA) 28 U.S.C. §1346 (b).

11. Liability of United States, 28 U.S. Code §2674.

12. *Kramer* v. *Lewisville Memorial Hospital,* 858 S.W.2d 397 (1993).

13. Texas Wrongful Death Act, Tex. Civ. Prac. & Rem. Code §§71.002 & 71.004.

14. Texas Survivorship Statute, Tex. Civ. Prac. & Rem. Code §71.021.

15. *Morlino* v. *Medical Center of Ocean County,* m706 A.2d 721 (1998).

16. *Physician's Desk Reference,* 52nd edition (Montvale, NJ: Medical Economics, 1998).

Chapter 66

Medical Records

Case

The medical director had received a call from the medical chief of staff pointing out that one of the emergency department (ED) physicians had been repeatedly cited by the medical records section for errors, inaccuracies, and delinquency. He had been suspended many times previously and placed on administrative suspension for 30 days at one point in the past. Any additional inadequacy would best be met by limiting hospital staff privileges.

The ED group found examples suggesting that the documentation was inaccurate regarding patients' demographic variables, such as age or sex. Some was still not completed up to 30 days after the event. The director planned to meet and counsel the physician and come up with a contingency coverage plan if he was suspended.

The director met with the physician the next day to discussed these findings. Thy physician's response was that it had to do with the new electronic health record (EHR) system. These errors were being made by the computer system and not by the physician himself. In addition, he stated the reason for the delay in completing some records was that the medical records section did not notify him when paper charts were ready, although their electronic documentation was completed in a timely fashion.

The director recognized the response was accurate in some respects, but suggested it was the physician's responsibility to see the records were completed accurately. They were signed off even though they were incorrect. If there was indeed a difficulty with record retrieval then that could be discussed with the administrative chain to help speed up the process.

There are detailed external guidelines based on recommendations of the Joint Commission and other regulatory agencies that specify the time for adequate medical record completion in outpatients, surgery, and inpatients.

Medical Approach

It is the responsibility of the physician to complete records accurately and in a timely fashion. Errors and inconsistencies need to be reconciled promptly. Seemingly minor errors such as assigning the wrong gender or age give the appearance of inattention to detail, imposing a distinct medicolegal risk. The Department of Health and Human Services (DHHS) Centers for Medicare and Medicaid Services (CMS) through its Interpretive Guidelines for Hospitals (42 C.F.R. 482.24 (c) (1) defines standards for medical record entries: "All patient medical record entries must be legible, complete, dated, timed and authenticated in written or electronic form by the person responsible for providing or evaluating the service provided, consistent with hospital policies and procedures" (Table 66.1).[1]

In addition, the deadlines imposed by the Joint Commission and external regulatory agencies are defined. Medical records need to be completed within a specific period, varying from 24 hours to a 15 to 30-day limit depending on the type of patient encounter, with the physician responsible for completion.

The patient's medical record is entrusted to the hospital and their health-care provider to ensure proper documentation occurs and is acknowledged and authenticated in a timely fashion.

For an EHR there must be proper policy and procedures in place to prevent alteration of record entries after they have been authenticated,[1] and the security features must be readily reviewable by outside surveyors. There must be an established procedure to countersign resident or non-physician notes according to medical staff bylaws. There must be a system that

Table 66.1 Medical record documentation requirements: S 482.24(c)(1)

1. Legible and clear, avoiding misinterpretation
2. Complete to identify, support, justify, and promote continuity of care plan
3. Dated, timed, and authenticated by the responsible party
4. Practitioner signs all written and verbal orders according to policy
5. Demonstrate authorship identification, security, and signature verification

Reference: Medical Records Service.[1]

Table 66.2 Electronic medical record requirements: S 482.24 (c)(1)

1. Procedure to prevent alteration after authentication
2. Security features should be readily reviewable
3. Established procedure to countersign orders
4. System requires review prior to authentication
5. Authentication and performance time (date stamp may be different)

Reference: Medical Records Service.[1]

Table 66.3 Clinical medical record document

1. Medical care and provider communication
2. Facilitate the payment process
3. Establish legal defense
4. Symptom surveillance, public health, research

Reference: Davidson et al.[2]

Table 66.4 Medical record functionality

1. Documentation of clinical findings
2. Record of test and imaging results
3. Computerized physician order entry (CPOE)
4. Clinical decision-making support

Reference: Mangalmurti et al.[3]

and research functions (Table 66.3). Mangalmurti et al. describe the core functionalities of the medical record to include documentation of clinical findings, recording of test and imaging results, computerized physician order entry (CPOE), and clinical decision-making support (Table 66.4).[3]

The Emergency Medicine Information Technology Consensus Conference offered ten general summary points discussing the information technology documentation interface.[4] First, every ED physician should be computer literate and every department should have high-speed internet access. Second, a departmental leader should be appointed. Third, there should be real-time data transfer capability. Fourth, data transfer should be available to support the needs of patients requiring care at other hospitals, Fifth, the clinical systems should be readily available with fast response time, high reliability, and usable interface. Sixth, hardware using wireless and portable technology should be ubiquitous. Seventh, the use of technology for education, management, and clinical care in emergency medicine should measurably improve, or at least not adversely affect, the overall quality of care as demonstrated by qualitative and quantitative analysis. Eighth, online decision support should be seamlessly integrated into all clinical systems. Ninth, emergency medicine training programs are encouraged to use simulation technology as an educational adjunct. Tenth, a data standard, not vendor standard, approach is the pathway to success (Table 66.5).

The relationship between the EHR and malpractice claims is controversial, with a suggestion that high-quality documentation decreases the likelihood of claims. Quinn et al. evaluated an analysis of 14.3% (27/189) physicians who had at least one malpractice claim.[5] Of these 51 claims, 49 came before EHR adoption and two after, with a relative risk of 0.16 (95% CI 0.04–0.71) They reported a six-fold claim reduction in claims after the introduction of an EHR system.

requires review prior to authentication, and does not permit an auto-authentication system. There must be a separate time and date stamp to contemporaneously verify review of an earlier electronically generated document (Table 66.2).

The physician-generated ED clinical document memorializes clinical observations and the decision-making process. Davidson et al.[2] offer four purposes of the clinical document including: (1) recording the medical care and provider communication; (2) providing a record for payment to the hospital and physician; (3) establishing legal defense from allegations of medical malpractice; and (4) offering a mechanism for symptom or disease surveillance, public health,

Table 66.5 Emergency Medicine Information Technology Consensus Conference: recommendations

1.	Computer literacy and department connectivity
2.	Appoint departmental leader
3.	Real-time capability of data transfer
4.	Data transfer to assist patients in external care
5.	Clinical systems should be readily available
6.	Hardware technology should be ubiquitous
7.	Technology should improve and not worsen outcome
8.	Online decision support should be integrated
9.	Emergency medicine training uses simulation technology
10.	Data, not vendor standard approach

Reference: Handler et al.[4]

The effect on office practice was reported by Virapongse et al. in 1140 respondents, in which 33.2% used an EMR.[6] Fewer physicians who utilized an EMR (6.1%) had a history of paid malpractice claims compared to those who did not (10.8%) (OR 0.54, 95% CI 0.33–0.86, $P = 0.01$). However, logistic regression analysis controlling for variables such as year of graduation, specialty, and practice effect saw this difference in malpractice claim lose significance (OR 0.69, 95% CI 0.40–1.20, $P = 0.18$).

Legal Analysis

The caselaw in this area is varied and diverse. In *Maryland State Board of Physicians* v. *Eist*, the treating physician had the records subpoenaed for three patients: the complainant's estranged wife and his two children.[7] In the course of an acrimonious divorce, the complainant alleged his family was overmedicated by the psychiatrist, as this physician had supported the patient's custody rights. In response to the filed complaint, the medical board issued a subpoena duces tecum compelling the physician to produce patient medical records without their consent. The board charged the physician with failing to cooperate with a lawful investigation in violation of the Maryland Code (1981, 2000 Repl. Vol. 2004 Supp.), section 14–404 (a) (33), but peer review supported his position.[8] In judicial review the circuit court reversed the board decision and remanded to the administrative-law judge for consideration, who supported the physician as well. The board again maintained their position that there was failure to cooperate, again reversed by

the circuit court, and affirmed by the Court of Special Appeals of Maryland.

In *Lofton* v. *Greico*, the decedent presented to the ED, where he required surgery. There was delay in consent with differing opinion on etiology, and the patient died before surgery could be completed.[9] The plaintiffs allege that additions to the hospital medical record relating to this consent were not made contemporaneously. The plaintiff argued it was not overburdening to produce the hospital record for review by a handwriting expert. CPLR §3101 (a) requires "full disclosure of all matter material and necessary to the prosecution or defense of an action."[10] The New York Supreme Court ordered that the Order To Show Cause (Mot. Seq. 01) pursuant to CPLR §§3101, 3120, and 3122 was granted to produce the records for inspection, non-destructive examination, and photographing by an expert.

Conclusion

There is a clear judicial predisposition to compel production of medical records in the appropriate circumstances. This order is typically entered into when the medical record contains information essential to the legal analysis. It may be released in this fashion, when a judicial request is lodged, typically with redaction of protected health information or masking precautions.

References

1. Medical Records Service. 42 C.F.R. 482.24 (c)(1), Conditions of Participation.

2. Davidson SJ, Zwemer FL, Nathanson LA, Sable KN, Khan ANGA. Where is the beef? The promise and the reality of clinical documentation. *Acad Emerg Med.* 2004;11(11):1127–1134. DOI:10.1197/j.aem.2004.08.004.

3. Mangalmurti SS, Murtagh L, Mello MM. Medical malpractice liability in the age of electronic health records. *N Engl J Med.* 2010;363(21):2060–2067.

4. Handler JA, Adams JG, Feled CF, Gillam M, Vozenilek J, Barthell EN, Davidson SJ. Emergency Medicine Information Technology Consensus Conference: executive summary. *Acad Emerg Med.* 2004;11(11):1112–1113.

5. Quinn MA, Kats AM, Kleinman K, Bates DW, Simon SR. The relationship between electronic health records and malpractice claims. *Arch Intern Med.* 2012;172(15):1187–1189. DOI:10.1001/archinternmed.2012.2371.

6. Virapongse A, Bates DW, Shi P, Jenter CA, Volk LA, Kleinman K et al. Electronic health records and malpractice claims in office practice. *Arch Intern Med.* 2008;168(21): 2362–2367. DOI:10.1001/archinte.168.21.2362.

7. *Maryland State Board of Medicine v. Eist. Court of Special Appeals of Maryland.* No. 329, Sept Term, 2006.

8. Maryland Code (1981, 2000 Rep.Vol., 2004 Supp.), Section 14–404 (a)(22).

9. *Lofton v. Grieco,* 2012 NY Slip Op 52003 (U).

10. New York Civil Practice Law and Rules §310. Scope of Disclosure.

Chapter 67

Medical Screening Exam

Case

The patient came in to the emergency department (ED) accompanied by his wife. He immediately asked if the facility was a stroke center. The triage nurse answered that they did not have a stroke designation, but they had the capability to take care of stroke patients and then transfer them. His wife said he was having some numbness, but that it got better. The waiting room was full, and patients were lined up to be triaged. The husband said as the facility wasn't a stroke center and he was feeling better now, they would drive downtown to the stroke center they had seen advertised.

The triage nurse reiterated that although the ED was busy, she would get the physician right away since this was an emergent condition, and urged him to stay. However, the husband said "No, I've seen the ads on TV and we're going to the stroke center." The triage nurse asked if they wanted an ambulance called, but they declined.

The remainder of the night was extremely busy. A week later the hospital received notice that a claim had been filed under the Emergency Medical Treatment and Labor Act (EMTALA). The allegation was that the patient had not had a proper medical screening exam (MSE), and should have been transferred to their hospital stroke unit directly rather than being allowed to drive themselves to the facility.

The physician responded that she was not informed of any of the discussions with this patient as the conversation had been with the triage nurse. The understanding was the nurse had offered transport, the patient and his wife declined, and said they would drive to the stroke center since he had felt better. Risk management pointed out that as an EMTALA claim had been filed they would have to generate a response, so the physician would be interviewed.

Medical Approach

There is a requirement that every patient who presents to the ED for emergency care, who has an emergency medical condition, should have an MSE performed by a qualified individual.[1] This is typically a physician-based exam and requires the standard diagnostics, therapeutics, and interventions that would be required for any patient evaluation with that set of circumstances. Some facilities empower an advanced practice provider (APP) to perform the MSE, and some very small or geographically isolated facilities allow a registered nurse (RN) to do it. This would require a hospital bylaws provision, and is very rarely encountered (Table 67.1). The Oregon State Board of Nursing states that the MSE is within the scope of RN practice if the following conditions are met defining the qualified individual (Table 67.2).[2] First, facility bylaws must designate the qualified individual and identify their role in performance. Second, there must be a protocol or algorithm that defines when a licensed independent practitioner who can diagnose and treat must be consulted. Third, the examiner must possess the knowledge and skill necessary to perform the MSE as identified by facility bylaws. Fourth, the examiner

Table 67.1 Medical screening exam

1.	Presents to ED
2.	Emergency medical condition
3.	Qualified medical person
4.	Complete medical evaluation
5.	Ensure stability or transfer to higher level of care

Reference: EMTALA.[1]

Table 67.2 Scope of practice for medical screening exam (MSE)

1.	Bylaws must designate the qualified examiner
2.	Protocol to contact licensed independent practitioner
3.	Knowledge and skill to perform exam
4.	Demonstrate competency to perform exam
5.	Monitor measurable outcome for quality improvement

Reference: Oregon State Board of Nursing.[2]

must demonstrate competency to perform the MSE prior to assignment. Fifth, the facility must evaluate measurable outcomes as part of the quality improvement process.

Routinely, the triage process does not constitute an adequate MSE. In this case, although the patient was counseled to stay, it appears the allegation is that a communication discrepancy allowed them to leave the facility without a physician evaluation, or the availability of transfer to a facility which would be more suitable in this circumstance.

Legal Analysis

In *Cleland* v. *Bronson Health Care Group*, the parents of a pediatric patient complained of their child's cramps and vomiting. The child was diagnosed with influenza, and ultimately succumbed to intussusception.[3] In addition to the medical negligence allegation, the plaintiff invoked the EMTALA medical screening requirement.[1] EMTALA requires the hospital to provide an "appropriate medical screening examination within the capability of the hospital's emergency department to any individual who comes to the ED to seek treatment." If the "hospital determines that the individual has an emergency medical condition, they must be stabilized before discharge or transfer" (42 U.S.C. §1395dd (b) (1) and (c) (1)). The district court held that the congressional intent behind this statute was unlikely to be used as a general malpractice action. They dismissed the complaint as only applying to uninsured patients. The United States Court of Appeals, Sixth Circuit differed in the rationale applying this screening to all patients, but affirmed the overall ruling that neither the screening nor stabilization obligations were breached.

In *Repp* v. *Anadarko Municipal Hospital*, the patient, who had a cardiac history, presented to the hospital after being seen earlier in the day and diagnosed with shingles.[4] The primary care physician

(PCP) was contacted, medications were administered, and the patient was discharged home where he succumbed allegedly to coronary artery disease. His family brought suit under EMTALA alleging deficiency in the medical screening process. The district court granted the physician defendant's motion to dismiss, claiming individual physicians could not be sued under EMTALA. As well, the hospital had a summary judgment granted since there was no dispute as to the material facts that suggested the EMTALA statute was violated. The United States Court of Appeals (USCA), Tenth Circuit affirmed, concluding the hospital had indeed met the screening obligations.

In *Bryant* v. *Adventist Health System/West*, a child with disability presented with fever and cough and was diagnosed with pneumonia.[5] He was administered antibiotics, allegedly without the full dose given, and was discharged home as he was felt to be more comfortable there. The family was recontacted as a lung abscess was noted. The patient was readmitted and it was acknowledged that the abscess was not noted initially. The family alleged an EMTALA claim for failure to properly screen for an emergency medical condition. The district court awarded defendant motion to dismiss, as the facility was not liable since the medical staff missed the condition. The USCA, Ninth Circuit affirmed the trial court decision as they found no credible claim of failure to screen.

In *Esperanza* v. *Sunrise Hospital*, the patient was transferred by ambulance to the ED allegedly "displaying suicidal and homicidal ideation" and was discharged after an evaluation.[6] He then re-presented with family members, was subsequently admitted with precautions to be evaluated as a psychiatric patient, was found unresponsive, and succumbed. The family filed suit alleging emergency care obligations were not met under CFR §489.24.[7] The district court compelled the defendant to comply with interrogatories and requests for production, specifically the "root cause analysis" report concerning the medical screening provided, in this case performed by the hospital safety committee according to NRS 439.875.[8]

Conclusion

The overall judicial trend is clear: the EMTALA medical screening criteria are not substituted for simple medical negligence criteria, but the screening information must be produced in order to reach that conclusion.

References

1. EMTALA 42 U.S.C. §1395 (a-d)).

2. Oregon State Board of Nursing. Role of the Registered Nurse in Performing Medical Screening Examinations Under the Emergency Medical Treatment and Active Labor Act. Board Policy Adopted February, 2005 and Revised September, 2013.

3. *Cleland* v. *Bronson Health Care Group, Inc.* 917 F.2d 266 (1990).

4. *Repp* v. *Anadarko Mun. Hosp.*, 43 F.3d 519 (1994).

5. *Bryant* v. *Adventist Health Systems/West*, 289 F.3d 1162 (2002).

6. *Esperanza* v. *Sunrise Hospital.* 2:10-CV-02228-PMP-PAL, 2:10-CV-01983-PMP-GWG (D. Nev. July 13, 2011).

7. 42 C.F.R. 489.24 – Special Responsibilities of Medicare Hospitals in Emergency Cases.

8. NRS Chapter 439: Administration of Public Health. Patient Safety Committee: Establishment; Composition; Meetings; Duties; Proceedings and Records Are Privileged.

Minor Consent

Case

The patient presented to the emergency department (ED) with frequent urination and burning and had been on the patient tracking board now for an hour. The physician had asked where the patient was, so that she could see her. The charge nurse said that she was still in triage since she was 16 years old and they couldn't get parental consent to have her treated. The physician suggested she should see the patient first, and the consent for care could be worked on later. The physician also pointed out that this may be an ostensible complaint that could be linked to request for other women's health services, which it is obligatory for the hospital to provide for a minor patient. The charge nurse said that the nursing administrator was already involved, and they should wait to try and find at least one of the parents. The physician again asked the nurse to bring the patient into the ED, as they would any other patient, and she was then evaluated. Her complaints included frequency and dysuria, and she had some sexually transmitted disease (STD) concerns as well. She was treated for infection and was also given some family planning services that she asked for.

The next day the provider received a call from nursing administration. They had concerns about the patient being seen before she was consented for care. Her mother had called back about a half an hour into the evaluation and consented when she came to pick her up. The physician again reiterated that her understanding of the process was that an emancipated minor, or one making adult decisions, can present for care and be seen without parental consent for particular disease states, of which this was one.

Medical Approach

Every patient who presents to the ED should have a prospective informed consent. However, consent for minor patients can be complicated. Minor patients often present without parental knowledge, but can still have disease states and conditions that require evaluation, diagnosis, and treatment. There is a margin of safety to allow for treatment of minors without parental consent for some conditions, particularly those relating to adolescent and juvenile sexual health issues.

Parental consent is generally desirable, but often a child would be more hesitant to present if the consent requirement was absolute. Most institutions have a structured process, in which an emancipated minor is able to present with a retrospective consent process involving the parent, to allow care to be delivered immediately with the consent required after the care has been provided.

The American Academy of Pediatrics (AAP) has stated that "a medical screening examination and any medical care necessary and likely to prevent imminent or significant harm to the pediatric patient with an emergency medical condition should not be withheld or delayed because of problems obtaining consent."[1] The goal of this policy statement is to provide guidance when parental consent is not available or not necessary, or where parental refusal places a child at risk of significant harm.

There are well-defined pediatric presentation scenarios: first, evaluation and treatment of the unaccompanied minor (Table 68.1).[2] The emergency exception rule presumes consent when an emergent condition exists, a parent or guardian is not available or is unable to consent, treatment cannot be safely delayed, and treatment is limited to the emergency condition (Table 68.2).

An alternative scenario is that the child may be an emancipated minor, essentially living as an adult, making adult decisions. Most states offer statutory exception to recognize those children who are married, economically self-sufficient, not living at home,

Table 68.1 AAP Consent for emergency medical services for children and adolescents

| 1. Evaluation and treatment of unaccompanied minor |
| 2. Emancipated minor criteria |
| 3. Non-urgent complaint with unauthorized caregiver |
| 4. Refusal of consent for emergency condition |
| 5. Consent and confidentiality |

Reference: American Academy of Pediatrics.[1]

Table 68.2 Minor consent emergency exception rule

| 1. Emergency medical condition exists |
| 2. Parent or guardian not available, or unable to consent |
| 3. Treatment cannot be safely delayed |
| 4. Limited to emergency condition |

Reference: American Academy of Pediatrics.[1]

Table 68.3 Emancipated "mature" minor criteria

| 1. Married |
| 2. Economically self-sufficient |
| 3. Not living at home |
| 4. Active duty military |
| 5. Pregnancy (some states) |
| 6. Parent (some states) |

Reference: American Academy of Pediatrics.[1]

Table 68.4 Minor consent general statutory exception

| 1. Sexually transmitted disease care |
| 2. Drug abuse treatment |
| 3. Mental health care |
| 4. Pregnancy |
| 5. Contraception |
| 6. Emancipation |

Reference: Sigman and O'Connor.[2]

active duty military, and in some states pregnant or already a parent (Table 68.3).[2]

In addition to statutory provisions, the "mature minor doctrine" is a common-law rule that permits a mature adolescent to make decisions concerning their health care without parental consent.[2] There are statutory exceptions to consent required for emergency care including STD care, drug treatment, mental health care, pregnancy, contraception, and emancipation. There is minimal legal risk in allowing adolescents older than 14 years of age, who demonstrate signs of maturity, to make adult-like health-care decisions (Table 68.4).

Alderson performed an evaluation of pediatric patients, who were to undergo elective orthopedic surgical procedures for chronic conditions, and their parents.[3] She evaluated 120 patients with mean age 8–15 years, and asked when they would be capable of making an informed decision. The parents (13.9 years) and children (14.0 years) provided a similar prediction of capability. There was a gender difference as well, with girls (13.1 years) and their parents (12.8 years) feeling they had better decision-making capability than boys (15.0 years) and their parents (14.9 years).

Another common scenario is a child with a non-urgent medical complaint presenting with someone who is not authorized to provide consent.[4] This is a complicated situation, in which a medical screening exam (MSE) needs to be performed. If an emergency medical condition is found, stabilizing care or transfer will need to be provided, while attempts are begun to obtain proper consent. The AAP has also authored a position paper on consent for non-urgent pediatric care, discussing the "consent by proxy" concept.[4] Here, they balance the child's access to medical care, parental responsibility, and family integrity against the provider's concerns for medicolegal liability. They recommend considering the care that needs to be provided, alerting the family or a responsible adult of intent to test or treat, and delaying all non-urgent care until consent is obtained.

The refusal of emergency evaluation and treatment by the legal guardian, when that care is necessary and helpful to the child, is particularly problematic.[4] Typically the minor child does not have the right to make a medical decision: the parent or legal guardian has that legally binding right. However, the parent or guardian is required to act in the best interest of the child. If they refuse the recommended care, the appropriate regulatory agencies, law enforcement, or judicial resources may intervene. The "in loco parentis" (in place of the parent) doctrine takes some responsibilities of the parent, often in the setting of school decisions, while the "in parens patriae" (parent of the nation) doctrine allows the state to intervene as legal guardian to make appropriate decisions, as in this case.

Consent and the right of confidentiality is often complicated in this setting, as protection from parental disclosure is not assured.[4] The balance is between adolescent confidentiality and parental responsibility. The child must understand that to maintain confidentiality, they need a secure means to receive care-related information or results, as well as taking financial responsibility for the visit to avoid the billing notice. From a federal perspective, the Family Planning Act of 1970 compels privacy in the setting of women's reproductive health care for minors.[5] However, it is essential that every practitioner be familiar with their state laws addressing minor confidentiality.

Legal Analysis

State-based statutes such as those found in California Family Code §6922–7002, Business and Professional Code §2397, and Penal Code §11711 address those medical services that can be consented for by minors with the associated confidentiality (Table 68.5).[6–8] Minors of any age can consent to pregnancy care, contraceptive services, abortion, emergency medical services, sexual assault evaluation, rape services for minors under 12 years of age, and a skeletal radiographic survey to diagnose child abuse or neglect. Minors 12 years of age or older can seek outpatient mental health services; diagnosis and treatment for infectious, contagious, or communicable disease or STD; AIDS/HIV testing and treatment; drug or alcohol abuse treatment; and rape services. Emancipated minors who are typically at least 14 years of age can seek general medical, dental, or psychiatric care.

Another area of concern is a child who presents with a divorced parent, in which custody and consent may be a concern. Parents who are married have the right to make decisions on behalf of their minor children.[9] According to California law, either parent acting alone can consent to mental health treatment of minor children. This area of health care is under significant scrutiny. It is usually advisable to seek the consent of both parents, although it is not legally necessary with an intact marriage. However, if the parents are divorced, their parental decision-making rights are often subject to court order. This responsibility should be decided by both parents beforehand to prevent uncertainty in an emergency situation.

In *Bellotti* v. *Baird*, four minors under the age of 18 wished to have abortions without informing

Table 68.5 Minor consent exception: California statutory exceptions

Any age
1. Pregnancy
2. Contraception
3. Abortion
4. Emergency medical services
5. Sexual Assault Services
6. Rape Services
7. Skeletal Survey
12 years of age or older
1. Outpatient mental health services
2. Diagnosis and treatment of infectious, contagious, communicable diseases
3. Diagnosis and treatment of sexually transmitted disease
4. AIDS/HIV testing and treatment
5. Drug and alcohol abuse treatment
6. Rape services
Minor emancipated 14 years, or minor 15 years
1. Medical
2. Dental
3. Psychiatric care

Reference: California Codes.[6–8]

their parents, and felt they were capable of giving informed consent.[10] The district court felt the minor patients were capable of giving informed consent, and questioned whether the state should be permitted to intervene. The district court enjoined several provisions of the abortion consent statute. They denied a motion by the appellants to abstain from deciding the issue pending authoritative construction of the statute by the Supreme Judicial Court of Massachusetts. The Supreme Court of the United States held that the court should have abstained, vacated the judgment, and remanded the cases so the relevant state law could be determined concerning consent. The underpinning of Supreme Court decision-making has always been to allow all avenues of resolution to be exhausted before it intervenes.

In *Caldwell* v. *Bechtol*, a high-school-aged patient had recurrent low back pain and multiple physician visits.[11] She was diagnosed with a herniated disc and prescribed a conservative treatment course.

Subsequently, she visited a licensed osteopath, underwent spinal manipulation, and had neurological compromise. The family alleged medical malpractice and battery for failure to obtain appropriate consent. The pertinent question addressed by the court is whether there was a "mature minor exception" to the common-law rule that requires parental consent for medical care. The trial court granted a directed verdict to the defendant on the medical malpractice count based on inadequacy of the expert report. The battery and consent issues were referred to the jury who returned a defense verdict after receiving a mature minor exception instruction. They felt that the patient, who was 5 months shy of capacity, had the appropriate level of maturity to make the appropriate decision regarding her care. The appeals court affirmed the directed verdict but reversed the battery consent issue as the "mature minor exception" had not been adopted by the state legislature. The Supreme Court of Tennessee reversed the decision on the issue of battery and reinstated the judgment of the trial court, recognizing the decision-making right of minors.

In *Tenenbaum* v. *Williams*, a caseworker removed a 5-year-old child from school and took her to the ED to be examined for abuse. No signs of abuse were found and the child was returned to her parents.[12] This emergency removal action was justified by the New York Social Services Law §417 and the New York Family Court Act §1024.[13,14] The parents brought suit alleging the medical evaluation was performed without their consent or judicial intervention, depriving the child of the Due Process clause of the Fourteenth Amendment and right to be free from unreasonable search and seizure under the Fourth Amendment applied to the states through the Fourteenth.[15,16] The United States Court of Appeals, Second Circuit affirmed the trial court judgment that the medical exam violated procedural due-process rights and unreasonable search and seizure, but remanded the triable issue of fact of how this applied to school removal.

Conclusion

There is a clear juridical predisposition to allow minors with an appropriate level of maturity to make independent medical decisions in carefully defined circumstances. The most crucial aspect of the minor informed consent quandary is to always err on the side of caution. Appropriate care should be provided in urgent or emergent situations, even as parental consent is being sought. It is also important to remember there are certain protected disease conditions in which medical care should be provided regardless of parental consent.

References

1. American Academy of Pediatrics Committee on Pediatric Emergency Medicine and Committee on Bioethics. Consent for emergency medical services for children and adolescents. *Pediatrics*. 2011;128(2):427–433. DOI:10.1542/peds.2011-1166.

2. Sigman GS, O'Connor C. Exploration for physicians of the mature minor doctrine. *J Pediatr*. 1991;119(4):520–525.

3. Alderson, P. *Children's Consent to Surgery* (Maidenhead, UK: Open University Press, 1993).

4. Berger GN, Committee on Medical Liability and Risk Management. Consent by proxy for nonurgent pediatric care. *Pediatrics*. 2010;126(5):1022–1031.

5. Family Planning Services and Population Research Act of 1970. Public Law 91-572-December 24, 1970.

6. California Family Code §6922 (a), 6924–6928, 6929 (b), 7002.

7. California Business and Professional Code §2397.

8. California Penal Code §11171.

9. Benitez BR. Consent for the treatment of minors with divorced parents. The Therapist; November/December 2001:1–3.

10. *Bellotti* v. *Baird*, 428 U.S. 132 (1976).

11. *Cardwell* v. *Bechtol*, 724 S.W.2d 739 (1987).

12. *Tenenbaum* v. *Williams*, 193 F.3d 581 (1999).

13. New York Social Services Law §417: Taking a Child into Protective Custody (2012).

14. New York Family Court Act §1024: Emergency Removal Without Court Order.

15. U.S. Const. Amend. XIV.

16. U.S. Const. Amend. IV.

Missed Illness and Injury

Case

The medical director had received an inquiry from a quality committee about a misread radiograph. One of the committee members suggested that the rate of missed illness or injury in the emergency department (ED) was higher than that of other specialties and physicians practicing in the facility. The director replied this was not the case. A literature review showed the overall missed illness or injury rate in the ED was significantly lower than anticipated, and certainly not greater than in other specialties. The areas of focus included missed imaging readings, medical diagnoses, and missed surgical illness.

The director pointed out the numerous issues with emergency medicine that may result in a perceived higher rate of error. These include a higher acuity patient population; rapid, irregular patient presentation; lack of primary care resources; and decreased follow-up care. He stated that at the next committee meeting he would present the available data looking at significant errors of omission in the practice of emergency medicine.

Medical Approach

There is a common assumption that error rates are higher in the ED than in other practice areas of the hospital or other specialties participating in that care, but this is not shown in the data.

Missed or delayed diagnoses are common, but this is an area we are beginning to study in the patient safety arena. Schiff et al. administered a survey at grand rounds presentations requesting a referral of three diagnostic errors, reporting 669 cases from 310 clinicians from 22 institutions.[1] Overall, they rated these errors as major in 28% (162), moderate in 41% (241), and minor or insignificant in 31% (180). The most common missed or delayed diagnosis was pulmonary embolism in 4.5% (26) of cases, drug reactions or

overdose in 4.5% (26), lung cancer in 3.9% (23), colorectal cancer in 3.3% (19), acute coronary syndrome in 3.1% (18), breast cancer in 3.1% (18), and stroke in 2.6% (15) (Table 69.1).

Further analysis found errors to occur most frequently in the testing phase, including failure to order, report, and follow up laboratory results in 44%; followed by clinical assessment errors, failure to consider or overweighting competing diagnosis in 32%; history taking in 10%, physical examination in 10%; and referral, consultation errors, and delays in 3% (Table 69.2).[1]

Early on, when the ED was staffed primarily by resident or less experienced physicians, the missed illness and injury rate was high. Lee and Bleetman in a review of the literature reported missed injury rates of 0.4 to 65%.[2] Missed illness and injury are preventable and have a multitude of implications for the patients and the providers.

Guly analyzed the records of 934 patients in a busy district ED, where 953 diagnostic errors were identified.[3] The majority of errors were identified as missed fractures in 77.8% of patients. The most common reasons for error cited included misread radiographs

Table 69.1 Most common missed or delayed diagnoses

	Condition	Incidence %, N = 669
1.	Pulmonary embolism	4.5 (26)
2.	Drug reaction or overdose	4.5 (26)
3.	Lung cancer	3.9 (23)
4.	Colorectal cancer	3.3 (19)
5.	Acute coronary syndrome	3.1 (18)
6.	Breast cancer	3.1 (18)
7.	Stroke	2.6 (15)

Reference: Schiff et al.[1]

Table 69.2 Medical error demographic profile

	Issue	Incidence (%)
1.	Testing phase	44
	Failure to order	
	Failure to report	
	Failure to follow up	
2.	Clinician assessment errors	32
	Failure to consider	
	Overweighting competitive diagnosis	
3.	History taking	10
4.	Physical examination	10
5.	Referral, consultation errors or delays	3

Reference: Schiff et al.[1]

Table 69.3 Process breakdowns in the diagnostic process

	Process	Incidence (%)
1.	Failure to order the proper test	58
2.	Perform adequate history and physical	42
3.	Incorrect interpretation of diagnostic test	37
4.	Failure to order appropriate consultation	33

Reference: Kachalia et al.[5]

Table 69.4 Factors contributing to missed diagnosis

	Factors	Incidence (%)
1.	Cognitive processing	96
2.	Patient-related	33
3.	Lack of appropriate supervision	30
4.	Inadequate handovers	24
5.	Excessive workload	23

Reference: Kachalia et al.[5]

(77.8%), and failure to perform the radiography itself (13.4%). Of the medical error cases, 2.3% (22) resulted in complaints or legal action, and 0.3% (3) of patients died. The authors concluded that most errors were made by physicians in training, and special focus on education was appropriate.

The trauma population is at especially high risk, requiring a cautious approach. Janjua et al. evaluated 206 trauma patients, in which 65% (134) had a total of 309 missed injuries.[4] The tertiary trauma survey, typically performed in the intensive care unit (ICU), detected 56% of all early missed injuries and 90% of clinically significant missed injuries at 24 hours. Most importantly, clinically significant missed injuries occurred in 9.7% (30) of cases, with complications in 3.5% (11) and death in 0.6% (2) patients. These authors identified 224 contributing errors, with most found in clinical assessment (55%, 123), followed by 37% (83) in radiology, patient-related factors in 6.2% (14), and 1.7% (4) related to technical errors.

It is crucial to recognize that the trauma secondary survey misses a significant proportion of injuries. The missed injury rate was increased significantly in patients who had been in a motor vehicle accident and had multiple injuries. Therefore, a careful tertiary survey performed on the ward or intensive care unit (ICU) is essential for superior trauma care.

Diagnostic errors in the ED are an important high-risk patient safety concern as well. Kachalia et al. reviewed 122 closed malpractice claims and identified 65% (79) of cases in which patients were harmed.[5]

They identified process breakdowns in the diagnostic process, including failure to order the proper test (58%), failure to perform adequate history and physical exam (42%), incorrect interpretation of a diagnostic test (37%), and failure to order the appropriate consultation (33%) (Table 69.3). The leading contributing factors to the missed diagnosis were cognitive factors identified in 96% of cases, patient-related factors in 34%, lack of appropriate supervision in 30%, inadequate handovers in 24%, and excessive workload in 23% (Table 69.4).

Missed ED diagnoses are complicated and multifactorial, with an average of two process breakdowns and three contributing factors per missed diagnosis. Areas of concern relating to missed injury or illness are focused first on radiology reading errors. The second area of concern is significant errors of omission regarding a medical diagnosis. Third, we focus on errors of omission, in which the primary illness or injury was missed. Fourth, errors of commission, such as falsely concluding that another disease entity was in play. Fifth, there is an examination of the treatment intervention, procedural process, or medication administration in an analysis of treatment intervention.

Legal Analysis

The Emergency Medical Treatment and Labor Act (EMTALA) is often invoked as the legal theory behind a missed illness or injury.[6] In *Reynolds v. Maine General Health*, the patient presented to the ED after a motor vehicle accident with significant lower extremity injuries.[7] The trauma evaluation consisted of a surgery consult with negative abdominal CT scan. The orthopedic evaluation found multiple fractures and operative fixation was required. During the postoperative discharge phase, the patient was discharged and within the week succumbed to a pulmonary embolism allegedly due to the right lower extremity fracture. The family testified and provided affidavits that when asked about allergies or medical problems, they told someone in the ED "with a white coat" there was a family history of clotting disorder. The family filed suit under an EMTALA (42 U.S.C. §1395), alleging the patient presented with an emergency medical condition (§1395dd (e) (1)); was not screened properly for deep venous thrombosis (DVT) (§1395dd (a)); and was not stabilized prior to discharge (§1395dd (b)).[6] The magistrate judge granted the defendant-appellee's motion for summary judgment, holding that there was no evidence of failure to screen, and the stabilization requirement was not activated as the patient was not known to be suffering from a DVT. The United States Court of Appeals, First Circuit affirmed the district court decision, granting defense summary judgment motion. They held that the appellant's claims of misdiagnosis and negligent treatment were not supported by any evidence of faulty process or disparate treatment consistent with an EMTALA theory.

In *Deberry v. Sherman Hospital Association*, the pediatric patient was taken to the ED by her mother with complaints of fever, rash, stiff neck, and her head tilted to the left.[8] She was discharged, worsened 2 days later and eventually admitted with a diagnosis of spinal meningitis and sequelae including deafness. The family filed a dual claim alleging an EMTALA violation for failure to adequately screen, as well as a medical negligence claim brought under the federal court's pendent jurisdiction.[6] (Pendent, or supplemental, jurisdiction allows a federal court jurisdiction to hear a closely related state-law claim, arising from the same nexus, in conjunction with the federal matter properly litigated before it.[9]) The hospital moved to dismiss for failing to state a claim upon which relief can be granted pursuant to the Federal Rules of Civil Procedure (FRCP).[10] The motion to dismiss tests the sufficiency of the complaint, and not the merits of the case. Under the "simplified notice pleading" of the FRCP, "the complaint should not be dismissed for failure to state a claim unless it appears beyond doubt that the plaintiff can prove no set of facts in support of the claim which would entitle to relief." *Conley v. Gibson*, 355 U.S. 41 (1957).[11] "Mere vagueness or lack of detail does not constitute sufficient grounds for a motion to dismiss." *Strauss v. City of Chicago*, 760 F.2d 765 (1986).[12] The defense alleged this was merely a state medical malpractice claim, not an EMTALA violation, and dismissal would preclude evaluation of the second pendent complaint. The district court denied this dismissal motion. The court supported a broad interpretation of EMTALA, holding that field preemption, in which the effect of state law in that area would be negated as well by the federal edict, which is disfavored by Congress and must be clearly stated through express language, was less likely than conflict preemption – the true intent, in their opinion. The Supremacy Clause of Article IV would have mandated the same conclusion if there was silence on the preemption issue, establishing that federal law takes precedence over state law, including the state constitution.[13] Therefore, the court held the initial claim should be dismissed, with the existent controversy precluding dismissal of the second as well.

Conclusion

The predominant theory underlying most medical malpractice claims is the failure to diagnose an acute medical condition, followed by failure to treat that condition, procedural errors, and failures of communication.

References

1. Schiff GD, Hasan O, Kim S, Abrams R, Cosby K, Lambert BL, et al. Diagnostic error in medicine: analysis of 583 physician-reported errors. *Arch Intern Med*. 2009;169(20):1881–1887. DOI:19.1001/archinternmed.2009.333.

2. Lee C. Commonly missed injuries in the accident and emergency department. *Trauma*. 2004;6(1):41–51. DOI:10.1191/1460408604ta298oa.

3. Guly HR. Diagnostic errors in an emergency department. *Emerg Med J*. 2001;18(4):263–269. DOI:10.1136/emj.18.4.263.

4. Janjua KJ, Sugrue M, Deane SA. Prospective evaluation of early missed injuries and the role of tertiary trauma survey. *J Trauma*. 1998;44(6):1000–1007.

5. Kachalia A, Gandhi TK, Puopolo AL, Yoon C, Thomas EJ, Griffey R, et al. Missed and delayed diagnoses in the emergency department: a study of closed malpractice claims from 4 liability insurers. *Ann Emerg Med*. 2007;49(2):196–205. DOI:10. 1016/ j.annemergmed.2006.06.035.

6. EMTALA, 42 U.S.C. §1395.

7. *Reynolds* v. *MaineGeneral Health*, 218 F.3d 78 (2000).

8. *Deberry* v. *Sherman Hospital Association*, 741 F. Supp. 1302 (1990).

9. 28 U.S. Code §1367 Supplemental Jurisdiction.

10. FRCP (12)(b)(6): Failure to State a Claim for Which Relief Can Be Granted.

11. *Conley* v. *Gibson*, 355 U.S. 41 (1957).

12. *Strauss* v. *City of Chicago*, 760 F.2d 765 (1985).

13. U.S. Constitution, Article VI, Para 2, Supremacy Clause.

Multiple Visits

Case

The patient had returned to the emergency depart-ment (ED) for the third time over the last few days. She had presented to the ED initially with nausea and urinary burning but did not have a fever. Since she was able to take medication orally she was started on an antibiotic (nitrofurantoin) and was discharged home. She then re-presented the next day with her symptoms slightly worse. She had a slight fever, but was able to take her medicine. The emergency physician switched her antibiotic to ciprofloxacin, which she was able to take before being discharged. She was sent home to follow up with her primary care physician (PCP).

She returned later that evening, which was when she was evaluated by the ED physician for the last time. This time she seemed worse than on her previ-ous visits. She had been taking her medicine, but had vomited her last dose of antibiotic that evening. On exam, she had clearly lateralized pain to her left back and had costovertebral angle tenderness. The phys-ician started her on intravenous antibiotics, ordered a CT scan to evaluate for pyelonephritis and infectious complications, and made plans for admission to the intensive care unit (ICU). The patient's CT scan came back revealing a perinephric abscess, and urology was consulted for surgical intervention.

The next week, the quality committee raised con-cerns about the patient presenting to the ED three times in a relatively short time frame and that she should have been considered for admission on the second visit. It appeared during the second visit that she was non-toxic, was switched to a more appropriate antibiotic choice, and her care was discussed with her PCP, who agreed to see her the next day.

Medical Approach

There is always a concern when a patient makes mul-tiple ED visits in a relatively short period of time. The classic emergency medicine adage suggests that, from a medicolegal perspective, three visits within 24 hours warrants a mandatory admission.

The "normal visit" demographic is hard to define, with significant site-specific variation. Brown reported on a ED cohort of 60,972 patients, in which one in five (22.1%) local residents had at least one ED visit in the previous 12 months; and one in three (30.1%) had two or more visits.[1] Multivariate analysis revealed that ongoing health needs, including significant accidents, number of health problems, and self-reported health status are the strongest determinants of ED use.

Repeat ED visits were analyzed in a statewide data-base by Cook et al. who reported on 780,074 patients with 1,370,607 distinct visits.[2] The repeat and serial patient group accounted for 33% of patients, who accounted for 62% of the ED visits. They tended to be younger, with smaller median ED charges per visit, with 30% persisting into the second year. The high-use group, who visited the ED at least five times annually, were more likely to present with minor complaints of sprains, back problems, and headaches and were more likely to self-pay for their health care.

The term "bounce-back" has been used to describe the short-term return visit to the ED. Pierce et al. reported on a 17,214 patient cohort with a 3% (569) incidence of patients who returned within 48 hours.[3] The majority (53%, 267) of repeat visits was associ-ated with patient-related factors. Physician-related factors were the primary reason for patient return in 18% (92), while 12% (60) returned with a new, unre-lated problem; problems with the public health sys-tem were the issue in 4% (18) of cases. There were consequences of the multiple visit process, as 19% (87) of patients required emergent hospitalization, with one-third (32.1%) attributed to physician error. Therefore, it is crucial that facilities have a prospec-tive quality improvement program to evaluate short-term returns.

A crucial part of the analysis is not just the unscheduled ED return, but also the readmission rate. Hu et al. evaluated 72-hour patient returns reporting a 3.1% return rate, in which 36% (147/413) were admitted, with an overall mortality rate of 4.1%.[4] However, half the cases (47.9%) attributed the return visit to an illness-based factor. The unscheduled return visit admissions were correlated with age, non-ambulatory status, high-grade triage, and underlying chronic disease. The independent predictors include age greater than 65 years (OR 2.2, CI 95% 1.4–3.5, high-grade triage (OR 2.1, CI 95% 1.3–3.2), and physician-based factors (OR 3.5, CI 95% 2.0–6.1) Interestingly, staff experience and ED crowding were not significant predictors of unscheduled ED return.

Another quality marker is the hospital readmission rate after an inpatient stay; however, tracking ED returns provides a higher level of refinement. Rising et al. evaluated a sample of 15,519 inpatient discharges, in which nearly one-quarter (23.8%, 3695) resulted in at least one ED visit within a 30-day period.[5] The ED return group had a readmission rate of slightly less than half (46%, 1873/4077). This finding certainly leaves us the opportunity to improve our care transitions, and interrupt the frequent readmission cycle.

Patients at age extremes are often at higher risk and should be monitored carefully. Allesandrini et al. evaluated return visits to the pediatric ED, reporting a figure of 3.5% (95% CI 3.3–3.6), similar to rates found in the general ED (2.4–3.4%).[6] The majority of the return visits were unscheduled (78.5%), 17% were scheduled returns, and 4% were direct callback patients. The most common diagnoses were infectious (45%), respiratory (16%), and trauma (16%) in the pediatric patients. The revisit patients were more likely to be younger than 2 years (RR 1.3 (1.2–1.5)), to be admitted to the hospital (RR, 1.3 (1.2–1.5)), and to be triaged as acute (RR 1.1 (1.0–1.2)). These authors recommended a more liberal callback system to reduce medical error and improve patient outcome.

A similar profile was defined among elderly patients returning to the ED by McCusker et al.[7] They identified a group of 1112 elderly patients (>65 years), in which 43.9% (492) made one or more return visits, 19.3% (216) returned early, and 7.5% (84) returned frequently within 30 days after discharge. Early returns were more likely than later returns to be for the same diagnosis ($P = 0.003$). Logistic regression analysis found that hospitalization within the previous 6 months, feeling depressed, and certain diagnosis

Table 70.1 Predictors of geriatric ED return

Early and frequent
1. Hospitalization within 6 months
2. Depression
3. Certain diagnosis
Early
4. Heart disease
5. Ever been married
6. Not drinking alcohol daily
Frequent
7. Diabetes
8. Recent ED visit
9. Lack of social support

Reference: McCusker et al.[7]

predicted early and frequent returns. History of heart disease, having ever been married, and not drinking alcohol daily, predicted early return, while a history of diabetes, a recent ED visit, and lack of support predicted frequent use. Return visits within the first month after discharge have both medical and social factors that can often be identified prospectively (Table 70.1).

Legal Analysis

In *Coppage* v. *Mann*, an incarcerated patient with multiple ED visits alleged medical negligence, violation of 42 U.S.C. §1983, under color of law rights deprivation provision, and his Eighth Amendment rights against cruel and unusual punishment by failing to diagnose and treat his cancer.[8–10] The patient had abdominal pain, low back pain, burning and discharge, and other pain complaints with approximately 50 health-care visits for this concern over a 6-month period. He was ultimately diagnosed with a spinal tumor with subsequent paraplegia. The trial court granted the defendant's motion for summary judgment, rejecting the Eighth Amendment and intentional tort claims related to restraint. However, the medical negligence claim survived the summary judgment motion and was justiciable.

In *Jackson* v. *East Bay Hospital*, the plaintiff presented to the ED for medical clearance for admission to a psychiatric facility.[11] He then returned to the ED 2 days later complaining of sore throat and vomiting and was recommended a mental health evaluation. He then returned the next evening in an agitated state and was transferred for psychiatric evaluation. There was a subsequent discharge after he was felt to be stabilized, and he succumbed to cardiac arrest allegedly from drug toxicity. His survivors filed EMTALA and California Health and Safety Code §1317 claims, requiring the health-care facilities to exercise reasonable care.[12,13] The district court granted summary judgment to the health-care facilities and this decision was affirmed by the United States Court of Appeals, Ninth Circuit.

Conclusion

As resources become more limited and more outpatient management plans are encouraged, these cases become more difficult to manage. It is clear that standards of care need to be followed, with safe diagnostic and treatment plans with a more conservative course on each revisit. In addition, a discussion with the patient's PCP to ensure continuity of care is essential. It is important to consider every return visit to be an independent evaluation, starting with a fresh look for additional diagnostic considerations and not falling prey to incorporation bias. One should certainly consider admission on a second visit and recognize that admission is probably required for a third return visit.

References

1. Brown EM, Goel V. Factors related to emergency department use: results from the Ontario Health Survey. *Ann Emerg Med.* 1994;24(6):1083–1091. DOI:10.1016/S0196-0644(94)70237-3.

2. Cook LJ, Knight S, Junkins EP, Mann NC, Dean JM, Olson LM. Repeat patients to the emergency department in a statewide database. *Acad Emerg Med.* 2004;11(3):256–263. DOI:10.1111/j.1553–2712.2004. tb02206.x.

3. Pierce JM, Kellerman AL, Oster C. "Bounces": an analysis of short-term return visits to a public hospital emergency department. *Ann Emerg Med.* 1990;19(7):752–757. DOI:10.1016/ S0196-0644(05)81698-1.

4. Hu KW, Lu YH, Lin HJ, Guo HR, Foo NP. Unscheduled return visits with and without admission post emergency department discharge. *J Emerg Med.* 2012;43(6):1110–1118. DOI:10.1016/ j.emergmed.2012.01.062.

5. Rising KL, White LF, Fernandez WG, Boutwell AE. Emergency department visits after hospital discharge: a missing part of the equation. *Ann Emerg Med.* 2013;62(2):145–150. DOI:10.1016/ j.annemergmed.2013.01.024.

6. Alessandrini EA, Lavelle JM, Glenfall SM, Jacobstein CR, Shaw KN. Return visits to the pediatric emergency department. *Pediatr Emerg Care.* 2004;20(3):168–171.

7. McCusker J, Cardin S, Bellavance F, Belzile E. Return to the emergency department among elders: patterns and predictors. *Acad Emerg Med.* 2000;7(3):249–259. DOI:10.1111/j.1553–2712.2000.tb01070.x.

8. *Coppage* v. *Mann*, 906 F. Supp. 1025 (1995).

9. 42 U.S.C. §1983 – Civil Action For Deprivation of Rights (1983).

10. U.S. Const Amend. VIII.

11. *Jackson* v. *East Bay Hospital*, 246 F.3d 1248 (2001).

12. EMTALA, 42 U.S.C. §1395.

13. California Health and Safety Code §1317: Emergency Services and Care.

Nursing

Case

In the emergency department (ED) the physician was caring for a young patient with diabetes, who had run out of insulin and been sick at home vomiting. His blood glucose was out of control. The initial blood glucose measurement was in excess of 500 mg/dL and he looked dehydrated. The physician administered 2 L of fluid and the patient's clinical status improved a little. He was on a large dose of insulin at home, more than 100 units a day of NPH (an intermediate-acting insulin). The nurse gave him an intravenous bolus of 10 units of regular insulin and started him on an infusion of 5 units per hour. A third liter of normal saline fluid was administered to follow.

The remainder of the workup was as one would expect for diabetic ketoacidosis (DKA). No sign of infection was identified, the urinalysis was normal, and he had no pneumonia. When the third liter of fluid was in, the physician asked the nurse if the insulin bolus had been administered. He then went on to the next patient as the ED was busy.

A little later, the physician was called urgently to the patient's room, and found him somnolent. They attended to the airway and he was arousable, but there was a clear decrease in his mental status. The nurse was asked again if she had given the insulin bolus. She said that she had and then exclaimed, "Oh my, I gave him too much insulin! I was supposed to give him 10 units tonight, but I think I gave him 100 units." The physician had already injected an ampoule of dextrose (D50) and the patient was beginning to come round. Since he was drowsy at that point the physician held the insulin infusion and asked the nurse to check his blood glucose level again in 15 minutes. He seemed OK during the rest of his ED stay. He was transferred to the medical intensive care unit without further incident, and seemed to be feeling a little better when he was heading upstairs.

Nine months later the ED received a call from risk management informing that the family had filed a lawsuit alleging insulin overdose and naming the physician as well. The response was that physician had written for the proper dose of insulin, but the error was a nursing medication administration issue. The physician order was indeed entered correctly, and a pharmacy fail-safe would be difficult, so the improvement focus was on education.

Medical Approach

These cases are often problematic: a single event may narrow down to one individual with potential culpability, but numerous people are named in the lawsuit. One legal strategy is to vindicate those providers that can be excluded from a procedural perspective, but if the allegations implicate another physician or provider then that is problematic as well.

The National Practitioner Data Bank Summary 2003–2012 reported the incidence of nursing malpractice and adverse action.[1] They defined a professional nurse classification to include registered nurses (RN), licensed practical nurses (LPN), licensed vocational nurses (LVN), nurse practitioners (NP), nurse anesthetists, nurse midwives, clinical nurse specialists, advanced nurse practitioners, and doctors of nursing practice. "All other practitioners" include all other health-care practitioners, non-health-care professionals, and non-specified professionals. Medical malpractice payments (147,870) accounted for 4.2% (6167) of the paid cases for nurses compared to 89.6% (132,513) for physicians and dentists and all other health-care practitioners in 6.2% (9190). Adverse action reports (330,782) affecting state licensure or privileges were found in 45.2% (149,505) of nurses compared to 18.3% (60,599) of physicians. There are historical and work cultural differences that police professional behavior differently, resulting in this discrepancy.

Table 71.1 Nursing Liability Exposure CAN HealthPro 2006–2010

Incidence (%)	Claim ($)
56.2	10,000–99,000
24.8	100,000–249,999
11.2	250,000–499,999
2.1	500,000–749,999
2.1	750,000–999,999
3.5	1,000,000 or over

Reference: Nurses Service Organization.[2]

Table 71.2 Decreased indemnity risk correlates

1. Early career mentor program
2. Decreased duration of practice
3. Continuing education
4. Early disclosure program
5. Electronic medical record
6. Management communication and support

Reference: Nurses Service Organization.[2]

Table 71.3 Nursing risk control strategies

1. Improve communication and interpersonal skills
2. Know and follow protocols
3. Continuing education to maintain competency
4. Thorough and accurate documentation

Reference: Nurses Service Organization.[2]

The Nurses Service Organization analyzed nurse license protection claims, and CNA HealthPro performed a joint analysis of nursing liability exposure from 2006 to 2010.[2] CNA HealthPro is the largest nurse liability insurer, with 600,000 policies in force and 516 closed claims in the 4-year time period. They found 91.9% of cases involved RN and 8.1% involved LPN/LVN. This finding was presumably due to differences in case complexity, and additional RN responsibilities. These were typically smaller claims with 56.2% in the $10,000–99,000 range, 24.8% in the $100,000–249,999 range, 11.2% in the $250,000–499,999 range, 2.1% in the $500,000–749,999 range, 2.1% in the $750,000–999,999 range and 3.5% claims for $1,000,000 or over (Table 71.1).

The specialties with the highest incidence of claims were medical/surgical, gerontology, and obstetrics, whereas the specialties with the highest indemnity were obstetrics, neurology/neurosurgery, and plastic/reconstructive surgery. The research group then considered accompanying nursing board complaints combined with paid defense claims. The majority of board decisions (50%) resulted in no action; 45.2% involved monitoring, further education or issuing a caution; and 4.8% resulted in revocation or surrender of license. In 2011 a nursing survey summarized that first, those with a mentor in their first 2 years had a deceased claim indemnity ($14,511 vs. $26,301); second, the incidence of claims increased with duration of practice, beginning at 11 years with the highest incidence in those working over 21 years; third, continuing education was associated with decreased average paid indemnity, and this effect was inversely proportional to the number of credit hours; fourth, an employer early disclosure policy resulted in a 50% decrease in average indemnity; fifth, indemnity was decreased when an electronic health record was

used exclusively; sixth, effective bidirectional communication with management, and an environment of employee support decreased indemnity as well (Table 71.2).

The Nurses Service Organization recommended nursing risk control strategies, to include: first, work to improve communication and interpersonal skills; second, knowing facility policies and adhering closely to them; third, maintaining nursing skill and competency through continuing education; fourth, ensuring thorough and accurate documentation in the patient care record (Table 71.3).

There has been a significant increase in the number of malpractice cases against nurses, which has been attributed to a number of defined factors.[2] First, as a result of cost-cutting efforts, the delegation of tasks to unlicensed assistive personnel has increased. This delegation should follow institutional standards or the state-based Nursing Practice Act. Second, there is greater early discharge for patients who had previously required more acute and intensive nursing care. Third, hospital downsizing and the nursing shortage have contributed to greater nursing workloads, potentially increasing the likelihood of error. Fourth, advances in technology require nurses to have knowledge of equipment capabilities, limitations, and safety features. Fifth, increased autonomy and responsibility of hospital nurses in the application of advanced nursing skills is associated with a greater risk of error. Sixth, better-informed consumers are more likely to

Table 71.4 Factors in increased nurse malpractice

1.	Greater task delegation to unlicensed personnel
2.	Facility early patient discharge
3.	Greater nursing workload
4.	Advances in technology
5.	Increased autonomy and responsibility
6.	Better informed consumers
7.	Expanded liability definitions

Reference: Croke.[3]

Table 71.5 Major categories of failure in nursing negligence

1.	Follow standards of care
2.	Use equipment in responsible manner
3.	Assess and monitor properly
4.	Communicate effectively
5.	Document properly
6.	Act as patient advocate

Reference: Croke.[3]

be aware of deviation in acceptable care, and malpractice issues. Seventh, expanded legal definitions of liability hold all medical professionals to a higher degree of accountability (Table 71.4).

Findings such as this may be associated with moral distress in registered nurses. Zuzaleo evaluated questionnaires submitted by 100 nurses defining morally distressing events.[3] These included working with staffing levels perceived as "unsafe," following family preference for care even though the nurse disagreed with the plan, continuing life support due to family wishes despite poor prognosis, and carrying out orders for perceived "unnecessary tests and treatments." The nurses sought support in their environment from management, requesting ethics input and continuing education.

Croke identified six areas of malpractice negligence risk, resulting from failure to follow care standards, use equipment in a responsible manner, assess and monitor, communicate effectively, document appropriately, and act as patient advocate (Table 71.5).[4]

Legal Analysis

In *Bass* v. *Barksdale*, a patient alleged blindness due to ethambutol prescribed in the public health department to treat tuberculosis.[5] Both the physician and charge nurse were sued, as clinic employees. The nurse wrote the prescriptions after discussion with the patient's primary care physician (PCP). The prescriptions were then signed by the clinic physician, who did not actually see the patient. The trial court held that the physician was the charge nurse's supervisor, but not her employer, so was not held responsible. However, the Court of Appeals of Tennessee, held that physicians are required to communicate and coordinate care, remanding for new trial.

Meadows v. *Patterson* defines the surgeon relationship, acknowledging the physician taking responsibility for nursing behavior in the operating room, but not on the postoperative surgical care ward.[6] They invoked the "res ipsa loquitur" doctrine applying to medical negligence. This requires that the event producing injury is under the defendant's control, occurrence does not happen if due care has been exercised, the facts of the injury afford sufficient evidence of responsibility, and the defense that injury was not due to want of care. Here, the patient injured his eye after the operative procedure was performed. The trial court felt the nurse was not the agent, and there was no respondeat superior relationship of the physician. The Court of Appeals of Tennessee concurred with the trial court, providing a directed verdict for the defense.

In *Koeniguer* v. *Eckrich*, the patient had urologic surgery and succumbed to multiorgan failure.[7] A significant proportion of the alleged negligence was directed at the nurse for not noting the patient's deterioration prior to discharge, noting an abnormal temperature, and failing to document her wound status. Most importantly, it is the responsibility of the nurse to refer significant change in patient status to the physician, as well as advocating for the patient by referring to the administrative chain of command, if the nurse feels that a different medical course is required. The trial court found the hospital did not prove its version of a summary judgment motion, in which the hospital suggested the physician's negligence exceeded that of the facility. This verdict was reversed by the Supreme Court of South Dakota and the case was remanded for jury consideration.

Conclusion

Typically, nurses are not involved in litigation unless they have clear liability, although this situation is changing. If they are involved, the agency relationship implicating the hospital as well as the nurse is much clearer than it is for a physician. Ideally, the goal of the health-care team is to prevent an episode like this from happening again via education, additional checks, or other "fail-safe" measures.

References

1. California Health and Safety Code §81317.

2. Nurses Service Organization. Understanding Nurse Liability, 2006–2010: A Three-Part Approach. *CNA HealthPro and Nurses Service Organization.* November 2011:1–64.

3. Zuzelo PR. Exploring the moral distress of registered nurses. *Nurs Ethics.* 2007;14(3):344–359. DOI:1177/ 0969733007075870.

4. Croke EM. Nurses, negligence and malpractice. *Am J Nurs.* 2003;103(9):54–68.

5. *Bass* v. *Barksdale*, 671 S.W.2d 476 (Tenn. Ct. App. 1984).

6. *Meadows* v. *Patterson*, 21 Tenn. App. 283 (Tenn. Ct. App. 1937).

7. *Koeniguer* v. *Eckrich*, 422 N.W. 2d 600 (1988).

Operations

Case

It was a particularly busy weekend in the emergency department (ED), in the middle of the flu season. There were extraordinary delays and trouble getting patients admitted. A significant number of patients were still boarding in the ED as well as a full waiting room through most of the weekend. The staff worked cooperatively to eventually move the remaining patients through the department, and said they couldn't remember such a busy time.

On Monday, the ED director received a call from the hospital's CEO, who said there were concerns about the weekend delays. There was an upcoming board meeting and she wanted to know if it was possible to give a short presentation on the operational efficiency of the ED. One of the board members had an interest in operational workflow and process and thought the topic would be of interest to the entire board.

Medical Approach

The ED is often prone to delays in care based on the obvious factors: irregular presentation, high acuity, decreased medical care continuity, and potential compliance issues. There are numerous suggestions for improvement. However, it is important to note that these interventions must be individualized to a particular location to be effective. There is also a growing consultancy industry that may offer operational suggestions and recommendations with varying degrees of effectiveness. They are most effective when they work cooperatively with the facility, integrating processes and seeking staff participation and a "champion" network.

The key to the analysis is to recognize the distinction between *efficacy*, which means reaching the desired endpoint under ideal conditions, and *effectiveness*, targeting the same endpoint but under real-world conditions.[1] This is balanced by an analysis of

efficiency: the ratio of resource input to work output. Obviously, in the ED the circumstances are often quite unpredictable, but our goal is to strive for the optimal balance of patient care outcome and experience.

One of the largest studies of ED throughput and related efficiency topics is by Zun, who identified 277 articles, of which 26 articles were evaluated as methodologically sound.[2] The studies were concentrated in five areas: techniques (38%), determinants (27%), laboratory (15%), triage (12%), and academic responsibilities (8%). They concluded that a combination of low patient inpatient census, in-room registration, point-of-care testing, and an urgent care area demonstrated improved patient throughput (Table 72.1).

Saunders studied ED patient movement, using a continuous observation time study to evaluate sources of delay in 1568 patients.[3] First, they defined the diagnostic and treatment interventions, and their impact on care. The time added for urinalysis was 45 minutes, procedures 63 minutes, radiographs 65 minutes, and blood work 126 minutes, compared to 31 minutes for those without intervention. The lower-acuity patients (the majority) had the shortest evaluation and treatment times, but the longest delay in ED processing time. There were fewer high-acuity patients, who had longer evaluation and treatment times but moved more quickly through the department. The inherent conclusion was that the majority of patients were of

Table 72.1 Factors associated with improved ED patient throughout

1.	Low inpatient census
2.	In-room registration
3.	Point-of-care testing
4.	Urgent care area

Reference: Zun.[2]

lower acuity, took longer to process, and can often be associated with lower satisfaction ratings.

Recurrent themes include improved communication and teamwork. Risser et al. evaluated a team building program based on successful aviation program ideology, creating small work teams.[4] This study evaluated 54 malpractice incidents, felt to be capable of improvement by better communication. They identified 8.8 teamwork failures occurring per case, with half of the deaths or permanent disabilities felt to be avoidable. Caregivers should improve teamwork skills to reduce error, improve care quality, and reduce litigation risk. This aviation concept of crew resource management has been used in the pediatric ED to improve communication and patient safety.[5] The ED practice dynamic benefits particularly from formal communication and medical team training to minimize errors and adverse events.

The ED's difficulties arise because it is often operating at full capacity, prone to surge dynamics and crowding situations. The concept of optimizing front-end operations has been instituted to improve quality and efficiency, while also addressing cost issues.[6] These interventions include immediate bedding, bedside registration, advanced triage protocols including triage-based care, physician/practitioner in triage (PIT), dedicated fast track (FT), patient tracking systems, wireless communication devices, kiosk self check-in, and personal health record technology (the use of "smart cards" and other mobile electronic archiving methods) (Table 72.2). These various possibilities should be evaluated and individualized for the particular institution.

The ED observation unit or rapid treatment unit has been an important part of the operation for years. Hostetler et al. reported on 5714 observation patients, in which 73% (4191) were discharged with an average length of stay of 14.92 hours.[8] The unit most commonly treated those with chest pain (26%) followed by abdominal pain (16%). Pediatric patients had shorter stays (11.2 hours) than geriatric patients (15.4 hours). The observation unit is a useful care adjunct in a number of departments.

PIT is a current intervention felt to be helpful to the ED operation. Imperato et al. evaluated 17,631 patients before (8620) and after (9011) implementation of a PIT program (Table 72.3).[9] The median time from registration to attending physician evaluation was reduced by 36 minutes (1:41 vs. 1:05, $P < 0.01$), while the median length of stay for all patients was reduced by 12 minutes (3:51 vs. 3:39, $P < 0.01$). Both the number of days on diversion (24 vs. 9 days) and total time on diversion (68.5 vs. 9 hours) were decreased ($P < 0.01$). However, there was no significant difference in the proportion of patients who left without being seen (1.5% vs. 1.3%).

Legal Analysis

In *Haynes* v. *Yale-New Haven Hospital*, the patient presented to the ED after a car accident, was taken to the operating room for significant orthopedic injury, had an emergent splenectomy but died during the

Table 72.2 Optimizing ED front-end operations

1.	Immediate bedding
2.	Bedside registration
3.	Advanced triage protocols – triage-based care
4.	Physician/practitioner in triage (PIT)
5.	Dedicated "fast track"
6.	Tracking systems
7.	Wireless communication devices
8.	Kiosk self check-in
9.	Personal health record technology – "smart cards"

Reference: Wiler et al.[6]

Table 72.3 Physician in Triage (PIT)

	Time interval	Improvement (min)	Significance ($P < 0.01$)
1.	Registration to evaluation	36	1.05 vs. 1.41
2.	Length of stay (LOS)	12	3.39. vs. 3.51
3.	Length without being seen	None	1.3. vs. 1.5 (%)
4.	Time on diversion	9 vs. 24 (days)	
		9 vs. 68.5 (hours)	

Reference: Imperato et al.[9]

procedure.[10] The plaintiff filed suit alleging a failure to meet the requisite standard of ED care. They cited the Connecticut Unfair Trade Practices Act (CUTPA), General Statutes §42-110a et seq.[11] The plaintiff also commented on operational issues, suggesting the ED was inadequately staffed and the staff present were inadequately trained and supported. They allege that as a certified trauma center, holding itself out as such, the facility was held to a particular standard. They also alleged there was failure to meet trauma center standards with respect to ED procedures in the care of patients with acute traumatic injury. The trial court granted the defendant's summary judgment motion, as the allegations were insufficient to sustain a CUTPA violation. They also concluded a medical malpractice claim cannot be recast as an unfair or deceptive trade practice claim affecting consumers. This decision was affirmed by the Supreme Court of Connecticut. They held that the representation to the public was that the providers were properly licensed and, by implication, will meet the applicable standard of care. If they fail to meet that standard of care and harm results, the remedy is one of standard malpractice. There were no unfair or deceptive practices.

In *Pulliam* v. *Coastal Emergency Services*, the patient presented to the ED complaining that her legs aching, after being diagnosed with influenza 2 days previously.[12] She was discharged with a muscle relaxant and instructions to rest. She returned that same day and transferred to the intensive care unit (ICU), where she succumbed allegedly to bacterial pneumonia and bacteremia. There was a contracted service to provide "professional and administrative services" on a full-time basis in the ED. The physicians would direct and supervise all medical services, participate in educational programs, and perform teaching functions. They would also provide the "Chief/Medical Director of the Department" to ensure medical direction in the continuing operation, assure the quality, safety and appropriateness of patient care, and see that the performance of the physicians was in accordance with the contract. The trial court jury returned a verdict in favor of the plaintiff against the treating ED physician and contracted group. The Supreme Court of Virginia held that a prima facie case was established that the business entity "which primarily renders health-care services" was within the definition of health-care provider in Virginia Code: Civil Immunity for Certain Health Care Professionals §8.01-581.15.[13] The trial court did not err in that the

Table 72.4 Operational benchmarks

	Parameter Proportion	Target %
1.	Leaving against medical advice	<1
2.	Leaving withour treatment	<1
		Time (min)
3.	Treatment room	<15
4.	Triage time	<5
5.	Physician to patient time	<30
6.	Presentation to departure time	<120

Reference: IASIS Healthcare.[14]

entity had carried its burden of proof. They were not just a "specialized employment service." Therefore, as health-care providers, the state statutory malpractice cap for the damage award applied.

In *IASIS Healthcare* v. *Apollo Physicians of Texas*, part of the litigation once again related to contractually stipulated operational performance guidelines.[14] The hospital system stipulated that the physician group would comply with and adhere to specific corporate quality standards (Table 72.4).

The group described these "benchmarks" as being worthy goals, but alleged that most fell outside of the doctor's control. Further, they suggested the facility attempted to insert their judgment ahead of the licensed physicians. The Court of Appeals of Texas, Thirteenth District held that the physician group did not elaborate on how the institution of benchmarks by the hospital facility constitutes the practice of medicine, and the judgment for Apollo was reversed taking nothing financially.

Conclusion

It is important to recognize that each ED is unique, but some combination of operational efficiency interventions should be instituted in every department to provide an optimum level of patient care balanced by efficiency.

References

1. Vukmir RB. *The Maximally Efficient and Optimally Effective Emergency Department* (Sewickley, PA: Dichotomy Press, 2015), pp. 1–2.

2. Zun LS. Analysis of the literature on emergency department throughput. *West J. Emerg Med.* 2009;10(2):104–109.

3. Saunders CE. Time Study of patient movement through the emergency department: sources of delay in relation to patient acuity. *Ann Emerg Med*. 1987;16(11):1244–1248. DOI:10.1016/ S0196-0644(87)80232-9.

4. Risser DT, Rice MM, Salisbury ML, Simon R, Jay GD, Berns SD, The MedTeams Research Consortium. The potential for improved teamwork to reduce medical errors in the emergency department. *Ann Emerg Med*. 1999;34(3):373–383. DOI:10.1016/ S0196-0644(99)70134-4.

5. Pruitt CM, Liebeit EL. Enhancing patient safety in the pediatric emergency department: teams, communication, and lessons from crew resource management. *Pediatr Emerg Care*. 2010;26(12):942–948. DOI:10.1097/PEC.0b013e3181fec9cf.

6. Wiler JL, Gentle C, Halfpenny JM, Heins A, Mehrotra A, Mikhail MG, File D. Optimizing emergency department front end operations. *Ann Emerg Med*. 2010;55(2):142–160. DOI:10.1016/ j.annemergmed.2009.05.021.

7. Nash K, Zachariah B, Nitschmann J, Psencik B. Evaluation of the fast track unit of a university emergency department. *J Emerg Nurs*. 2007;33(1):14–20. DOI. 10.1016/j.jen.2006.08.003.

8. Hostetler B, Leikin JB, Timmons JA, Hanashiro PK, Kissane K. Patterns of use of an emergency department-based observation unit. *Am J Ther*. 2002;9(6):499–502.

9. Imperato J, Morris DS, Binder D, Fischer C, Patrick J, Sanchez LD, Setnik G. Physician in triage improves emergency department patient throughput. *Intern Emerg Med*. 2012;7(5):457–462. DOI:10.1007/ s11739-012-0839-0.

10. *Haynes* v. *Yale-New Haven Hospital*, 243 Conn. 17 (1997).

11. Connecticut Unfair Trade Practices Act (CUTPA), General Statutes §42-110a et seq. (11).

12. *Pulliam* v. *Coastal Emergency Services*, 509 S.E.2d 307 (1999).

13. Code of Virginia §8.01–581.15, Limitation on Recovery in Certain Medical Malpractice Actions (2006).

14. *IASIS Healthcare* v. *Apollo Physicians*, Case No.13-10-00173-CV (TX. Court of App. 13, October 20, 2011).

Organ Donation

Case

The patient had a cardiac arrest at home and the paramedics had made an attempt to resuscitate. There was an initial return of spontaneous circulation and resuscitative efforts were then continued in the emergency department (ED) for another 20 minutes without success. The staff called the code to end the resuscitation event, and broke off to speak with the family in the waiting room. This outcome was something the family had anticipated, as the patient's care and course had been discussed, and they knew what had been done by the paramedics and in the ED. The ED physician let the family know that the patient's primary care physician (PCP) would be contacted and that chaplain services were available. She then suggested there was one more issue to discuss, which was organ donation. The patient's daughter spoke up and said she remembered her father commenting favorably on the concept, but he had never got around to the driver licensing bureau to make that change. The family was sure it would be fine and could be discussed with the organ donation group. Soon the organ recovery network would come and speak about the issue with them.

The ED physician continued with the rest of her shift, finished her documentation, and then left for home. The next day the ED director received a call from the quality department to the effect that they had been contacted by the organ recovery network, who reported they had discussed organ donation with the family but had been unsuccessful in getting the family to agree to it. They suggested that only an organ recovery professional should speak to the patient's family about this.

Medical Approach

The organ donation and recovery network has undergone significant changes in recent years. Transplantation medicine programs have grown significantly, and the organ donation solicitation approach has increased in sophistication. Ideally, patients have a pre-stated wish about what they would want done. If not, then one should discuss with the family the "substituted judgment" argument in which the relative is asked to consider the patient's preference if they could speak for themselves.

Despite general public support for organ donation and transplantation, there has been a shortage of organs for transplantation for some time. The legislative process can prove complex at times, and success rates may be improved by more efficient donation processes. Matas favors a "presumed consent" model rather than a "requested consent" model, more common in Europe.[1] However, this strategy is not consistent with the medical informed consent model.

The challenges of organ donation and transplantation often involve the ED, beginning with the question of brain death. The most crucial distinction is between procuring organs in heart-beating donors, the neurologic standard of death, and non-heart-beating donors, the circulatory–respiratory standard of death.[2] The standards clearly should not give the appearance of an active life-ending intervention in the setting of organ procurement.

Public perception of the donor process was studied by Manninen et al. who reported on 2056 respondents, in which 94% had heard of transplantation, but only 19% carried donor cards.[3] They were potentially more likely to donate organs of a relative (53%) than their own (50%), and more likely to donate kidneys (50%) than other organs, such as skin (40%). Most (58%) felt that family should not be able to override a valid donor card, but did not support the concept of presumed consent (7%).

There is a discrepancy between public support for organ donation and actual behavior, with approximately half of the families declining consent for donation in DeJong et al.'s evaluation.[4] They interviewed

Table 73.1 Factors associated with organ donation consent

1.	Beliefs and attitudes concerning organ donation
2.	Family aware of deceased's wishes
3.	Family satisfaction with hospital care
4.	Specifics of donation request process
5.	Family understanding of brain death

Reference: DeJong et al.[4]

Table 73.2 Hierarchy of organ donation consent

1.	Spouse
2.	Adult son or daughter
3.	Either parent
4.	Adult brother or sister
5.	Guardian
6.	Authorized or obligated to dispose

Reference: Uniform Anatomical Gift Act.[7]

families of 164 medically suitable donor candidates and identified factors associated with consent (Table 73.1). First, the characteristics of the patient and family beliefs and attitudes about organ donation and transplantation are predicted. Second, whether the family is aware of the deceased's wishes concerning organ donation. Third, the family's satisfaction with the hospital care their relative received. Fourth, the specific aspects of the donation request process having impact. Fifth, the family's understanding of the of the brain death process has additional impact on the donation process.

Legal Analysis

In *Strachan* v. *John F. Kennedy Memorial Hospital*, a patient who presented to the ED had a self-inflicted cerebral gunshot wound, and quickly progressed to a brain-dead state.[5] The family was approached for organ donation and they declined. Their son met brain death criteria, and support was withdrawn after EEG tests 24 hours apart. The care personnel had varying opinions and thoughts about the support withdrawal process, but the physician agreed as long as the family signed a written consent. Later the family alleged emotional distress due to delay in burial and to discontinuation of life support without standardized procedures and protocols for the process. The trial court initially awarded damages to the family but the Superior Court of New Jersey reversed the ruling, stating there was no breach of any duty by the hospital.

In *Kelly-Nevils* v. *Detroit Receiving Hospital*, the patient again had a self-inflicted gunshot wound, and was declared brain dead.[6] A person identifying himself as the patient's brother, providing his correct birthdate, stated he was the only relative and signed the organ donation consent form. As it turned out, the patient was survived by his mother with whom he resided, and had no brother. The mother filed suit, alleging negligence in the donation process. The question was one of good faith compliance with the

Uniform Anatomical Gift Act (UAGA) which guides the organ donation process, passed in 1968 and 1987 and revised most recently in 2006.[7] Twenty states incorporated the Act in 2007, including Michigan (MCL 333.10101-3 et seq., MSA 14.15 (10101–3) et seq.).[8,9] The Act specifies that:

> Any of the following persons, in order of priority stated, when persons in prior classes are not available at the time of death, and in the absence of actual notice of contrary indications by the decedent or actual notice of opposition by a member of the same or a prior class, may give all or any physical part of the decedent's body for any purpose specified in Section 10103: including spouse, adult son or daughter, either parent, adult brother or sister, guardian or any other person authorized to dispose of the body (Table 73.2).

The circuit court ruled that the defendant acted in good faith and was entitled to immunity under the UAGA, and the Michigan Court of Appeals concurred.

In *Colavito* v. *New York Organ Donor Network*, the patient's widow sought a directed organ donation to her husband's long-time friend.[10] The directed kidney was declined due to a structural defect and the remaining organ was requested, but was already assigned to another patient by the organ-sharing network. In addition, there were some histocompatibility issues with the donated organ. The question arises of whether a property right exists for the organ intended for donation. The trial court awarded a summary judgment motion to the organ-sharing network. The New York Court of Appeals ruled that the property right did not exist, so a claim filed for a tort of conversion did not exist.

Conclusion

In the early days of transplantation, the issue or organ donation was raised by the attending physician who would have presided over end-of-life care. However, in a number of areas the organ donation network is now the group that is empowered to make this first contact and the suggestion is that physicians, nurses, and other health-care professionals should leave the discussion to those with specialist training and education in this area. Organ donation networks feel this increases their success tremendously, and it is worth the time and effort to postpone decision-making until the organ recovery professional arrives.

References

1. Matas AJ, Veith FJ. Presumed consent for organ retrieval. *Theoret Med*. 1984;5(2):155–166.

2. Rady MY, Verheijde JL, McGregor JL. Scientific, legal and ethical challenges of end-of-life organ procurement in emergency medicine. *Resuscitation*. 2010;81(9);1068–1078. DOI:10.1016/j.resuscitation.2010.05.007.

3. Manninen DL, Evans RW. Public attitudes and behavior regarding organ donation. *JAMA*. 1985;253(21):3111–3115. DOI:10.1001/jama.1985.03350450083026.

4. DeJong W, Franz HG, Wolfe SM, Nathan H, Payne D, Reitsma W, Beasley C. Requesting organ donation: an interview study of donor and nondonor families. *Am J Crit Care*. 1998;7(1):13–23.

5. *Strachan* v. *John F. Kennedy Hospital*. 209 N.J. Super. 300 (1986).

6. *Kelly-Nevils* v. *Detroit Receiving Hospital*. 207 Mich. App. 410 (1994).

7. Uniform Anatomical Gift Act (2006). National Conference of Commissioners on Uniform State Laws. January 12, 2008.

8. Michigan Public Health Code. Act 368 of 1978. Revised Uniform Anatomical Gift Law. 333.10101-3.

9. Michigan Determination of Death Act (Excerpt) Act 90 of 1992. 333.1031-33.

10. *Colavito* v. *New York Organ Donor Network*. 8 N.Y. 3d 43 (2006).

Overcrowding

Case

The waiting room was packed. It was a particularly busy time of year: everyone seemed to have a gastrointestinal illness, and the hospital was already full. The average emergency department (ED) wait was a little over 4 hours. The physician had already activated all the available interim measures: the backup ED physician had been called in, nurses were staying over, the floor teams were activating their discharge protocols. But the influx of patients was just too great, the numbers were still overwhelming.

The physician contacted the on-call administrator and discussed diversion of emergency medical services (EMS) patients to other hospitals if the situation didn't start to turn around. The ED remained busy throughout the weekend, but by Monday it was back to its normal level of activity.

At the next medical executive committee meeting, the quality director suggested the amount of ED overcrowding was a safety risk, and wanted to know what the plan might be to address the issue. Other medical staff members commented that it was a particularly busy weekend from their perspective as well. They thought the teamwork between physicians and nurses went well. They asked administration about additional staffing, but were told that was not possible in the current budgetary cycle. The provider team would continue to work cooperatively with their current level of resources and augmented programs to address the overcrowding issue.

Medical Approach

The overcrowding problem is a pervasive part of emergency medicine, particularly in areas with fewer resources, decreased primary care, fewer consultants, and more difficult bed availability. The problem is often sporadic, making it hard to address on the basis of staff considerations alone. In the most extreme circumstances, it has been suggested that this overcrowding issue may manifest as a constructive violation of the Emergency Medical Treatment and Labor Act (EMTALA) by preventing adequate medical screening.[1] Although this is only a theoretical possibility, it may be helpful to think about overcrowding in this way.

Overcrowding in the ED is a long-standing and complex problem, based on many interrelated issues. It has many consequences, including placing the patient at risk for poor outcome, prolonged pain and suffering, prolonged waits, dissatisfaction, ambulance diversion, decreased physician productivity, increased medical staff frustration, and the potential for violence (Table 74.1).[2] It is an emerging threat to patient safety and public health, as described by Trzeciak who identifies key findings from a comprehensive literature review.[3] First, the ED is a vital component of the health-care "safety net." Second, overcrowding of the ED treatment area threatens public health by compromising patient safety and affecting the reliability of the entire emergency care system. Third, although complex, the main causative issue is inadequate capacity for a population with increasing severity of illness. Fourth, potential solutions for the overcrowding

Table 74.1 Effects of ED overcrowding

1.	Poor outcome
2.	Prolonged pain and suffering
3.	Prolonged waits
4.	Patient dissatisfaction
5.	Ambulance diversion
6.	Decreased physician productivity
7.	Medical staff frustration
8.	Potential for violence

Reference: Derlet and Richards.[2]

Table 74.2 Impact of overcrowding

1. Vital component of health-care safety net
2. Compromises patient safety, public health and emergency system reliability
3. Inadequate capacity for increasing disease severity
4. Multidisciplinary system-wide solution

Reference: Trzeciak and Rivers.[3]

Table 74.3 NEDOCS calculator: census effects on crowding

Institutional constants
1. Number of ED beds
2. Number of hospital beds
ED Variables
3. Total ED patients
4. Total admissions
5. Number of critical care patients (ventilators, 1:1 nursing)
6. Longest admission time (hours)
7. Waiting room time of last patient placed in bed (hours)

Reference: Weiss et al.[4]

Table 74.4 Factors related to overcrowding

1. Downsizing of hospital capacity
2. ED closures
3. Increased ED volume
4. Increased number of uninsured patients
5. Declining reimbursement for uncompensated care
6. Providision of routine care
7. Barriers to inpatient admission

Reference: Olshaker and Rathlev.[6]

crisis will require multidisciplinary system-wide support (Table 74.2).

In the National ED Overcrowding Study (NEDOCS), Weiss et al. studied ED overcrowding in academic medical centers.[4] They assessed the status of eight academic medical centers and found overcrowding to occur at a mean of 35%, with a range of 12–73% of cases. Two facilities experienced overcrowding more than 50% of the time. The NEDOCS calculator was developed to estimate census effects based on institutional constants (number of ED beds and number of hospital beds) and ED variables (total ED patients, total admissions, number of ED ventilators, longest admission time, and waiting room time of last patient placed in bed) (Table 74.3). Categories were defined as not busy (00–20), busy (20–60), extremely busy (60–100), overcrowded (100–140), severely overcrowded (140–180), and dangerously overcrowded (180–200). Comparison of objective and outcome data defined a correlation coefficient (R^2) of 0.49 ($P < 0.001$), described as a "good correlation" between variables.

The effects of overcrowding are significant when entry overload can ultimately result in ambulance diversion. Fatovich and Hirsch reported on 141 cases of ambulance bypass with a mean duration of 187 minutes (range 35–995 minutes).[5] Ambulance diversion occurred most commonly on Monday (28%), mid afternoon or evening shift, with entry block the most common (30.4%) reason for activation. During the diversion period, the ED was at 174% (40) capacity, with 61% (14) of patients waiting to be seen, 39% (9) in the hall, and 30% (7) still waiting for admission. Ambulance bypass was associated with a presentation rate of 10 patients, or 44% capacity, presenting for >2 hours (OR 6.2, 95% CI 4.3–8.5). Obviously, the more routine care is provided in this setting, the less episodic, emergency care can be provided.

The overcrowding problem is pervasive, reported in almost every state and by 91% of ED directors.[6] The problem is related to downsizing of hospital capacity, significant number of ED closures, increased ED volume, increase in the uninsured population, declining reimbursement for uncompensated care, and the cyclical use of the ED by those without urgent conditions (Table 74.4). The most significant contributing factor is inability to admit patients to an inpatient bed.

Another clear area for improvement is the availability of primary care resources. Grumbach et al. evaluated 700 patients waiting for ED care at a public hospital.[7] Nearly half (45%) of patients cited barriers to primary care access as their primary reason to use the ED for care. Only 13% of those waiting for care had medical conditions that were appropriate for the ED. Those with a regular source of primary care had more appropriate ED use than those who did not. Most importantly, 38% would accept a visit to a primary care physician within 3 days as an acceptable alternative to their ED visit.

The most important issue is the effect of over-crowding on patient outcome. Bernstein and the Society for Academic Emergency Medicine ED Crowding Task Force identified 369 articles, in which 11% (41) met inclusion criteria.[8] However, study quality was modest, with single-institution observational studies and no randomized clinical trials. ED crowding was associated with increased risk of in-hospital mortality, prolonged treatment times for patients with pneumonia or acute pain, and a higher likelihood of leaving without being seen or against medical advice. However, there was no difference in time to ST elevation myocardial infarction (STEMI) reperfusion, and insufficient data to comment on patient satisfaction.

Likewise, the correlation with overcrowding and mortality appears to be sustained. Richardson evaluated a stratified cohort of 66,608 patients. The mean occupancy was obviously higher for overcrowded shifts (21.6 vs. 16.4 patients).[9] The 10-day mortality was higher in the overcrowding group (0.42% vs. 0.31%, $P = 0.025$), and the relative risk of death was 1.34 (95% CI 1.04–1.72) After controlling for variables, this effect was 13 deaths per year.

Legal Analysis

This can often be an emotional area of emergency medicine practice. In *Genova* v. *Banner Health*, the ED physician had allegedly raised issues of department overcrowding in what was perceived to be a reactionary way, citing a "captain of the ship" analogy.[10] The physician alleged the overcrowding was based on financial considerations, and the hospital alleged the physician's reaction was unprofessional. The physician filed suit, alleging the overcrowded ED conditions were an EMTALA violation.[1] The trial court granted a summary judgment motion for the defendants. The United States Court of Appeals, Tenth Circuit concurred with this decision, stating this sort of private action was not the intent of the EMTALA statute.

Issues of ED staffing or overcrowding often figure in a potential malpractice claim. In *Jersey City Medical Center* v. *Halstead*, it was alleged that bed space was at a premium with 90–98% hospital occupancy.[11] The hospital stated that standard procedure calls for an occupancy rate of not more than 85% to be able to meet emergent needs. The high occupancy rate often manifested as ED bed boarding, delay in admission, postponing of elective surgery and admission to a unit not accustomed to that patient type. The hospital

utilization review committee thought the patient in question could be cared for in a nursing home and she was to be discharged. The hospital sought a mandatory injunction requiring the patient's removal from the hospital. The Superior Court of New Jersey held that the facility has the moral duty to reserve its accommodations for persons who need medical and hospital care. It would be a deviation from its purposes to act as a nursing home for elderly people who do not need acute care. In fact, the cited overcrowding presents a danger for those patients who truly need emergency care. The motion for summary judgment was granted to the facility; the patient's ongoing presence constituted a trespass that would incur damages. However, no action was taken 6 months after the utilization review committee decision.

In *Perry* v. *Owensboro Health*, the patient presented to the ED on two separate occasions complaining of a wound, fever, nausea, vomiting, diarrhea, and an elevated while blood cell count.[12] She was evaluated and discharged twice, was allegedly in pain, and died at home. The plaintiff alleged an EMTALA violation for failure to adequately screen, diagnose, treat, and transfer.[1] The plaintiff also argued improper motive, alleging that an ED overcrowding situation existed and was possibly involved in the patient's discharge after her first ED visit. The trial court granted the defendant's motion for judgment on the pleadings as the complaint failed to state a claim upon which relief can be granted by EMTALA. The district court found any speculative argument concerning improper motivation relating to overcrowding to be insufficient. The plaintiff's remaining state-law claims were dismissed without prejudice.

In *Stock* v. *Harborview Medical Center*, a patient who was found unconscious behind the wheel of her vehicle was intubated and taken to the hospital.[13] She had a small intraventricular hemorrhage and an elevated blood alcohol concentration and was admitted to the intensive care unit (ICU). She was released a few days later, and subsequently filed suit for alleged negligence. Among numerous other claims, she alleged that facility overcrowding compelled her admission to a pediatric ICU, where she felt she would not get proper care as an adult.

The trial court granted summary judgment and dismissed her claim for failing to provide pre-suit notice (RCW 4.92.100) and lack of expert testimony to support her claims.[14] The Court of Appeals of

Washington, Division One held that she indeed failed to provide proper notice of her lawsuit, as well as lacking any expert testimony evidence showing a standard of care deviation. No genuine issue of material fact existed.

Conclusion

Numerous suggestions for operational improvement have been made and many studies performed, but the benefits are often short-lived and unique to the site in question. The key is a local approach with team participation including nurses, physicians, and administrative support. This should be augmented by the adoption of alternative, innovative approaches using externally benchmarked interventions.

References

1. EMTALA, 42 U.S.C. §1395.

2. Derlet RW, Richards JR. Overcrowding in the nation's emergency departments: complex causes and disturbing effects. *Ann Emerg Med.* 2000;35(1):63–68. DOI:10.1016/S0196-0644(00).

3. Trzeciak S, Rivers EP. Emergency department overcrowding in the United States: an emerging threat to patient safety and public health. *Emerg Med J.* 2003;20(5):402–405. DOI:10.1136/emj.20.5.402.

4. Weiss SJ, Derlet R, Arndahl J, Ernst AA, Richards J, Fernandez-Frankelton M, et al. Estimating the degree of emergency department overcrowding in academic medical centers: results of the National ED Overcrowding Study (NEDOCS). *Acad Emerg Med.* 2004;11(1):38–50. DOI:10.1197/j.aem.2003.07.017.

5. Fatovich DM, Hirsch RL. Entry overload, emergency department overcrowding, and ambulance bypass. *Emerg Med. J.* 2003;20(5):406–409. DOI:10.1136/emj.20.5.406.

6. Olshaker JS, Rathlev NK. Emergency department overcrowding and ambulance diversion: the impact and potential solutions of extended boarding of admitted patients in the emergency department. *J Emerg. Med.* 2006;30(3):351–356. DOI:10.1016/j.jemermed.2005.05.023.

7. Grumbach K, Keane D, Bindman A. Primary care and public emergency department overcrowding. *Am J Public Health.* 1993;83(3):372–378. DOI:10.2105/AJPH.83.3.372.

8. Bernstein SL, Aronsky D, Duseja R, Epstein S, Handel D, Hwang U, et al. and SAEM ED Crowding Task Force. The effect of emergency department crowding on clinically oriented outcomes. *Acad Emerg Med.* 2009;16(1):1–10. DOI.10.1111/j.1553-2712.2008.00295.x/full.

9. Richardson DB. Increase in patient mortality at 10 days associated with emergency department overcrowding. *Med J Aust.* 2006;184(5):213–216.

10. *Genova* v. *Banner Health*, 734 F.3d 1095 (2013).

11. Jersey City Medical Center, 404 A.2d 44 (1979).

12. *Perry* v. *Owensboro Health*, 4:14-CV-00046-JHM, July 20, 2015.

13. *Stock* v. *Harborview Medical Center*, No. 71768-5-I.

14. RCW 4.92.100 Tortious Conduct of State or its Agents – Presentment and Filing of Claim Requisite to Suit.

Pain Control/Medication

Case

The patient came to the emergency department (ED) frequently. He had numerous pain complaints – low back pain, dental pain, headache, kidney stone pain, ankle injury – but only rarely was any organic pathology found. The testing, diagnostics, and exams could vary considerably, depending on how familiar the providers were with the patient, but it had been some time since any pathology was indeed found.

This time he presented with flank pain and said he had another kidney stone. His urinalysis was noted to be trace positive for blood, which was not uncommon. The CT scan was normal with no evidence of kidney stone or other pathology. He was to be discharged home to his primary care provider (PCP), and he asked for something for the pain on discharge. He had numerous analgesic allergies, so he was discharged with a prescription for naproxen. This was not one of the allergies that he had reported on registration, but he quickly said that it upset his stomach. He was prescribed paracetamol (acetaminophen) on discharge but again raised concerns over his pain. He insisted that the ED staff was obligated to prescribe oxyco-done/paracetamol (Percocet), which was his usual request. There was discussion with the attending physician, the charge nurse, and the patient advocate. The patient's PCP was called as well. She confirmed that the current treatment course was entirely appropriate and that the patient was in the process of transferring to another physician over the same issue.

The patient stated emphatically that the ED was obliged to prescribe pain medicine and that Percocet was his medication of choice because that was the only thing that had worked in the past. He was referred to a PCP as well as the pain center and was discharged home after an injectable analgesic and a prescription for Tylenol.

The next day the patient advocate called because the patient had complained he had not received his usual pain medication on presentation. The patient's medical record was independently reviewed, and his treatment pathway was found to be entirely appropriate. This pathway had been reviewed numerous times previously, always coming to the same conclusion.

Medical Approach

All patients who present to the ED receive the same comprehensive history, physical exam, and whatever diagnostic testing and type of medication that may be warranted. But the choice of analgesic medication has become significantly more complicated as the number of external agencies with opinions on the subject has increased exponentially.

The concern has been raised that pain control is inadequate in some emergency settings. Rupp and Delaney in 2004 reviewed ED pain management practices and suggested inconsistency and inadequacy affecting multiple demographic groups due to multiple factors (Table 75.1).[1] First, there is a lack of educational emphasis on pain management in medical school, nursing, and postgraduate training programs. Second, clinical quality management programs evaluating pain management practice are inadequate. Third, there is a lack of rigorous studies of populations with special analgesia needs such as geriatric or pediatric patients. Fourth, attitudes of clinicians to opioid analgesics result in inappropriate diagnosis of drug-seeking behavior and misdirected concerns about addiction, even in those with painful conditions requesting relief. Fifth, "opiophobia," inappropriate concerns about opioid safety compared with non-steroidal anti-inflammatory drugs (NSAIDs), results in their underuse. Sixth, there are under-appreciated gender and cultural differences in pain reporting by

Table 75.1 Potential factors related to inadequate analgesia

1.	Lack of pain management education
2.	Lack of quality management programs
3.	Paucity of studies in populations with special needs (pediatric and geriatric)
4.	Inappropriate clinician attitudes, drug-seeking labels, and addiction concerns
5.	"Opiophobia": inappropriate opioid safety concerns
6.	Unappreciated gender and cultural differences impacting pain reporting
7.	Racial and ethnic stereotyping bias on pain interpretation

Reference: Rupp and Delaney.[1]

patients and interpretation by providers. Seventh, extrinsic bias related to racial and ethnic stereotypes causes disbelief of pain reporting.

The *Morbidity and Mortality Weekly Report* (MMWR) profiled ED visits involving non-medical use of selected prescription drugs.[2] The Drug Abuse Warning Network defines the non-medical use of medication at higher than the recommended dose, taking a medication prescribed for another patient, drug-facilitated assault, or misuse or abuse, all of which must be documented in the medical record.[3] They analyzed 1.6–2.0 million ED visits from 2004 to 2008, where there was a 111% increase in non-medical use of opioid analgesics and an 89% increase in benzodiazepine use. The fastest growing group was in the 21–29-year age range, and 25% of all patients who presented to the ED were admitted.

One of the concerns is that chronic pain patients incorrectly self-report their drug use during evaluation. Fishbain et al. obtained toxicology testing for drugs in 226 patients, which were negative in 53.5% (121) and positive in 46.5% (1054). There were 8.4% of patients with illicit drugs in their urine samples, 6.2% cannabis, and 2.2% cocaine. Likewise, 8.8% (20) patients provided incorrect self-report information about current drug use, most frequently involving illicit drugs. The misreporting group was more likely to be younger, on workers compensation, with a polysubstance abuse diagnosis.

One suggested interventional approach is the prescription monitoring program (PMP) for chronic pain management irregularities.[5] The designated prescription drug abuse behaviors include doctor shopping, drug theft, feigned pain symptoms to gain health-care access, drug sharing, prescription forgery, and improper prescription practices. In the 38 states that had a monitoring program it was felt to decrease the availability of the diverted prescription medication supply, and decrease the time required for law enforcement to conduct investigations. However, some feel that although prescribing practice is changed, the actual rate of abuse may not be decreased.

Another common concern is the liability associated with prescribing controlled substances.[6] Ideally, the patient has an acute condition and pain is adequately controlled until the patient makes a complete recovery. The initial high-risk area is when the physician overprescribes, or prescribes off protocol, making them liable for licensing board or regulatory agency report. As well, a potential lawsuit alleges the physician should have known this practice would predispose the patient to addiction. More recently, the concern is under-treatment of pain with again a regulatory agency report, and the potential for litigation alleging negligent prescribing practice precipitating needless suffering.

Legal Analysis

In *O'Donnell* v. *Barnhart*, the patient had residual disability after an automobile accident.[7] The ED evaluation used radiographic and MRI examinations to reveal no fractures and dislocations, although mild degenerative disease was present. The ED physician discharged the patient, prescribing rest, a cervical collar, and medications. The patient then made multiple primary and specialty care visits, where it was suggested that there was no objective basis for symptoms. Over a 5-year period, she made over 50 office visits or phone calls relating to various pain syndromes, and was referred to a pain management service for intractable pain. She declined to participate in pain management programs, and there was other alleged non-compliance.

The administrative-law judge (ALJ) recommended additional evaluations, which she attended in a wheelchair, keeping her hat and sunglasses on for the duration of the exam. Benefits were denied, and a request to appear before the Appeals Council was declined. The United States Court of Appeals (USCA), Eighth Circuit reversed the judgment of the district court and remanded to the Commissioner for further proceedings. They acknowledged the established non-compliance with treatment recommendations, but felt the rationale could have been investigated further.

In *Carradine* v. *Barnhart*, the claimant alleged severe and disabling pain making a productive occupation difficult.[8]

The ALJ found that the available physical and psychological medical findings did not support her allegations of suffering from debilitating pain, and that her pain complaints were unreliable. This decision was upheld by the district court and affirmed by the USCA, Seventh Circuit.

Clinicians are surprised to find that the criteria for disability determination, in the setting of pain, focus as much on subjective as objective findings:

> Once the claimant produces medical evidence of an underlying impairment, the Commissioner may not discredit the claimant's testimony as to subjective symptoms merely because they are unsupported by objective evidence.[9]

Conclusion

These cases are best handled with a combination of primary care and a specific case management protocol for chronic recurrent pain and a referral to the pain service itself. This is more helpful to the patient than sporadic episodic courses of analgesics prescribed by acute care providers. The key here is the continuum of care, involving the same group or practitioner to be most effective.

References

1. Rupp T, Delaney KA. Inadequate analgesia in emergency medicine. *Ann Emerg Med*. 2004;43(3):494–503. DOI:10.1016/j.annemergmed.2003.11.019.

2. Cai R, Crane E, Poneleit K. Emergency department visits involving nonmedical use of selected prescription drugs-united states, 2004–2008. *MMWR* 2010;59(23):705–709.

3. Drug Abuse Warning Network, 2007: National Estimates of Drug-Related Emergency Department Visits. (Rockville, MD: U.S. Department of Health and Human Services, Office of Applied Studies, May 2010).

4. Fishbain DA, Cutler RB, Rosomoff HL, Rosomoff RS. Validity of self-reported drug use in chronic pain patients. *Clin J Pain*. 1999;15(3):184–191.

5. Wang J, Christo PJ. The influence of prescription monitoring programs on chronic pain management. *Pain Physician*. 2009;12(3):507–515.

6. Nist JB. Liability for overprescription of controlled substances: can it be justified in light of the current practice of undertreating pain? *J Leg Med*. 2002;23(1):85–113.

7. O'Donnell MJ, Barnhart JB, 318 F.3d 811 (2003).

8. *Carradine* v. *Barnhart*, 360 F.3d 751 (2004).

9. *Lester* v. *Chater*, 81 F.3d 821 (1996).

Chapter 76

Patient Satisfaction

Case

Another group of consultants was coming through the emergency department (ED) on one of its busiest days in recent memory. These consultants were targeting improvements in customer service and patient satisfaction. Two other consulting groups had visited the department in the past year, and the department's customer service scores were quite good by industry comparison.

The consultants seemed pleasant enough and made a number of suggestions to the staff implying that customer service scores were associated with medical malpractice experiences. One of the physicians questioned this. He thought it was partially true, but there wasn't a simple relationship between customer service and medicolegal experience.

The hospital's new patient experience coordinator was there as well, and she outlined the hospital's goals and objectives. She also stated there was a clear correlation between customer service and adverse medical events and medical errors. The consultants were asked to provide some evidence for this assessment. They said they did not have that available currently but would send it later.

The ED made recommendations to the hospital administration and suggested they would do their best to implement those suggestions that were important from a patient care perspective.

Medical Approach

The patient experience is a very important part of the emergency health-care delivery system. This experience ties directly to customer service and patient satisfaction. A host of correlations have been found, including the interface with medicolegal experience, efficiency, adverse events, and return hospital visits, but currently the evidence is variable regarding correlation to objective outcome measures.

Patient satisfaction in emergency medicine was studied by Taylor and Benger who performed a systematic review and identified seven controlled intervention studies.[1] The most frequently identified factors strongly correlated with patient satisfaction were interpersonal skills and staff attitudes, provision of information and explanation, and perceived waiting times (Table 76.1). There was some correlation with age and race, but it was less consistent. The triage category was strongly associated, but this may have been related to less waiting time. Key interventions to improve satisfaction address staff attitudinal skills, increase communication, and reduce perceived waiting times.

The ED complaint demographic was profiled by Taylor et al. who reported on 2419 ED patients generating 3418 complaints from 36 facilities, which was 15.4% of the hospital total.[2] The complaints were communicated by telephone in 47.8% (1157) cases and by letter in 34.3% (829). Interestingly, most (63.1%, 1526) complaints were made by someone other than the patient. The highest complaint rates were from patients who were female, born in non-English-speaking countries, and at age extremes, either very young or old.

First, the major category of concern related to patient treatment (33.4%, 1141), predominantly treatment felt to be inadequate (28.8%, 329) or inadequate

Table 76.1 Factors identified in ED customer satisfaction

1.	Interpersonal skills
2.	Staff attitudes
3.	Provision of information
4.	Adequate explanation
5.	Perceived waiting time

Reference: Taylor and Benger.[1]

diagnosis (21.8%, 249). Second came issues related to communication (31.6%, 1079), with the majority of cases (41.1%, 444) relating to poor staff attitude, discourtesy, and rudeness. Third, 11.9% (407) of issues related to delay in treatment (Table 76.2).

The overall resolution was satisfactory in the majority of cases (73.6%, 2516), usually by explanation or apology. Remedial action was taken in 3.2% (109) of cases, 1.7% (59) resulted in procedure or policy change, and compensation was paid in only 0.23% (8).

The ED patient interaction can be problematic since there is no prior relationship, interactions are brief, and the environment can be hectic at times.

Cydulka et al. evaluated the administrative databases from 34 EDs in eight states merged with patient satisfaction data.[3] They evaluated 2,462,617 patient interactions with an overall complaint incidence of 0.015% (375) and a 0.002% (61) rate of risk management episodes. Those providers in the lowest quartile of patient satisfaction were almost twice as likely to have a complaint (OR 1.84; 95% CI 1.29–2.63) as those in the highest. Satisfaction scores were not correlated with subsequent risk management episodes. However, complaints were more strongly associated with risk management episodes. Those providers receiving two or more complaints per quarter were 4.13 times (95% CI 1.12–15.2) more likely to have a risk management episode.

The presence of adverse events (AE), and their disclosure is associated with patient's ratings of care quality. Lopez et al. identified 603 patients with 845 AEs, in which 40% were disclosed to the patient (Table 76.3).[4] Those AEs that required additional treatment, in patients who were in good health, were more likely to be disclosed. The AEs not likely to be disclosed were preventable, or still affecting the patient at time of survey. Higher care quality ratings were associated with disclosure of preventable or non-preventable events the patients felt they were able to protect themselves from. Care quality ratings were lower when events were preventable, increased discomfort, or were still affecting the patient.

The next step in the analysis is to evaluate the association between patient satisfaction and malpractice lawsuits. Stelfox et al. evaluated 353 physicians correlating customer service ratings by tertile to risk management episodes (Table 76.4).[5] Decreases in patient satisfaction survey scores were associated with increased rates of unsolicited complaints and risk

Table 76.2 Adverse event disclosure and patient care ratings

Status	Likelihood	
	OR	95% CI
Disclosed		
1. Required additional treatment	1.64	1.16–2.32
2. Affected those in good health	2.04	1.29–3.24
Not disclosed		
3. Preventable	0.58	0.41–0.83
4. Still affected	0.49	0.31–0.78
Higher quality rating		
5. Protect themselves	2.04	1.39–2.99
Lower quality rating		
6. Preventable	0.55	0.40–0.76
7. Cause of discomfort	0.62	0.46–0.86
8. Adverse effect still present	0.68	0.46–0.98

Reference: Taylor et al.[2]

Table 76.3 Patient satisfaction, complaints, and lawsuits

Satisfaction		Tertile			Comparison
100,000 visits	**High**	**Middle**	**Low**		
1. Unsolicited complaints	200	243	492		P < 0.0001
2. Risk management episodes	29	43	56		P < 0.007
Malpractice rates					**%RR, 95% CI, P**
	0				
		26			1.26, 0.72–2.18, 0.41
			110		2.10, 1.13–3.90, 0.019

Reference: Lopez et al.[4]

Table 76.4 ED service complaints

Issue	Incidence (%)
1. Inadequate treatment	33.4
Treatment	
Diagnosis	
2. Communication	31.6
Staff attitude	
Discourtesy	
Rudeness	
3. Delay in treatment	11.9

Reference: Taylor et al.[2]

management episodes ($P = 0.007$). Compared to the highest rating, the middle tertile had malpractice lawsuit rates 26% higher ($P = 0.41$), and the lowest tertile 110% higher ($P = 0.019$). The authors concluded that prospectively distributed customer service questionnaires have validity.

The experience is that medical malpractice exposure is concentrated in a small portion of physicians. Hickson et al. evaluated 645 general and specialist physicians comparing unsolicited patient complaints and risk management events.[6] They found that both patient complaints and risk management events were higher in surgeons than non-surgeons: 32% (137/426) of non-surgeons had at least one risk management filing, compared to two-thirds or 63% (137/219) of surgeons ($x^2 = 54.7$, $P < 0.001$) However, both complaint and risk management data were correlated with clinician activity. Logistic regression with data adjusted for clinical activity found that risk management reports, file opening with expenditure, and lawsuits were significantly related to total number of patient complaints.

Legal Analysis

In *Pegram* v. *Herdich*, the physician representing a clinic and health maintenance organization (HMO) evaluated the patient for abdominal pain and found a mass.[7] The physician is alleged to have ordered an ultrasound examination to be performed not at the local hospital but rather at an affiliated clinic, allegedly after an 8-day delay. The patient subsequently ruptured her appendix with resulting peritonitis. The patient sued the facility and clinic for medical malpractice, and added two subsequent claims alleging state law fraud counts. They alleged that HMOs are better served by rewarding both quality of care and patient satisfaction. The legal question raised is whether the decisions made by an HMO acting through its physician employees are fiduciary acts within the meaning of the Employee Retirement Income Security Act of 1974 (ERISA).[8] The malpractice counts were tried by jury with a financial recovery for the patient. However, the ERISA claim was dismissed, and appealed to the United States Court of Appeals, Seventh Circuit. The appeal court held that the clinic was acting as a fiduciary, although the offering of financial incentives does not automatically give rise to that breach. The US Supreme Court of the United States granted certiorari, and reversed the appeal court decision. The fiduciary responsibility under ERISA provides that the discharge of duties with respect to the plan is "solely in the interest of the participants and beneficiaries – for the exclusive benefits of the beneficiaries and to defray reasonable expenses of the plan." [9] They held that mixed eligibility decisions by HMO physicians are not fiduciary decisions under ERISA.

Conclusion

The advent of the "patient experience" perspective has supplanted "customer service" as the newest frame of reference to address this important issue. Focus on this cornerstone issue is crucial to the provision of optimal medical care.

References

1. Taylor C, Benger JR. Patient satisfaction in emergency medicine. *Emerg Med J*. 2004;21(5):528–532. DOI:10.1136//emj.2002.003723.

2. Taylor DM, Wolfe R, Cameron PA. Complaints from emergency department patients largely result from treatment and communication problems. *Emerg Med*. 2002;14(1):43–49. DOI:10.1046/j.1442–2026.2002.00284.x.

3. Cydulka RK, Tamayo-Sarver J, Gage A, Bagnoli D. Association of patient satisfaction with complaints and risk management among emergency physicians. *J Emerg Med*. 2011;41(4):405–411. DOI:10.1016/j.jemermed.2010.10.021.

4. Lopez L, Weismann JS, Schneider EC, Weingart SN, Cohen AP, Epstein AM. Disclosure of hospital adverse events and its association with patients' ratings of the quality of care. *Arch Intern Med*. 2009;169(20):1888–1894. DOI:10.1001/archintmed.2009.387.

5.   Stelfox HT, Gandi TK, Orav EJ, Gustafson ML. The relation of patient satisfaction with complaints against physicians and malpractice lawsuits. *Am J Med.* 2005;118(10):1126–1133. DOI:10.1016/j.amjmed.2005.01.060.

6.   Hickson GB, Federspiel CF, Pichert JW, Miller CS, Gauld-Jaeger J, Bost P. Patient complaints and malpractice risk. *JAMA.* 2002;287(22):2951–2957. DOI:10.1001/jama.287.22.2951.

7.   *Pegram* v. *Herdrich,* 530 U.S. 211 (2000).

8.   Employee Retirement Income Security Act of 1974 (ERISA) 29 U.S.C. §1001 et seq. (1994).

9.   29 U.S. Code §1104 – Fiduciary Duties.

Pediatric Abuse

Case

When she presented to the emergency department (ED) the child's mother said she wasn't acting right. She was normally an active 10-month-old, she didn't have a fever, but seemed less active than usual. Her appetite was decreased as well. She had no recent cough or cold illness and had no diarrhea or vomiting, but just seemed listless.

The child had no other health history and had been immunized appropriately. The physician asked about her care circumstances, and was told she was cared for in a daycare center. But her mother said sometimes her friends watched her as well occasionally, if she could not get a sitter.

The provider performed a urinalysis, which was normal, and ordered a chest radiograph because of the recent cough. On the chest radiograph, they noticed two left-sided anterior rib fractures. The child's mother was asked again if there had been any issues at home recently, any falls or trauma. She said she didn't know of any, but couldn't be sure. The physician performed a skeletal survey and found a proximal fibula fracture as well.

A history that did not fit the presentation and the presence of two fractures was a cause of concern. The child was admitted to the pediatric service who began a suspected child abuse evaluation. Child Protective Services was also consulted to begin a suspected child abuse and neglect evaluation.

Medical Approach

In the ED, the message is to always be suspicious of child abuse or neglect. In younger children, the presentation will often be subtle, as it was with this case. A significant finding was noted, which was then followed up with a more general screen and skeletal survey for other injuries. Finding a second injury indicated the child was clearly at risk for abuse or neglect, requiring admission to the hospital system and further workup and inquiry to evaluate the likelihood of abuse.

As of 2013, all 50 states and five territories have some sort of mandatory child abuse or neglect reporting law.[1] The majority of states (48) designate specific reporting requirements for medical, educational, law enforcement, social service, mental health, and administrative professionals, while 18 states require any person, including lay people, to make the report.

Health-care reporting requirements often involve the primary care community. Flaherty et al. evaluated 85 providers in 17 clinical practices.[2] They reported 56% (48) of the providers felt they had treated a potentially abused child in the last year, estimated to be 152 children in total. There were 8% (7) of providers who did not report 5% (7) of potential abuse cases. Providers who had post-residency training in pediatric abuse were more likely to report.

Unrecognized child abuse is problematic as a leading cause of morbidity or mortality. King et al. identified 44 pediatric homicide deaths, in which 84% (37) of victims were younger than 4 years of age.[3] Cause of death in this group was blunt head injury (57%), blunt torso injury (13%), gunshot wound (11%), fire (8%), drowning (8%), and poisoning (3%). Fractures were particularly common, found in 24% (9), in which most (78%, 7) fractures were at different stages of healing. Most importantly, 30% (11) of children had documented non-routine health-care visits during the previous year with 19% (7) occurring in the month before their death.

The standard for child abuse diagnosis should be the pediatric ED. Keshavarz et al. reviewed 106 reported suspected child abuse cases reporting physical abuse in 55%, neglect in 30%, and sexual abuse in 15%.[4] The suspected perpetrator was the mother in 41% and the father in 21% of cases and the mean patient age was 6.4 years. There was an average of 4.6

previous ED visits and 69% presented for care between 5 p.m. and 9 a.m. Physical abuse cases had bruises in 25% of cases, but sexual abuse cases typically had no physical findings at the time of presentation. After completion of the external review 46% (49) cases were found to be valid, 34% (36) undetermined, and 20% (21) unfounded. The majority of cases of both physical and sexual abuse did not have physical evidence on presentation.

Forensic evidence is particularly difficult in cases of pediatric sexual assault. Christian et al. reviewed the records of 273 children less than 10 years of age evaluated in the ED.[5] For those who presented within 24 hours there was a 90% rate of recovery of forensic evidence, and for those examined within 44 hours of their assault the recovery rate was 25%. The majority (64%) of evidence was found on clothing or linen, while a minority (23%) of children had forensic evidence of a genital injury. This population requires a high level of suspicion for proper diagnosis and intervention.

The delay in diagnosis with pediatric abuse can be especially problematic. Ravichandiran et al. reported on 258 pediatric patients aged less than 3 years with abusive fractures.[6] They found that one-fifth (20.9%, 54) of patients had at least one previous clinical visit at which the alleged abuse was missed. The median time to correct diagnosis was 8 days, with a range of 1 to 160 days. Independent predictors of missed abuse were male gender, extremity versus axial fracture location, presentation to primary care versus ED, and general to pediatric ED.

An area of some uncertainty is the interface of information disclosure and the pediatric abuse process. The Health Insurance Portability and Accountability Act (HIPAA) permits disclosure of information without legal guardian authorization in matters that affect the treatment of, and medical intervention for, the child and the intervention and investigation of matters that relate to abuse or neglect, public health, and safety.[7,8] HIPAA also regulates release of information to the legal guardian of the child for situations when disclosure may jeopardize the safety of the child. In addition, HIPAA allows disclosure of protected health information (PHI) without legal guardian authorization in the setting of reported suspected child abuse or neglect. Information can be released to law enforcement if they are a designated authority and part of the child abuse investigation process.

Legal Analysis

In *Deshaney* v. *Winnebago County Department of Social Services*, the abused minor through his guardian sued the respondents, the county social service agency, for not removing him from a dangerous living situation.[9] The child was allegedly beaten and permanently injured by his father, and the department had received previous reports of abuse. The petitioner sued, alleging he was deprived of his Fourteenth Amendment rights afforded by the Due Process clause.[10] The mother and child brought suit invoking 42 U.S. Code §1983 – Civil Action For Deprivation of Rights, allowing personal recovery for a constitutional issue.[11] The district court granted judgment to the respondents, which was affirmed by the United States Court of Appeals, Seventh Circuit. The Supreme Court of the United States felt that the obligation to shift the liability to the state may have merit, but is not supported by expanding the Due Process clause of the Fourteenth Amendment.

In *State of North Carolina* v. *Grover*, the issue of expert testimony in pediatric abuse cases was reviewed.[12] This case centered around the alleged sexual abuse, resulting in felony child abuse of minor children. The issue addressed by the court was from the defendant's appeal, suggesting that since there were no physical signs of abuse, the pediatric nurse practitioner and social service expert opinions should be dismissed. The trial court declined this argument, but this decision was overruled by the North Carolina Court of Appeals recommending a new trial for the defendant. They held that, "the state was required to lay a sufficient foundation to show that the opinion expressed by [the experts] was really based on [their] special expertise, or stated differently, that [the experts were] in a better position than the jury to have an opinion on the subject."[13]

Likewise, in *State of Minnesota* v. *Scacchetti*, the appellant was convicted of alleged sexual misconduct and assault of a child.[14] The child had allegedly suffered both physical and sexual abuse. The child, who was 3.5 years of age at the time, was incompetent to testify, so the pediatric nurse practitioner was required to testify as an expert witness. She testified the child had sexual knowledge beyond her age, and based on her experience, the child had been abused. The defendant was convicted by the trial court, and the conviction was affirmed by the appeal court. He appealed to the Supreme Court of Minnesota, the petition was granted and remanded to the appeal court for reconsideration.

The Sixth Amendment of the United States Constitution ensures the defendant's right "to be confronted with the witnesses against him."[15] Until this time the Roberts Test had held, "where an unavailable witness's statements were admissible if they bore adequate indicia of reliability." The evidence was reliable if it fell within a firmly rooted hearsay exception or bore "particularized guarantees of trustworthiness."[16] The Supreme Court rejected this premise in *Crawford* v. *Washington*, explaining, "the principal evil at which the Confrontation Clause was directed was the civil-law mode of criminal procedure, and particularly its use of ex-parte examinations as evidence against the accused."[17] Therefore, when a witness is unavailable, testimonial statements made by the witness are inadmissible at the defendant's trial, unless the defendant has the opportunity to cross-examine the witness.

Conclusion

We all recognize that emergency physicians and other licensed professionals have an obligatory reporting requirement in relation to suspected child abuse. Failure to report results in civil or criminal liability for the health-care provider. Our goal is always to err on the side of caution in a non-confrontational way. Hospital admission often proves to be a way to achieve that endpoint without further confrontation, allowing our objective workup to be completed as well.

References

1. National Conference of State Legislatures. Mandatory Reporting of Child Abuse and Neglect. 2013 Introduced State Legislation. September 20, 2015.

2. Flaherty EG, Sage R, Binns HJ. Mattson CL, Christoffei KK and the Pediatric Practice Research Group. Health care providers's experience reporting child abuse in the primary care setting. *Arch Pediatr Adolesc Med*. 2000;154(5):489–493. DOI.10.1001/archpedi.154.5.489.

3. King WK, Kiesel EL, Simon HK. Child abuse fatalities: are we missing opportunities for intervention? *Ped Emerg Care*. 2006;22(4):211–214. DOI:10.1097/01.pec.0000208.180.94166.dd.

4. Keshavarz R, Kawashima R, Low C. Child abuse and neglect presentations to a pediatric emergency department. *J Emerg Med*. 2002;23(4):341–345. DOI:10.1016/S0736-4679(02)00575-9.

5. Christian CW, Lavelle JM, De Jong AR, Loiselle J, Brenner L, Joffe M. Forensic evidence findings in prepubertal victims of sexual assault. *Pediatrics*. 2000;106(1):100–104.

6. Ravichandiran N, Schuh S, Bejuk M, Al-Harthy N, Shouldice M, Au H, Boutis K. Delayed identification of pediatric abuse-related fractures. *Pediatrics*. 2010;125(1):60–66. DOI:10.1542/peds.2008–3794.

7. Health Insurance Portability and Accountability Act of 1996 (HIPAA), Title XI, Pub. L. 104–191, 110 Stat. 1936 (August 21, 1996), codified as 42 U.S.C. 1301 et seq.

8. American Academy of Pediatrics: Committee on Child Abuse and Neglect. Child abuse, confidentiality and the Health Insurance Portability and Accountability Act. *Pediatrics*. 2010;125(1):197–201. DOI:10.1542/Peds.2009–2864.

9. *Deshaney* v. *Winnebago County Department of Social Services*, 489 U.S. 189 (1989).

10. U.S. Const. Amend. IV.

11. 42 U.S. Code §1983–Civil Action For Deprivation of Rights.

12. *State* v. *Grover*, 543 S.E.2d 179 (2001).

13. *State* v. *Trent*, 320 N.C. 610, 614, 359 S.E.2d 463, 465 (1987).

14. *State of Minnesota* v. *Sacchetti*, 711 N.W.2d 508 (2006).

15. U.S. Const. Amend VI.

16. *Ohio* v. *Roberts*, 448 U.S. 56, 100 S.Ct. 2531, 65 L. Ed.2d 597 (1980).

17. *Crawford* v. *Washington*, 541 U.S. 36 (2004).

Chapter 78

Peer Review

Case

The quality committee contacted the emergency department (ED) regarding a case it had referred for peer review for one of the physicians in the practice. The allegation was that a patient had been mismanaged in the ED and the wrong therapeutic plan had been instituted. The physician involved offered to contribute her own review of the case. The quality committee had already begun their review and welcomed the ED input, but wanted a response from the physician personally as well. They were hoping to have this information before the next committee meeting.

Participation in the process was to let the treating physician know that a concern had been raised. The quality committee's decision stated that the care was appropriate, and they would provide some articles in support of that position. In any event, one member of the committee stated, "the utility of peer review for individual case analysis has not been proven." In fact, some research suggests peer review may not be reliable at all, and the committee member offered to provide that information as well. The committee chair suggested that although this may be true, perhaps the information could be presented at a later time, when the committee did not have a case under scrutiny. This is probably the proper administrative approach.

Medical Approach

From a historical perspective the use of hospital-based peer review has been the standard practice. Here, a physician, ideally of a similar practice specialty and circumstance, reviews the case compared to evidence-based standards. In practice, however, often a physician of the same specialty cannot be identified, or if they are identified they may work in a similar or competitive group. Therefore, the physician under review often raises issues of competitive disadvantage when care is reviewed by another staff member.

The hospital peer review process is one of the cornerstones of medical care quality, taking its place along with the facility credentialing and privileging process, specialty board certification, state medical licensure board certification, professional society monitoring, governmental regulatory agency oversight, and medical malpractice litigation (Tables 78.1 and 78.2).

The crux of the review process rests with the medical record itself. O'Neill et al. questioned the

Table 78.1 Cornerstones of medical care quality

1.	Peer review process
2.	Facility credentialing and privileging
3.	Specialty board certification
4.	State medical licensure
5.	Professional society monitoring
6.	Governmental agency oversight
7.	Medical malpractice litigation

Table 78.2 Peer review protection privilege parameters: balancing public and private interests

1.	Should create and maintain records
2.	Record dedicated solely to pursuit of safety
3.	Excludes original source information
4.	Excludes dual source information
5.	Chartered patient safety organization (PSO)
6.	Organization uses patient safety evaluation system (PSES)
7.	Patient safety work product (PSWP) cannot be shared with non-approved entities
8.	Records must be safely and securely sequestered from inspection
9.	Analysis utilized for education and patient care improvement
10.	Excludes information dedicated to facility or individual licensing requirements

reliability of physician self-reporting compared to structured medical record review to identify adverse medical events in an analysis of 3416 admissions.[1] The physician reporting mechanism identified nearly the same number of adverse events (AE) as the structured review method of analysis (2.8%, 89 vs. 2.7%, 85). However, the physician identification method defined more preventable events (62.5 vs. 32%, $P = 0.003$), and could be performed at one-third of the cost ($15,000 vs. $54,000). This finding was related to the use of house staff as the physician reviewers.

The next step of the analysis is to predict the concurrence of physician opinion in chart review. Localio et al. performed an observational study of 7533 pairs of structured implicit reviews from medical records, in which subjective opinions are formulated based on clinical guidelines, by 127 physicians.[2] There was concurrence in the identification of an AE between two physicians in 10% (757) of medical record reviews. However, there was extreme disagreement about the occurrence of an AE in 12.9% (971) of the physician reviews. There was greatest agreement for specific disease conditions such as wound infection cases. As well, physicians with greater experience with record review increased the level of concordance. There was less agreement with more general concerns, such as failure to diagnose or treat. Even with standardization of the sample, the incidence of an individual physician finding evidence of an AE still varied widely, from 9.9 to 43.7% ($P < 0.001$), raising concerns for external validity.

Likewise, the routine clinical audit process has been evaluated as a peer review method. McKay et al. evaluated 1002 audit submissions and judged 55% (552) to be satisfactory in the care provided by general practitioners.[3] Longer practice experience was more likely to generate a satisfactory peer review. The decrease in the proportion of acceptable peer review may as well be related to difficulty with the audit methodology, as with the care provided.

Lastly, the agreement in expert opinion in medical malpractice review is examined. Posner et al. allowed a team of anesthesiologists to review 103 malpractice claims, each independently reviewed by two physicians.[4] Most (83%, 25) had previous experience as an expert witness, 53% (16) practiced in an academic setting, 30% (9) in private practice with teaching, and 17% (5) in private practice. They had been in practice for a median of 16 years with a range of 5 to 41 years.

They reviewed care as appropriate in 62% (64) of the claims and disagreed in 38% (39). However, overall they suggested care was appropriate in 27%, less than appropriate in 32%, and impossible to decide in 3% of cases. The level of agreement was suboptimal in the barely above chance to poor range ($\kappa = 0.37$; 95% CI 0.22–0.52), with 0.40 required for good and 0.75 for excellent agreement.

Legal Analysis

In *Roach* v. *Springfield Clinic*, a question was raised concerning an alleged anesthesia delay in the care of an obstetrics patient.[5] The trial court sustained the Memorial Medical Center motion to prevent the nurse anesthetist from testifying, based on the privileged nature of the communication. They concluded it was inadmissible under Section 8–2102 and privileged under Section 8–210 of the Code of Civil Procedure:

> All information, interviews, reports, statements, memoranda for other data … of committees of licensed or accredited hospitals or their medical staffs, including Patient Care Audit Committees, Medical Care Evaluation Committees, Utilization Review Committees, Credential Committees and Executive Committees (but not the medical records pertaining to the patient), used in the course of internal quality control or of medical study for the purpose of reducing morbidity or mortality, or for improving patient care, shall be privileged, strictly confidential and shall be used only for medical research, evaluation and improvement of quality care, or granting limiting or revoking staff privileges, except that in any hospital proceeding to decide upon a physician's staff privileges, or in any judicial review thereof, the claim of confidentiality shall not be invoked to deny such physician access to or use data upon which such a decision was based.[6]

The appellate court affirmed, as the information was privileged, used for "staff of an accredited hospital … used in course of internal quality control … for the purpose of improving patient care." The Supreme Court of Illinois affirmed in part and reversed in part, remanding for reconsidering the denial motion as the conversation concerning care did not appear to be related to an official peer review committee meeting.

In *Virmani* v. *Novant Health*, the hospital appealed an order of the district court denying a protective order and compelling the physician's motion to produce medical peer review records.[7] The physician allegedly had a patient care complication, resulting in an extensive peer review evaluation. The initial review lasted 5 months and reviewed over 100 cases, allegedly finding that 25% of this physician's cases were felt to be problematic, resulting in a termination of staff privileges. This finding was echoed by a second, separate peer review committee. Novant argued the district court erred in refusing to recognize privilege of medical peer review. Federal Rule of Evidence 501, which governs privilege in federal courts, provides that, with certain specific exceptions, privilege "shall be governed by the principles of the common law as they may be interpreted by the courts of the United States in light of reason or experience." [8] The United States Court of Appeals, Fourth Circuit held that the interest in obtaining probative evidence in a discrimination action outweighs the interest in continuing to recognize the medical peer-review privilege. The balance of these two interests requires the patient care event be sent for external peer review, which can be a costly and time-consuming process, but eliminates the potential bias of an on-site review. In addition, even eliminating the possibility of bias, it is suggested that the review process may not be objective. Even an unaligned remote reviewer may issue a suboptimal opinion based on the nature of the review process itself, which is often subjective, where objective data may be lacking.

There has clearly been a recent trend toward loss of protection for patient safety activities. For example, in *Reginelli* v. *Boggs*, the patient presented to the ED with chest pain and alleged negligent care by the physician resulting in long-term cardiac sequelae.[9] During the course of discovery, it became apparent that the management company physician supervisor monitored performance data for the ED physician group. The trial court issued an order to compel production of the "complete performance file" pertaining to the defendant physician. The defendants appealed the release of the performance file, asserting the file was privileged as peer review protected by the Pennsylvania Peer Review Protection Act (PRPA).[10] The court acknowledged the PRPA requirement that official proceedings of the quality review committee are to be held in confidence. However, for the privilege to be maintained there was a two-pronged test: this required the parties asserting the privilege to prove that (1) the privilege was properly invoked, and (2) that privilege is limited to matters that have maintained their privacy. The Superior Court of

Pennsylvania in a non-precedential decision affirmed the trial court's disclosure decision. They held that privilege could not be granted: (1) the hospital could not claim privilege for performance records it did not create or maintain; (2) the management company and physician could not claim privilege as independent contractors as they are not afforded protection under the Act; (3) any privilege that potentially existed was lost when the performance record was shared from group to hospital. The decision regarding peer review protections was then appealed to the Supreme Court of Pennsylvania.[11]

In *Charles* v. *Southern Baptist Hospital of Florida*, the question was whether records specifically relating to "adverse medical incidents" are governed by state or federal statute.[12] The hospital participated in the state patient safety organization (PSO), and provided reports to the state as mandated. In this case, it had produced occurrence reports through the hospital patient safety evaluation system, which had not yet been referred to the PSO. The Florida voters approved Amendment 7, codified as Article X, Section 25 of the Florida Constitution, which provides "a right to have access to any records made or received in the course of business by a healthcare facility or provider relating to any adverse medical incident."[13] The Patient Safety and Quality Improvement Act of 2005 established privilege protections that are "the foundation to furthering the overall goal of the statute to develop a national system for analyzing and learning for patient safety events."[14] The Florida Supreme Court held that the Federal Safety Act does not, nor was it intended to, preempt or provide a shield from a state-based statute to compel production. Therefore, adverse medical incident reports made in conjunction with state law cannot be classified as protected, privileged work products.

Conclusion

Recent legislation has brought about great changes in the realm of patient safety and risk management. In the interim, maintaining stringent information management and protection protocol for the PSO can help to ensure ongoing confidentiality (see Table 78.2). This will ensure protection from being compelled to divulge peer review work product in an extrinsic judicial proceeding.

References

1. O'Neil AC, Petersen LA, Cook EF, Bates DW, Lee TH, Brennan TA. Physician reporting compared with medical-record review to identify adverse medical events. *Ann Intern Med*. 1993;119(5):370–376. DOI:10.7326/0003-4819-119-5-199309001-00004.

2. Localio AR, Weaver SL, Landis JR, Lawthers AG, Brennan TA, Hebert L, Sharp TJ. Identifying adverse events caused by medical care: degree of physician agreement in a retrospective chart review. *Ann Intern Med*. 1996;125(6):457–464. DOI:10.7326/0003-4819-125-6-199609150-00005.

3. McKay J, Bowie P, Lough M. Variations in the ability of general medical practitioners to apply two methods of clinical audit: a five-year study of assessment by peer review. *J Eval Clin Pract*. 12(6):622–629. DOI:10.1111/j.1365-2753.2005.00630.x.

4. Posner KL, Caplan RA, Cheney FW. Variation in expert opinion in medical malpractice review. *Anesthesiology*. 1996;85(5):1049–1054.

5. *Roach* v. *Springfield Clinic*, 623 N.E.2d 246 (1993).

6. Code of Civil Procedure §8-2101, 2 (735 ICLS 5/8-2101) (West 1992).

7. *Virmani* v. *Novant Health Inc.*, 259 F.3d 284 (2001).

8. Federal Rules of Evidence. Rule 501. Privilege in General.

9. *Reginelli* v. *Boggs*, Nos. 1584 WDA 2014, 1585 WDA 2014.

10. Pennsylvania Peer Review Statute, 63 P.S. §425.1 et seq.

11. *Reginelli* v. *Boggs*, 141 A.3d 440 (2016).

12. *Charles* v. *Southern Baptist Hospital of Florida, Inc.*, No. SC15-2180, January 31, 2017.

13. Florida Constitution, Art. X, §25.

14. Patient Safety and Quality Act of 2005. *Pub.L.* 109-41, 42 U.S.C. ch. 6A subch. VII part C.

Chapter 79

Policy/Procedure

Case

The patient had come to the emergency department (ED) presenting with acute chest pain. It was clear from the first EKG that there was an ST elevation myocardial infarction (STEMI). The interventional cardiologist was called, and the ED physician completed the history and physical exam and gave routine cardiac admission orders. The nurse said not to worry because they had a protocol for that. She proceeded to implement the cardiac protocol which included administration of oxygen, an intravenous start, aspirin and nitroglycerin infusion, and a dose of clopidogrel (Plavix).

The interventional cardiology physician was on his way in, and the nurses were ready to call for transport of the patient to the cardiac cath lab. At that point the ED physician was asked to review the medications, as nursing had implemented the policy in the physician's name. The physician inquired about the medication dosing, because the Plavix dosage was clearly out of date. The patient was given the correct dose for a cardiac percutaneous intervention (PCI). She was then transferred to the cath lab, the procedure went well, and she was eventually discharged home. At the next departmental meeting, the STEMI policy was reviewed. The ED physician asked when was the last time it had been updated, and apparently the protocol had last been reviewed 4 years previously.

Medical Approach

The Institute of Medicine in a classic treatise defines the six domains of quality of care (Table 79.1).[1] First, care should be safe, resulting in greater benefit than harm. Second, effective care is based on scientific knowledge providing service to those most likely to benefit. Third, the goal is patient-centered care, incorporating individual needs and preferences. Fourth, the care should be timely, reducing waits and

harmful delays. Fifth, efficient care delivers quality while avoiding waste. Sixth, care should not vary in quality based on the individual or circumstances.

It is clear that the presence of rules, policy, procedural guidelines, and treatment protocols ensures an appropriate standard of care, while allowing for individual variation. Using a checklist helps to ensure all health-care provider staff are caring for their patients properly.

A clinical decision rule is a sequence of algorithmic choices dictating the proper diagnosis and treatment of a medical or surgical condition. A *policy* is a general statement describing goals, objectives, and implementation, while a *guideline* is typically a step-by-step intervention list that involves the mechanics of achieving the goal and endpoint of the policy. Lastly, a *protocol* is typically a procedure list that is focused on medications and pre-rehearsed steps to arrive at the proper point in patient care.

It is important to recognize the difference between *practice guidelines*, which are physician-orchestrated medical directives, and *clinical pathways*, which are multidisciplinary, involving all aspects of the health-care delivery process.[2] Practice guidelines demonstrate improved quality of care, and are developed as best practice standards. Clinical pathways have been proven to reduce length of stay, complications, and cost of care, while increasing patient satisfaction.

Table 79.1 The six domains of care quality of care

1.	Safety
2.	Effectiveness
3.	Patient-centered
4.	Timely
5.	Efficient
6.	Equitable

Reference: Institute of Medicine[1]

Table 79.2 Clinical practice guidelines: impressions

Impression	Incidence (%)
Positive	
1. Favorable effect	75 (66–83)
2. Educational tools	71 (63–79)
3. Improve quality	70 (69–80)
Negative	
4. Impractical and rigid	30 (23–36)
5. Reduced autonomy	34 (22–47)
6. Increase litigation	41 (32–49)
7. Intended to cut costs	53 (39–66)

Reference: Farquhar et al.[3]

Table 79.3 Clinical guidelines and medicolegal interface

1. High-risk events
2. Widely accepted
3. System-wide integration
4. Clear and easily interpreted

Reference: Garnick et al.[5]

Clinician's attitudes to clinical practice guidelines have been studied by Farquhar et al., who evaluated 30 studies with 11,611 responses (Table 79.2).[3] Clinicians agreed there were positive aspect to clinical guidelines (mean 75%, range 66–83%), they were good educational tools (71%, 63–79%), and intended to improve quality (70%, 69–80%). However, they cited negatives as well, considering guidelines impractical and too rigid to apply to individual patients (30%, 23–36%), reducing physician autonomy and oversimplifying medicine (34%, 22–47%), likely to increase litigation (41%, 32–49%), and intended to cut health-care costs (52.8%, 39–66%). Providers feel that although clinical practice guidelines are associated with high satisfaction, they are also associated with practicality concerns.

The key to successful implementation of guidelines is to factor an update plan. Shekelle et al. evaluated 17 US Agency Healthcare Research and Quality (AHRQ) clinical guidelines.[4] They found 46.2% (7) required major revision, 35.3% (6) required a minor update, 17.6% (3) were judged to be currently valid, and for 5.8% (1) no decision could be made. Survival analysis indicated that half of the guidelines evaluated were outdated in 5.8 years (95% CI, 5.0–6.6 years) but the majority (90%) were still valid after 3.6 years (95% CI, 2.6–4.6 years). This resulted in the recommendation to update clinical guidelines every 3 years.

The obvious question is whether clinical guidelines favorably affect medical malpractice exposure. For practice guidelines to be most effective there are four crucial factors (Table 79.3).[5] First, they should be developed for conditions or procedures that address high-risk events or circumstances. Second, they should be widely accepted by the medical profession. Third, they should be capable of system-wide integration. Fourth, they should be clear and easily interpreted in the clinical and legal settings.

However, there are legal risks with clinical practice guidelines. There are concerns that they are more often used in an inculpatory than an exculpatory fashion.[6] This can occur even though limiting language in the form of a disclaimer is often added to address liability. As well, physician contributors should consider future legal repercussions in the use of clinical practice guidelines. There is a difference between "best practice," which we aspire to provide, and "average care," which is used to set legal standards. Remember, the legal standard is that performed by the average practitioner in similar circumstances.

The inculpatory nature of the guidelines was defined by Hyam et al. reporting on 259 claims, of which 17 involved practice guidelines.[7] Initial analysis found that 70.6% (12) of guidelines implicated physician error, 23.5% (4) exonerated the physician, and in 5.9% (1) no conclusion was reached. Later an attorney survey reported that once suit was initiated, guidelines again were used more often in an inculpatory (54%) fashion than in an exculpatory (23%) fashion. Guidelines were more often used by more experienced attorneys with the majority of their practice involved with medical malpractice.

Legal Analysis

In *Washington* v. *Washington Hospital*, the patient underwent elective gynecological surgery, had alleged difficulty with endotracheal ventilation, and suffered cerebral anoxia.[8] The trial court awarded summary judgment to the defendants, and the family appealed based on loss of consortium. The court recognized the American Association of Anesthesiology Standards for Basic Intraoperative Monitoring, which "encouraged" the use of monitoring, as well as a scientific journal article that stated that, "monitoring end-tidal CO_2 is an emerging standard and is strongly preferred."

The standard of due care necessarily embodies "what a reasonably prudent hospital would do." [9] The court concluded that although "emerging standards" were not conclusive, reasonable jurors would conclude that monitors were required as recommendations of similar prudent hospitals were consistent. However, the District of Columbia Court of Appeals was bound by precedent holding such loss of consortium claims unrecognizable, and the original judgment was affirmed.

In *Levine* v. *Rosen*, the patient filed suit for failure to diagnose breast cancer after symptoms consistent with this diagnosis were allegedly discussed with the physician on two occasions.[10] The jury returned a unanimous verdict for the defense, which was reversed on appeal. The Supreme Court of Pennsylvania affirmed the appellate court decision and remanded for a new trial. They felt that both the "irrelevant considerations" and the "two schools of thought" instruction were improper and may have influenced outcome. The "two schools of thought" doctrine provides complete defense when the prescribed treatment or procedure has been approved by one group of medical experts, even though another group recommends a different approach.[11] However, this doctrine only applies if there are alternative treatments, which was not the case for diagnosis of physical symptoms. The court held that, "where competent medical authority is divided, a physician will not be held responsible if in the exercise of his judgment he followed a course of treatment advocated by a considerable number of recognized and respected professionals in his given area of expertise." In this case, there was evidence that there were some proponents of yearly mammography screening and others who recommended "regular" screening.

In *Moore* v. *Baker*, the patient underwent carotid endarterectomy at the behest of the neurosurgeon to prevent the onset of stroke.[12] The patient had a postoperative complication and suffered a stroke. The patient sued, alleging there was an alternative medicine approach utilizing chelation therapy, with lower risk, that the physician could have offered. The trial court granted summary judgment in favor of the defendant as this alternative therapy is "not generally recognized, or acceptable." The United States Court of Appeals, Eleventh Circuit affirmed, holding that the mainstream medical community does not recognize or accept the alternative therapy suggested by the patient in preference to the surgical intervention.

In *Frakes* v. *Cardiology Consultants*, the patient had an episode of chest pain and dizziness, with a normal rest EKG. He was admitted to the hospital and evaluated by the cardiologist, who ordered an exercise treadmill EKG.[13] The stress test was allegedly stopped for severe chest pain, although there were no EKG changes. The patient was discharged home and died a few days later. The jury returned a verdict for the defense and an appeal followed. The plaintiff alleged that a table showing stress test interpretation parameters to diagnose coronary artery disease, which the defendant complied with, should not have been submitted to the jury. The plaintiff alleged the table would not have survived the hearsay exemption, should it have been admitted as evidence before jury instruction. The Court of Appeals of Tennessee affirmed the trial court verdict, as they felt that the clinical guideline was appropriately shared.

Conclusion

Remember that initially there is a lot of enthusiasm and buy-in because a clinical practice guideline is typically assembled by a multidisciplinary team. But it is crucial to remember these guidelines should be revisited annually and rewritten regularly – every 2 to 3 years, as a general rule. In addition, they pose additional medicolegal liability and are more often used in an inculpatory rather than an exculpatory fashion.

References

1. Institute of Medicine. *Crossing The Quality Chasm: A New Health System for the 21st Century. The Six Domains of Health Care Quality* (Washington D.C., National Academy Press, 2001).

2. Wetland DE. Why use clinical pathways rather than practice guidelines? *Am J Surg.* 1997;174(6):592–595. DOI:10.1016/S0002-9610(97)00196-7.

3. Farquhar CM, Kofa EW, Slutsky JR. Clinician's attitudes to clinical practice guidelines: a systematic review. *Med J Aust.* 2002;177(9):502–506.

4. Shekelle PG, Ortiz E, Rhodes S, Morton SC, Eccles MP, Grimshaw JM, Woolf SH. Validity of the agency for healthcare research and quality clinical practice guidelines. *JAMA.* 2001;28(12):1461–1467. DOI:10.1001/jama.286.12.1461.

5. Garnick DW, Hendricks AM, Brennan TA. Can practice guidelines reduce the number and costs of malpractice claims? *JAMA.* 1991;266(20):2856–2860. DOI:10.1001/jama.1991.03470200068037.

6. Moses RE, Feld AD. Legal risks of clinical practice guidelines. *Am J Gastroenterol.* 2008;103(1):7–11. DOI:10.1111/j.1572–0241.2007.01399.x.

7. Hyams AL, Brandenberg JA, Lipsitz SR, Shapiro DW, Brennen TA. Practice guidelines and malpractice litigation: a two-way street. *Ann Intern Med.* 1995;122(6):450–455. DOI:10.7326/0003-4819-122-6-199503150-00008.

8. *Washington* v. *Washington Hosp. Center,* 579 A.2d 177 (1990).

9. *Meek* v. *Shepard,* 484 A.2d 579, 580 (D.C. 1984).

10. *Levine* v. *Rosen,* 532 Pa.512. (1992).

11. *Jones* v. *Chidester,* 531 Pa. 31 (1992).

12. *Moore* v. *Baker,* 989 F.2d. 1129 (1993).

13. *Frakes* v. *Cardiology Consultants,* 597 (Tenn Ct App 1997).

Pregnancy

Case

The medics brought in a young woman who had been involved in a moderate-speed motor vehicle collision. She was 21 years old, was not wearing a seat belt, and was 14 weeks pregnant. In the emergency department (ED) the standard trauma protocol was followed, substituting ultrasound for CT scan. The conventional trauma screening laboratory tests were normal. There were no signs of bleeding or electrolyte abnormalities. A routine trauma urine was sent off, and the urine drug screen was positive for three separate controlled substances. She was admitted presumptively to the trauma service for observation overnight. There were no further findings, so the patient was discharged home with a recommendation to continue prenatal vitamins and stop smoking. She was offered counseling for substance use and some outpatient treatment programs.

That next week the ED physician was contacted by the patient advocate who stated the patient's mother had raised concerns about the drug screening. She said her daughter was not informed of the drug testing, and would not have consented to it.

In discussion with the patient advocate, the ED physician pointed out that there is a standard trauma protocol that, from a medical perspective, is in the patient's best interest. Part of the protocol in case of a motor vehicle accident is a drug and alcohol screen, which unfortunately was positive in this case. The case is further complicated by the fact the patient was in the second trimester of pregnancy, which raised additional psychosocial concerns about subjecting her unborn child to this hazard.

Medical Approach

The issue raised is complicated in that the patient being evaluated is actually two patients: mother and fetus. There is a standard screening protocol for numerous disease conditions and this is a standard of care in these circumstances. Normally, a positive finding would not be such a significant issue. However, with pregnancy it raises additional concerns about the psychosocial interventions that may be required. But in most cases, as long as the testing is medically necessary and is done in the best interest of the unborn child, consent is typically not required for testing in pregnancy.

The management of pregnant patients in the ED is often a cause of concern, requiring careful intervention and special care. Triage of the pregnant patient in the ED requires us to treat both patients at all times, although the mother's care is prioritized. The Pennsylvania Patient Safety Authority estimates that in half of the cases of pregnant patients presenting to the ED, there is ineffective communication between the ED and obstetric staff.[1] Optimal care can only be achieved by a systematic approach to care that involves open communication between the emergency and obstetric services. Obstetric care in the ED requires a risk reduction strategy that includes policies and procedures to ensure proper care, including triage and assessment. This approach focuses on the presenting complaint, gestational age, availability of testing and consultants, and fetal monitoring capability (Table 80.1).

Table 80.1 Care of the pregnant patient in the ED

1.	Systematic approach to triage and assessment
2.	Presenting complaint
3.	Baby's gestational age
4.	Testing availability
5.	Consultant availability
6.	Fetal monitoring capability

Reference: Pennsylvania Patient Safety Authority[1]

One of the most controversial issues in ED management is maternal drug use and its potential effect on the unborn child. Illicit drug use during pregnancy occurs nationwide, with higher rates in selected subgroups.[2] Substance abuse is often associated with poverty, substance use in the family, and family violence. Perinatal drug abusers experience poorer birth outcomes, chaotic home environments, and child removal with ongoing substance abuse.

Chasnoff et al. evaluated 715 women, who attended both public health clinics and private obstetric offices, and provided toxicological screening for illicit drugs.[3] The overall prevalence of the positive urine screening was 14.8%, 13.1% in private offices and 16.3% in the clinics. There were 18.6% (133) of patients reported for substance abuse during pregnancy. Programs targeting parental abstinence, facilitated by child care, parenting classes, and vocational training allow children to remain in the house with their parents.

The sensitivity of urine drug testing is always a question in these circumstances. Grekin et al. utilized an anonymous brief clinical screening protocol in 300 low-income postpartum women.[4] Overall a positive toxicological screen was found in 24%, but 19% of those with a positive screen denied drug use. This clinical screening protocol was of limited utility in this pregnant population.

An obvious concern is the effect of maternal drug use on the newborn. Osterloh and Lee performed paired sample analysis of 19.2% (601) of women and 15.3% (339) of newborns admitted.[5] The urine drug screens were positive for one drug in 68.2% of mothers and 63.1% of babies, for more than one drug in 38.8% and 21.1%, and positive for cocaine 45.8% and 41.6%. In mother–newborn pairs (191), there was an 84% concordance for cocaine, 67% for methadone, but much less (<21%) for other drugs.

This raises the specter of neonatal drug withdrawal, as commented on by the Committee on Drugs and the Committee on the Fetus and Newborn.[6] Maternal use of drugs during pregnancy can result in transient neonatal effects consistent with withdrawal or more sustained adverse effects. There are treatment protocols for weaning from narcotics or benzodiazepines, or blunting the hyperadrenergic effects of stimulants.

The Society of Obstetricians and Gynecologists of Canada Maternal–Fetal Medicine, Family Physicians, and Medicolegal Committees have published a

Table 80.2 Substance use in pregnancy

1. All pregnant women should be screened for substance use (III-A)
2. Urine screening preferred (II-A)
3. Informed consent should be obtained (III-B)
4. Caregivers should be familiar with regulations (III-A)

Reference: Society of Obstetricians and Gynecologists of Canada.[7]

consensus document on substance use in pregnancy, with recommendations for testing.[7] First, all pregnant women, and those of childbearing age should be screened periodically for alcohol, tobacco, and illicit drug use (III-A). Second, when testing for substance use is clinically indicated, urine drug screening is the preferred method. (II-2A). Third, informed consent should be obtained from the woman before maternal drug toxicology testing is ordered (III-B). Fourth, policy and legal requirements with respect to drug testing of newborns may vary by jurisdiction, and caregivers should be familiar with the regulations in their region (III-A) (Table 80.2).

Legal Analysis

There is a tense balance between the rights of the mother and the unborn child in relation to illicit drug use. In *Troy* v. *San Diego County Department of Social Services*, the mother and child tested positive for amphetamines and opiates.[8] A petition was filed to remove the child from the mother's custody, as she was alleged to be unable to protect him. It was awarded and the child was placed with his grandmother. The mother's demurrer to the amended petition was overruled. The Court of Appeals of California, Fourth District affirmed the trial court decision, as they held that the expert opinion alleged neonatal harm to be more likely from drug exposure than from premature delivery.

Likewise, in *In the Interest of W.E.C.*, the mother had an alleged history of heavy alcohol use through early pregnancy and then, after delivery, had an acute bout of intoxication requiring an emergency room visit.[9] Her newly born twins had special care needs, and the trial court terminated the mother's parental rights. She appealed, stating that privileged information was admitted. The Court of Appeals of Texas, Fort Worth affirmed the trial court's ruling that clear and convincing evidence exists to establish burden of proof to terminate parental rights.

However, in *Ferguson* v. *City of Charleston* the state hospital's performance of a diagnostic test to obtain evidence of criminal conduct for law enforcement purposes was held to be an unreasonable search if not consented.[10] The facility originally performed a screening exam for substance use in patients in their prenatal clinic to refer them to substance abuse programs. However, they were contacted by law enforcement to assist in prosecution of postpartum patients who had exposed their child to illicit drugs. The Supreme Court of the United States granted certiorari, concluding, as the United States Court of Appeals, Fourth Circuit had done, that the search was performed without informed consent. This testing qualifies as "search and seizure" within the guidelines of the Fourth Amendment.[11] The judgment was reversed and case remanded to address the consent issue. The court attempts to strike a balance between the rights of the child and those of the mother within reason, especially related to consent and the law enforcement interface.

Conclusion

The legal interface must always recognize obligations to two patients – both mother and child. However, the primary patient focus, whether mother or child, may vary based on disease condition and prevailing circumstances. The baby may be protected if the mother has placed her child at risk, whereas the mother may be the primary focus if her health is placed at risk.

References

1. Pennsylvania Patient Safety Authority. Triage of the obstetrics patient in the emergency department: is there only one patient? *Pa Patient Saf Advis*. 2008;5(3):85–89.

2. Howell EM, Heiser N, Harrington M. A review of recent findings on substance abuse treatment for pregnant women. *J Subst Abuse Treat*. 1999;16(3):195–219. DOI:10.1016/S0740-5472(98)00032-4.

3. Chasnoff IJ, Landress HJ, Barrett ME. The prevalence of illicit-drug or alcohol use during pregnancy and discrepancies in mandatory reporting in Pinellas County, Florida. *N Engl J Med*. 1990;322(17):1202–1206.

4. Grekin ER, Svikis DS, Lam P, Connors V, LeBreton JM, Streiner DL, et al. Drug use during pregnancy: validating the drug abuse screening test against psychological measures. *Psychol Addict Behav*. 2010;24(4):719–723. DOI:10.1037/a0021741.

5. Osterloh JD, Lee BL. Urine drug screening in mothers and newborns. *Am J Dis Child*. 1989;143(7):791–793. DOI:10.1001/archpedi.1989.02150190041017.

6. Hudak ML, Tan RC, American Academy of Pediatrics. The Committee on Drugs, the Committee on Fetus and Newborn. Neonatal drug withdrawal. *Pediatrics*. 2012;129(2):e540–e560. DOI:10.1542/Peds.2011-3212.

7. Society of Obstetricians and Gynecologists of Canada. Substance use in pregnancy. *J Obstet Gynaecol Can*. 2011;33(4):367–384.

8. *Troy D.* v. *San Diego County Department of Social Services*, 215 Cal. App. 3d 889 (1989).

9. In the Interest of W.E.C., 110 S.W. 3D 231 (2003).

10. Ferguson v. *City of Charleston*, 532 U.S. 67 (2001).

11. U.S. Const. Amend. IV.

Chapter 81

Prescription Writing

Case

The triage nurse called the physician's office to say someone was asking for him at the front desk of the emergency department (ED). When the ED physician went to the desk he found the pastor's wife from his local church waiting there. She asked if he could refill a prescription for her husband's stomach medicine, which she thought was famotidine (Pepcid). The physician was hesitant to do this, but the pastor had always been helpful at the hospital and had been quite a comfort in time of need. The physician asked the pastor's wife what symptoms he was having and she said it was his usual gastric reflux. The physician quickly wrote a prescription for a week's supply of Pepcid, but emphasized that the pastor needed to be seen by his own doctor for follow-up.

Three weeks later as the physician was coming in for his shift, he was told the pastor had suffered a cardiac arrest at home. The paramedics had responded, but were unable to resuscitate him. The physician offered condolences, saying again that the pastor had been a positive influence on the facility, and had been helpful over the years.

Six months later the physician was contacted by the hospital's legal department who told him they were in receipt of a lawsuit in which he was named, along with the pastor's primary care physician (PCP), as being allegedly responsible for his demise. The pastor had seen his PCP as instructed by the ED physician, but one of the points in the pleading was that he had a prescription written from the ED for Pepcid. The hospital's legal department wanted to know when he was seen in the ED. The physician could only say he wasn't seen officially, but that a prescription had been written for him unofficially at his wife's request, and that he had been encouraged to see his PCP. The legal department recommended that an incident report be filled out based on the fact that the patient had not been registered in the department, nor was he actually present to make a request to be seen, or receive advice directly.

Medical Approach

This is not an uncommon scenario, when the physician is "curbside consulted" to write a prescription for a patient unofficially for a friend or acquaintance, a family member of a work colleague, or the colleague themselves. We all recognize this is a problematic thing to do. However, when confronted with the scenario, we recognize it is something that would be viewed as being a positive or charitable interaction, friendly and helpful.

A number of authorities have commented on nonstandard prescribing of medication. The Centers for Disease Control (CDC) reviews the public health law as it applies to prescription writing requirements.[1] Overall, 41 states and the District of Columbia require an examination of the patient as the basis for prescribing and dispensing medication. Most examination laws require a physical examination when prescribing or dispensing a controlled substance. Many states prohibit the use of electronic questionnaires as the sole basis for prescribing.

The Federation of State Medical Boards (FSMB) has published a summary of state-by-state internet prescribing language recommendations and requirements.[2] They recommend establishing a proper physician–patient relationship, obtaining a reliable medical history, conducting an appropriate physical examination, and establishing a diagnosis before prescribing medication (Table 81.1). An online questionnaire does not meet these requirements. Failure to follow these guidelines may be classified as unprofessional conduct. The FSMB clarifies exceptions to include admission orders for a newly hospitalized patient, prescribing for a patient related to an on-call

Table 81.1 FSMB proper prescribing recommendations

1.	Establish proper patient–physician relationship
2.	Obtain reliable medical history
3.	Conduct appropriate physical examination
4.	Establish a proper diagnosis

Reference: Federation of State Medical Boards.[2]

Table 81.2 AMA self-treatment or treatment of immediate family members (Opinion 8.19)

1.	Professional objectivity may be compromised
2.	Fail to perform proper history or physical
3.	Treat problems beyond training
4.	Taint other family relationships
5.	Concerns over autonomy and consent
6.	Feel obligated to provide care
7.	Emergency or short-term care may be appropriate
8.	Controlled substances (I, II, IV) are prohibited

Reference: American Medical Association.[3]

Table 81.3 Non-standard prescription requests

	Issue	Incidence (%)
	N = 982	
1.	Relative request	75.7
	Spouse	51.2
2.	Self-prescribed	48.6
3.	Asked colleague	48.1

Reference: Walter et al.[6]

responsibility for another physician, and continuing short-term medication prior to the first appointment.

The advent of telemedicine has obliged some states to revisit their internet prescribing policy, making general recommendations. If they do permit electronic prescribing, the electronic examination must meet the standards of care. The interaction must be reliably documented and proper records kept. If a computer interface is used, it must disclose the practitioner's medical license and the state board address and telephone number. Intermediaries may be utilized to obtain vital signs and other medical information.

Another area of significant discussion is the area of self-prescribing or prescribing for family members. The American Medical Association's Code of Medical Ethics Opinion 8.19 (1993) states that "physicians generally should not treat themselves or members of their immediate families" (Table 81.2).[3] First, professional objectivity may be compromised, in which personal feelings may unduly influence care. Second, physicians may fail to probe sensitive areas during medical history or be reluctant to perform intimate parts of the exam. Third, they may be inclined to treat problems and conditions beyond their training. Fourth, if there is an untoward medical outcome, this may taint other family personal relationships. Fifth, there are concerns over patient autonomy and informed consent, in

which the patient may be reluctant to express wishes and preferences. Sixth, the physician may feel obligated to provide care even if they are uncomfortable providing that care. Seventh, providing emergency or short-term routine care may be acceptable. Eighth, except in an emergency, it is not appropriate to write prescriptions for controlled substances (Schedules I, II, IV) for oneself or family members. This opinion has been incorporated by state boards of medicine, such as New Hampshire, which endorsed this recommendation for its licensees.[4] They emphasize the family treatment exception for short-term conditions and situations.

Other professional societies, such as the College of Physicians and Surgeons of Ontario, also address the treating of self and family members in their Policy 7-06.[5] First, they establish an exception for a minor condition or emergency situation and when another qualified provider is not available. Second, they recommend the highest caution in treating a spouse or romantic or sexual partner. Third, physicians should not prescribe controlled substances or for those who have the potential for habituation or addiction. Fourth, self-treatment is undesirable except for minor conditions, or emergency situations when there is no other qualified medical provider available.

This practice of self-prescribing, curbside consulting a colleague, or prescribing to friends or family has been profiled by Walter et al. reporting on the practice of 1086 pediatricians with a 44% (430/982) response rate.[6] Almost half (48.6%, 198/407) of respondents had self-prescribed and an equal proportion (48.1%, 198/411) had requested a prescription from a colleague. Three-quarters (75.7%, 325/429) of providers had been asked by a relative for a prescription. Their spouse had asked for a prescription in half (51%, 186/363) of cases (Table 81.3). Most of them (86%, 343/397) had refused to provide a prescription to a friend

Table 81.4 Refusal to provide non-standard prescription

	Issue	Incidence (%)
1.	Outside of their expertise	88
2.	Patient needs to be their own physician	70
3.	Not medically indicated	69
4.	Physical exam required	65

Reference: Walter et al.[6]

or family member at least once. They cited their rationale as follows. First, the provider felt the request was outside of the provider's expertise (88%). Second, there was the perception of the patient's need to be their own physician (70%). Third, they felt the medication was not medically indicated (69%). Fourth, they felt a physical exam was required before a prescription could be provided (65%) (Table 81.4).

Legal Analysis

In *United States* v. *Moore*, a physician who was registered and licensed to distribute controlled substances was alleged to "knowingly and unlawfully" dispense methadone.[7] The legal question raised was whether a person who is properly registered under the Controlled Substances Act can then be prosecuted for misuse, violating 21 U.S.C. §841 (a) (1).[8] The physician was alleged not to have properly evaluated, examined the patient, or administered medicine in a supervised fashion. The appeal court held that the physician had acted wrongfully, but felt §§842 and 843 of the Act were applicable with less severe penalties.[8] The Supreme Court of the United States reversed and held that registered physicians can be prosecuted under §841 of the Act, when their activities fall out of a professional scope of practice.

In *Kirk* v. *Michael Reese Hospital*, the plaintiff alleged he was negligently prescribed medication that diminished his mental and physical capabilities without being informed of the side effects.[9] This "failure to warn" was manifest in the lack of warning relating to ability to safely operate an automobile. The trial court dismissed the multiple plaintiff complaints against the physician, hospitals, and drug companies. The appeal court reversed the dismissals and remanded

for further proceedings. The Supreme Court of Illinois reversed and reinstituted the trial court rulings, on the grounds that holding the hospital responsible for all harmful acts committed by patients would be "an unreasonable burden on the facility."

Conclusion

The bottom-line recommendations are clear. No patient should be evaluated in the ED without a chart being generated in the medical record, even if at some point the cost can be negated or minimized. It is required from the medicolegal perspective that a chart be appropriately documented and recorded to note the encounter. Obviously, if the patient is not present in person a prescription should not be written unless there is an established client–patient relationship.

References

1. Prescription Drug Physical Examination Requirements. Office for State, Tribal, Local and Territorial Support Centers for Disease Control and Prevention. January 29, 2015.

2. Federation of State Medical Boards. Internet Prescribing Language State-by-State Overview. January 26, 2012.

3. AMA Code of Medical Ethics, Opinion 8.19: Self-Treatment or Treatment of Immediate Family Members. June 1993.

4. New Hampshire Board of Medicine Board News and Policies. Guidelines for Self-Prescribing and Prescribing for Family Members. 8.19 Self-Treatment of Immediate Family Members. State of New Hampshire. 2008.

5. College of Physicians and Surgeons of Ontario. Treating Self and Family Members. Policy 7-06. November 2001.

6. Walter JK, Lang CW, Ross LF. When physicians forego the doctor-patient relationship, should they elect to self-prescribe or curbside? An empirical and ethical analysis. *J Med Ethics*. 2010;36(1):19–23. DOI:10.1136/me.2009.032169.

7. *United States* v. *Moore*, 423 U.S. 122 (1975).

8. 21 U.S. Code Subchapter I – Control and Enforcement. Part A. Introductory Provisions §§801, Part D Offenses and Penalties §§841 (a)(1).

9. *Kirk* v. *Michael Reese Hospital and Medical Center*, 513 N.E. 2d 387 (Ill. 1987).

Privacy

Case

The patient presented to the emergency department (ED) with a gastrointestinal (GI) hemorrhage. She had previously had an episode and this one seemed to be similar, with bleeding from the rectum for the last 3 days. She was not especially symptomatic, but the bleeding seemed persistent. The standard workup was ordered and her hemoglobin and hematocrit were 10 g/dL and 30% respectively, on the borderline for being low in a female patient. The physician needed to perform a digital rectal exam, which was positive for fecal occult blood. It was especially noisy in the ED that day, and the physician had to pull the curtain to finish discussing the results with the patient. There was a lot of discussion about another patient who was coming in, and the physician also heard bits and pieces of a staff personal conversation accompanied by some laughter.

The patient's primary care physician (PCP) was called and the patient was admitted to the hospital. The physician reminded the ED staff that at least unofficially there should be a "noise discipline" policy in the department – the quieter the better. The ED director received a call the next day as this patient had raised a concern about privacy. She felt that as she could easily overhear conversations from the staff, they could equally well overhear the discussion about her care. She felt the department could do a better job with patient privacy. The staff agreed and discussed the noise discipline policy, ensuring patient confidentiality was maintained throughout their ED visit.

Medical Approach

Going to the ED these days is often associated with noise and clamor because that's what people see on TV. In real life we should strive for noise discipline in the ED, trying to maintain a quiet and relaxing atmosphere for the patients and staff. This is especially important at night, because sleep deprivation can be an issue for patients.

Overcrowding in the ED is associated with increased risk of patient harm, delay in care provision, compromised privacy and confidentiality, impaired communication, and diminished access to care.[1] A significant proportion of issues raised about privacy, confidentiality, and impaired communication emanate from the overcrowding issue.

The fundamental concept of privacy between patient and physician involves more than simple confidentiality. Parrott et al. evaluated 427 patients and the privacy perceptions associated with the physician–patient dyad.[2] The authors stress the multidimensional and situational nature of privacy. Confidentiality is not just a monodimensional issue focused only on information transfer. It has both informational and psychological realms of privacy, and has a direct impact on interview techniques, especially in sensitive areas such as sexual history.

The patient's perception of privacy is crucially important. Nayeli and Aghajani reported on a questionnaire of 360 patients, in which 50.6% stated that the degree to which their privacy was respected was weak or average.[3] There was significant correlation between respect of privacy and the patient's satisfaction about various aspects of the process.

Karro et al. reported on 1169 patients, in which 20.1% (235) returned questionnaires concerning their perceptions of privacy in the ED.[4] Overall, almost half (45%, 105) of patients reported a total of 159 privacy incidents. A definite breach of privacy was noted by 33% (78) of patients, while 35% (81) felt there was at least a likely confidentiality breach (Table 82.1). The patients found that 41% (96) reported overhearing another patient–staff conversation, while 15% (36) felt their conversations with staff were overheard, and 11% (27) experienced or observed inappropriate exposure of body parts. There

Table 82.1 Patient impression of privacy incidents

Incident	Incidence (%)
N = 105	(95% CI)
General	
1. Definite (78)	33% (28–36%)
2. Probable (81)	35% (29–37%)
Specific	
3. Overheard patient–staff conversations (96)	41% (35–47%)
4. Their conversations overheard (36)	15% (11–21%)
5. Body part exposure (27)	11% (6–14%)
6. Privacy expectations not met (24)	10% (6–14%)
7. Withheld information (10)	4% (2–7%)
8. Refused exam (2)	0.8%
Associated	
9. Length of stay	P < 0.01
10. Curtains vs. cubicles	P < 0.05

Reference: Karro et al.[4]

Table 82.2 Patient's perception of privacy

Factors	Significance
	OR
Negative	
1. Personal information overheard by others	0.6273
2. Overhearing others' personal information	0.5521
3. Inappropriate conversation of providers	0.5992
4. Seen by irrelevant persons	0.6337
Positive	
5. Privacy for physical exam	1.6091
6. Provider's respect for privacy	4.3455

Reference: Lin and Lin[8]

were 10% (24) of patients who stated their privacy expectations were not met. This was significant enough that 4% (10) of patients withheld history from the staff so it was not overheard. As well, 0.8% (2) of patients refused part of the physical exam, to avoid inappropriate exposure. The likelihood of privacy incidents was greater the longer the ED stay (P < 0.01). Lastly, the use of curtains versus a structured cubicle was associated with a greater incidence of privacy breach (P < 0.05).

Patient confidentiality and privacy rights are clearly related to structural design features of the ED. Olsen and Sabin evaluated a convenience sample of ED patients, who reported that 36% overheard other patient conversations, and 1.6% of these were felt to be inappropriate or unprofessional.[5] Interestingly, they noted similar rates in either a curtained space or a walled room. The curtained spaces allowed conversation from the adjacent space to be overheard; while the walled rooms allowed more noise from the hallway and nurses' station to be heard. However, the patients felt more comfortable relating their history in a walled examination room. This same research group headed by Olsen then compared their results after an ED renovation.[6] The rate of overheard conversation decreased from 36% to 14% after the renovation. This beneficial effect was felt to be the result of using walled examination areas, as well as increasing the size

of each treatment space from 375 square feet (35 m²) to 564 square feet (52 m²). They recommended considering these factors in any new renovation projects.

The curtained versus walled examination room comparison was also studied by Barlas et al., who conducted a structured interview of 108 ED patients.[7] Those treated in curtained areas felt they could overhear others. As well, they thought others could overhear them, see them, hear personal information, and view their personal areas (P < 0.04) and perceived an overall decreased sense of privacy (P < 0.01). However, the majority (82.5%) of patients reported "a lot of" or "complete" respect for privacy by the staff, and 92.6% experienced as much privacy as expected. Clearly, ED design has an impact on the patient's auditory and visual privacy in the treatment areas.

The patient's perception of privacy has a significant association with satisfaction about their care. Lin and Lin evaluated 364 patients, in which 86% (313) completed a questionnaire concerning their perception of ED privacy.[8] Factors that can adversely affect the patient's perception of privacy include personal information heard by others (OR 0.6273), overhearing the personal history of others (0.5521), unintentionally hearing inappropriate conversations from other health-care staff (0.5992), or being seen by irrelevant persons (0.6337). Factors that improve the perception of privacy include space provided for privacy during the physical exam (OR 1.6091) and the provider's respect for the patient's privacy (OR 4.3455) (Table 82.2).

Patient characteristics that predicted lower ratings for perception of privacy include older age, hallway treatment area, and longer length of stay. Patient satisfaction was strongly predicted by the perception of privacy (OR 8.4545) and the majority (75%) of patients felt privacy played a crucial role in their health care.

An observation of confidentiality and privacy breaches and a patient exit survey was performed by Mlinek and Pierce.[9] They found the frequency of breach was dependent on room location or design. Breaches in the waiting room and triage occurred in more than 53% of the patients. Breaches near the nursing station and physician work area ranged from 3 to 24 per hour and 1.5 to 3.4 per patient per hour. A frequently mentioned area of concern is the confidentiality of the patient tracking board. Interestingly, an exit interview with patient and family members found that only 2% (2/100) noticed the status board at all, and none could remember any specific details.

Legal Analysis

Privacy concerns are often the center of controversy in criminal matters. In *Estelle Warden* v. *McGuire*, the defendant and his wife brought their infant daughter to the ED with numerous contusions and she succumbed to significant blunt traumatic injury shortly after arrival.[10] The father was charged with second-degree murder after an inconsistent history of the child's injuries. The issue raised was related in part to an overheard conversation in the ED, where the mother ascribed responsibility for the injuries to the father. He was convicted by the trial court, and unsuccessfully challenged the appeal in state court. He then sought federal relief under a habeas theory, stating his confinement was improper or unlawful. This concept was first embodied in the Magna Carta imposed on King John by feudal landowners in 1215.

> "No free man shall be seized, imprisoned, disseized, outlawed, exiled or injured in any way. Nor will we enter on him or send him except by the lawful judgment of his peers, or by the law of the land."[11]

This evolved into the modern concept of due process of law. The writ of habeas corpus compels the custodian to produce the prisoner at a particular time and place, where a state or federal court may rule on the legality of the detention.[12] The defendant raised issues of inadmissible evidence, such as the witness overhearing a protected conversation, as well as an

erroneous jury instruction. The United States Court of Appeals (USCA), Ninth Circuit set aside his conviction in *McGuire* v. *Estelle*.[13] However, the Supreme Court of the United States reversed, holding that the USCA exceeded the scope of federal habeas review of state cases.

In *State of Oregon* v. *Cromb*, a patient was being treated in the ED after a car accident, when a police officer walked into the treatment area.[14] He observed the defendant's vital signs, and the medical staff's diagnosis and obtained a urine sample for chemical testing.[15] The patient was indicted by the grand jury for multiple offenses including driving under the influence of intoxicants (DUI).[15] The defendant filed a motion to suppress the urine toxicology sample, asserting the officer's warrantless observations in the ED violated his Fourth Amendment to the United States Constitution, right to be free from unreasonable search and seizure, and Article I, Section 9 of the Oregon Constitution.[16,17] The trial court denied the motion, and he was convicted based on the previous conditional guilty plea. He appealed the denial of his motion to suppress. The Court of Appeals of Oregon affirmed the trial court judgment, holding the officer was there in an official capacity, and had probable cause to obtain the sample result. They did acknowledge that the officer entered the patient's treatment room, but felt there was no protected privacy interest for the patient there.

In *United States* v. *Eide*, the defendant was employed as a pharmacist at the Veterans Administration Medical Center. Police were summoned to a car due to alleged witnessed drug use[18] and the defendant was taken to the ED by his supervisor for evaluation. Allegedly, his speech was impaired and he appeared incoherent. In the ED he consented to a urinalysis for toxicological screening, which was allegedly positive. The defendant stated he was informed this would be confidential. However, the supervisor testified that this confidentiality applied to the treatment only, and not the overall situation. No ED report was made, and the urine sample was sent as "John Doe." The defendant alleged this was done to "ensure maximum confidentiality," while the facility alleged it was due to the fact he was not a veteran or eligible to receive care there. A pharmacy audit demonstrated irregularities and potential tampering. The focus again shifted to the defendant, who received his Miranda rights at that point.[19] The trial court convicted him for various drug-related crimes, and he appealed alleging an improper denial of his motion to suppress. He theorized the ED record should be suppressed since his statements were involuntary and he was not Mirandized. As well, the urine result should be excluded based on the Confidentiality of Alcohol and Drug Abuse Patient Records.[20] The USCA, Ninth Circuit affirmed the trial court rulings, save for the refusal to suppress evidence obtained in violation of 42 U.S.C. §290ee-3, and remanded for further proceedings. They held that he was indeed a patient afforded testing confidentiality, in contradistinction to the trial court which felt that since he was not a "patient," the privilege did not apply.

In *Estate of William Behringer M.D.* v. *Medical Center at Princeton*, the patient was a physician presenting for care at the institution in which he practiced.[21] He was diagnosed with an acute medical illness, and allegedly the information became known within the institution without his consent. The plaintiff alleged a breach in the maintenance of medical confidentiality, and a violation of the New Jersey Law Against Discrimination regarding his subsequent work restrictions.[22] The Superior Court of New Jersey held that there was indeed a breach in confidentiality associated with the release of his medical information. However, the burden was not met in the discrimination claim, as the balance with the potential for patient harm dictated a prudent course for the facility.

However, there is an obligation to protect the health of care providers as well. In *Johnson* v. *West Virginia University Hospitals*, the appellee was a police officer employed at the hospital, where he assisted with the care of an unruly patient.[23] The patient needed to be restrained, and the officer was bitten by the patient in the process. He filed suit alleging the facility was negligent in not informing him of the patient's health status related to potential exposure. The trial court held that the facility had the obligation to inform providers of care hazards according to the rules and regulations of the hospital. The defendant facility appealed the verdict. The Supreme Court of Appeals of West Virginia upheld the trial court decision, but reduced the jury award by 5% for the appellee's contributory negligence.

Conclusion

Most importantly, we should take every step to ensure patients' privacy is protected, and that well-meaning side conversations are not audible in public areas of the ED. Creating the atmosphere of a comfortable and quiet patient care environment in the midst of a busy emergency center is often difficult. It may require a financial investment and the support of administration.

References

1. Moskop JC, Sklar DP, Geiderman JM, Schears RM, Bookman KJ. Emergency department crowding, part 1 – concept, causes and moral consequences. *Ann Emerg Med.* 2009;53(5):605–611. DOI:10.1016/j.annemergmed.2008.09.019.

2. Parrot R, Burgoon JK, Burgoon M, LePoire BA. Privacy between physicians and patients: more than a matter of confidentiality. *Soc Sci Med.* 1989;29(12):1381–1385. DOI:10.1016/0277-9536(89)90239-6.

3. Nayeri ND, Aghajani M. Patients' privacy and satisfaction in the emergency department: a descriptive analytical study. *Nurs Ethics.* 2010;17(2):167–177. DOI:10.1177/0969733009355377.

4. Karro J, Dent AW, Farish S. Patient perceptions of privacy infringements in an emergency department. *Emerg Med Australas.* 2005;17(2):117–123. DOI:10.1111/2005.17.issue-2/issuetoc.

5. Olsen JC, Sabin BR. Emergency department patient perceptions of privacy and confidentiality. *J Emerg Med.* 2003;25(3):329–333. DOI:10.1016/S0736-4679(03)00216-6.

6. Olsen JC, Cutcliffe B, O'Brien BC. Emergency department design and patient perceptions of privacy and confidentiality. *J Emerg Med.* 2008;35(3):317–320. DOI:1016/j.emergmed.2007.10.029.

7. Barlas D, Sama AE, Ward MF, Lesser ML. Comparison of the auditory and visual privacy of emergency department treatment areas with curtains versus those with solid walls. *Ann Emerg Med.* 2001;38(2):135–139. DOI:10.1067/mem.2001.115441.

8. Lin YK, Lin CJ. Factors predicting patients' perception of privacy and satisfaction for emergency care. *Emerg Med J.* 2011;28(7):604–608. DOI:10.1136/emj.2010.093807.

9. Mlinek EJ, Pierce J. Confidentiality and privacy breaches in a university hospital emergency department. *Acad Emerg Med.* 1997;4(12):1142–1146. DOI:10.1111/acem.1997.4.issue-12/issue-12/issuestoc.

10. *Estelle Warden* v. *McGuire*, 502 U.S. 62 (1991).

11. Habeas Corpus, legal-dictionary.thefreedictionary.com. Accessed March 6, 2016.

12. 28 U.S.C. §2241: Petition for a Writ of Habeas Corpus.

13. *McGuire* v. *Estelle,* 902 F.2d 749 (1990).

14. *State of Oregon* v. *Cromb*, 185 P.3d 1120 (2008).

15. Oregon Revised Statutes S 813.010, 140 Driving Under the Influence of Intoxicants, Chemical Test with Consent.

16. U.S. Const. Amend. IV.

17. Oregon Constitution, Article I, Section 9: Unreasonable Searches or Seizures.

18. *United States* v. *Eide*, 875 F.2d 1429 (1989).

19. *Miranda* v. *Arizona*, 384 U.S. 436 (1966).

20. 42 U.S.C. §290ee-3: Confidentiality of Alcohol and Drug Abuse Patient Records.

21. *Estate of William Behringer, MD* v. *The Medical Center at Princeton*, 592 A. 2d 1251 (1991).

22. New Jersey Law Against Discrimination, N.J.S.A 10:5-1 et seq.

23. *Johnson* v. *West Virginia University Hospital*, 413 S.E.2d 889 (1991).

Professional Boundary Issues

Case

There had been a lot of discussion in the emergency department (ED) recently regarding this physician's behavior. He was said to have some relationship issues at home, and it seemed like some of that stress was manifesting itself in the workplace. The physician had always been friendly with female colleagues, but it seemed to have gone overboard recently. Some of the staff felt he was making inappropriate comments when joking in the workplace, and outright persistent dating requests that were unwanted.

This was brought to the attention of hospital administration who arranged an informal outreach session involving a staff member with whom the physician had a close relationship. His behavior seemed to settle down for a bit, but then reverted and was even more aggressive than before. Administration was then left without any option as an employee filed a complaint relating to his behavior. He was referred to a more formal internal committee consisting of administrative and physician representatives, but he did not accept their concerns and suggested he was misunderstood in the workplace. They asked him to attend counseling and he said he would think about it, but everyone in the room knew that would not happen.

Two weeks later another complaint was filed. This one went beyond the point of verbal harassment; the complainant alleged a physical altercation of a sexual nature that was inappropriate and undesired. The physician was put on leave pending further investigation.

Medical Approach

The most critical concern is a professional boundary violation in the physician–patient sexual relationship. These cases of sexual boundary violations that occur in the workplace are truly problematic. They typically start slowly with personality traits that are initially observed as just being overly friendly and

are generally accepted over time. Often times, there is a work–home stressor that then precipitates more aggressive behavior.

Gabbard and Nadelson summarized the professional boundary relationship and potential violations.[1] Professional boundaries "are the parameters that describe the limits of a fiduciary relationship in which one person, a patient, entrusts their welfare to another, a physician, to whom a fee is paid for the provision of that service." The most extreme form of boundary violation involves sexual contact; however, there are other behaviors that exploit the inherent patient–physician power differential. These prohibited interactions include dual relationships, business transactions, certain gifts and services, some language use, some types of physical contact, time and duration of appointments, location of appointments, mishandling of fees, and misuse of the physical examination (Table 83.1).

The American Medical Association Council on Ethical and Judicial Affairs stated that "sexual contact or romantic relationships concurrent with the patient–physician relationship may be unethical."[2]

Table 83.1 Physician professional boundary violations

1.	Sexual contact
2.	Dual relationships
3.	Business transactions
4.	Certain gifts or services
5.	Some language use
6.	Types of physical contact
7.	Time and duration of appointments
8.	Location of appointments
9.	Mishandling of fees
10.	Misuse of physical exam

Reference: Gabbard[1]

Table 83.2 AMA prohibited boundary behaviors

1. Personality disorder – predatory, repetitive seduction
2. Sex for "therapeutic" purpose
3. Physical exam abuse
4. Asking patient on a "date"
5. Long-standing relationship evolution
6. Isolated practitioner exposure
7. Contact while medicated
8. Sexual harassment comments

Reference: American Medical Association[2]

They offer these suggestions as boundary violations. First, physicians with personality disorder who systematically attempt to seduce patients in a predatory fashion. Second, those who purport that sex can have a therapeutic purpose. Third, those who implement a routine physical exam procedure, such as a breast or genital exam when it is not indicated or in an inappropriate, eroticized manner. Fourth, situations in which the physician asks the patient on a date in the office or ED visit. Fifth, a long-standing physician–patient relationship evolves from infatuation to a relationship. Sixth, isolated situations in which the only physician in town dates a patient as there are no other social options. Seventh, cases in which a patient is touched inappropriately or raped in an office or operative setting, where medication or anesthesia may be used. Eighth, sexual harassment cases in which suggestive or inappropriate comments are made (Table 83.2).

Gartell et al. surveyed 10,000 physicians on the subject of physician–patient sexual contact, with a 19% response rate.[3] Of the 1891 responders, 9% acknowledged sexual contact with at least one patient, which could predict a 2% incidence in the entire group. The respondents reported 23% of patients had sexual contact with at least one other physician, and 63% thought this contact was "always harmful." Almost all (94%) of the responding physicians opposed contact with current patients and 37% with former patients. More than half of respondents (56%) stated that physician–patient sexual contact had never been addressed in their training, while only 3% had participated in a continuing education course. This issue needs to be addressed with clear and enforceable ethics codes and preventive and continuing education programs.

The problem affects both genders: female physicians may be sexually harassed by male or female patients. Phillips and Schneider mailed random surveys to 599 female licensed family physicians in Canada with a 79% (422) response rate.[4] More than 75% of the respondents reported sexual harassment by a patient at some point in their careers. These events occurred most often in their own offices by their own patients. However, in the ED or clinic setting the unknown patient presents a proportionately higher risk. This problem occurs more frequently than predicted and should be addressed by education and professional development.

The phenomenon of sexual harassment may begin early in medical training. Komaroy et al. surveyed 133 internal medicine residents with a 62% (82) response rate – 60% (49) men and 40% (22) women.[5] However, the majority of cases (73%, 24) were reported by women while 22% (11) of men reported at least once episode of sexual harassment in training. Women were more likely to report physical harassment, typically by someone of higher professional status. The majority of women (79%, 190) and 45% (5) of men thought the experience created a hostile work environment or interfered with work performance. The reporting rate was minimal, with only 2.4% (2) of women and none of the men reporting. The women cited a lack of confidence in obtaining assistance, and the men felt they would handle the matter themselves.

Sexual harassment in the nursing workplace has also been well described. Kaye et al. surveyed 188 critical care nurses in which half (46%) of the respondents felt they had been sexually harassed at the hospital.[6] The most common behaviors were offensive sexual remarks (56%), unwanted physical contact (53%), unwanted non-verbal attention (27%), requests for dates (16%), and sexual propositions (9%). The alleged harassment was perpetrated by physicians (82%), coworkers (20%), and immediate supervisors (7%). The majority of incidents (69%) were not reported. Education, training, protocols, policies, or procedures to address this behavior were not available to most nurses (80%). There is little protocol-driven guidance for this very common problem.

There should be surveillance for sexual addiction in potential exploitation behavior. Irons and Schneider reported their experience with the intensive, multidisciplinary assessment of 137 health-care professionals, predominantly (85%) physicians, almost all male (97%), referred by state licensing boards with allegations of professional sexual impropriety.[7] They postulated an addictive feature underlay, in which 54% were diagnosed with Psychosexual Disorder

With Addictive Features, and 31% were chemically dependent. Those who had a sexual addiction had a higher prevalence of chemical dependence (38%) than those who did not (21%). They found that two-thirds (66%) were determined to be sexually exploitative, while 68% were impaired or potentially impaired, and required at least temporary withdrawal from professional work. Sexual addiction is present in two-thirds of sexually exploitive health-care professionals, as well as concurrent chemical dependence in one-third.

The Vanderbilt Comprehensive Assessment Program for Professionals (V-CAP) was used as the research base by Roback et al. for an evaluation of 88 physicians referred for misconduct.[8] They attempted to profile behavioral offenses with direct therapy and prognosis for remediation. The physicians were referred for three groups of offenses: (1) sexual boundary violations; (2) disruptive behavior; (3) other misconduct. Their evaluation consisted of the Minnesota Multiphasic Personality Inventory (MMPI-2) and Personality Assessment Inventory (PAI).[9,10] The sexual boundary violator category generated the greatest percentage of profiles indicative of character pathology on both personality scales. Therefore, it is the sexual boundary violator that poses the greatest theoretic challenge, and the greatest risk of reoffending.

Legal Analysis

In *O'Connor* v. *Ortega*, a male physician and psychiatrist was responsible for training young physicians in psychiatry.[11] Several issues were attributed to the defendant including allegedly coercing resident contributions for a computer, sexually harassing two female hospital employees, and taking inappropriate disciplinary action against a resident. He was placed on administrative leave, and personal items suggesting a potential relationship with a former resident physician were allegedly identified when his office contents were inventoried. The defendant filed suit under 42 U.S.C. §1983 concerning the Fourth Amendment rights against unreasonable search and seizure.[12,13] The district court concluded the search was proper because of the need to secure state property. The United States Court of Appeals (USCA), Ninth Circuit affirmed in part and reversed in part, concluding that the inventory process was for those leaving or terminated. They concluded the defendant held a reasonable expectation of privacy, and the search was deemed

unreasonable with a remand to district court for damages. The Supreme Court of the United States granted certiorari, reversed and remanded to the USCA. The Supreme Court held that there was a privacy right at stake, but search and seizure may be reasonable at its inception in light of the allegations of this case. On remand, the district court should determine the justification for search and seizure and evaluate the reasonableness and scope to determine the admissibility of evidence.

In *Fisher* v. *San Pedro Peninsula Hospital*, a surgical nurse employed by the hospital alleged she was the subject of sexual harassment, offensive touching, and injury by a physician in authority.[14] This behavior was repetitive and apparently corroborated by two other employees. However, allegedly the facility subjected her to retaliation, did not report to external regulatory bodies, or did little to restrict this offensive behavior. The plaintiff filed a claim for environmental sexual harassment under the California Fair Employment Housing Act (FEHA).[15]

> Sexual harassment creates a hostile, offensive, oppressive, or intimidating work environment and deprives its victim of her statutory right to work in a place free of discrimination, when the sexually harassing conduct sufficiently offends, humiliates, distresses, or intrudes upon its victim, so as to disrupt her emotional tranquility in the workplace, affect her ability to perform her job as usual, or otherwise interferes with an undermines her personal sense of well-being. (*DFEH* v. *Bee Hive Answering Service*, FEHC No. 84-16 at pp. 18–19.).[16]

The trial court dismissed her complaint after defendant's demurrers were sustained without leave to amend. It was not enough to plead that a pattern of activity existed, but that "sexual harassment permeated the workplace." She filed a second amended complaint, and the Court of Appeals of California, Second District held that she had not pled a valid sexual harassment claim. They held that it was not proven the alleged contact was either "systematic or pervasive" toward other women, with an established pattern of abuse. However, they did reverse and remand to amend their cause of action, as the analysis is one of first impression.

In *Kopp* v. *Samaritan Health System*, the complainant was a long-term technician employee with supervisory responsibilities, with excellent evaluations.[17] The facility had a physician provider who had held various executive and committee positions and an important clinical position generating significant revenue for the hospital. It was alleged that he was responsible for numerous verbally assaultive events involving other female employees. The plaintiff alleged the verbal and physical abuse, coupled with the hospital's inability to curtail this conduct, amounted to hostile-environment sexual harassment.[18] The district court held the evidence was not sufficient to sustain a finding that the alleged abuse was gender based. The USCA, Eighth Circuit disagreed and reversed the decision. The evidence available to the district court, viewed in the light most favorable to the non-moving party, the plaintiff in this case, was sufficient to withstand the defendant's motion for summary judgment. There appeared to be evidence of a sustained pattern with general awareness.

Conclusion

These issues tend to be persistent and refractory to informal methods of resolution. Interventions include a corrective pathway with guidelines defining the behavior involved, and work-related restrictions. The presence of chaperones and other behavioral interventions can be useful. However, an educational approach such as an assessment course to deal with sexual boundary violations is the most helpful, going beyond the usual continuing medical education and requiring provider participation and self-assessment. These courses are highly effective and straddle the boundary between passive education and active therapeutic intervention.

References

1. Gabbard GO, Nadelson C. Professional boundaries in the physician-patient relationship. *JAMA*. 1995;273(18):1445–1459.

2. American Medical Association, Council on Ethical and Judicial Affairs. Sexual misconduct in the practice of medicine. *JAMA*. 1991;266(19):2741–2745.

3. Gartrell NK, Milliken N, Goodson WH, Thiemann S, Lo B. Physician-patient sexual contact. Prevalence and problems. *West J Med*. 1992;157(2):139–143.

4. Phillips SP, Schneider MS. Sexual harassment of female doctors by patients. *N Engl J Med*. 1993;329(26):1936–1939.

5. Komaromy M, Bindman AB, Haber RJ, Sande MA. Sexual harassment in medical training. *N Engl J Med*. 1993;328(5):322–326.

6. Kaye J, Donald CG, Merker S. Sexual harassment of critical care nurses: a costly workplace issue. *Am J Crit Care*. 1994;3(6):409–415.

7. Irons RR, Schneider JR. Sexual addiction: significant factor in sexual exploitation by health care professionals. *Sex Addict Compulsivity*. 1994;1(3):198–214. DOI:10.1080/107201694084000043.

8. Roback HB, Strassberg D, Iannelli RJ, Reid Finlayson AJ, Blanco M, Neufeld R. Problematic physicians: a comparison of personality profiles by offence type. *Can J Psychiatry*. 2007;52(5):315–22.

9. Butcher JN, Graham JR, Ben-Porath YS, Tellegen A, Dahlstrom WG, Kaemmer B. *Minnesota Multiphasic Personality Inventory (MMPI-2) PsychCorp* (Minneapolis, MN: University of Minnesota Press, 2001).

10. Morey LC. *Personality Assessment Inventory (PAI), Professional manual* (Lutz, FL: Psychological Assessment Resources, 1991).

11. *O'Connor* v. *Ortega*, 480 U.S. 709 (1987).

12. 42 U.S. Code §1983–Civil Action for Deprivation of Rights.

13. U.S. Const. Amend. IV.

14. *Fisher* v. *San Pedro Peninsula Hospital*, 214 Cal. App.3d 590 (1989).

15. California Government Code §12900 et seq.: Fair Employment Housing Act (FEHA).

16. *DFEH* v. *Bee Hive Answering Service, FEHC No. 84–16. (1984).*

17. *Kopp* v. *Samaritan Health System, 13 F.3d 264 (1993).*

18. *Title VII, 42 U.S.C. §2000e-2 (a)(1) – Unlawful Employment Practices.*

Chapter 84

Protected Health Information

Case

The patient had come in to the emergency department (ED) with chest pain. The symptoms were fairly standard: substernal location, left arm radiation, shortness of breath, and nausea. He immediately had an EKG and was given aspirin and oxygen. An intravenous line was established and nitroglycerin was administered. The EKG showed some subtle ST changes, and the ED physician called the interventional cardiologist who was on call that day.

The cardiologist went over the history, the physical exam findings, and the EKG. The ED physician discussed the EKG with her, and was concerned about some subtle findings. The cardiologist asked what the troponin level was, and the ED physician said that although the point-of-care test was negative at this point he still had concerns. The cardiologist said she wanted to look at the EKG, but she was currently traveling between facilities. She asked the ED physician if he could snap a picture, and send it to her. The ED physician expressed his concern about sending health information in this way, but the cardiologist said that she had no other option to view the EKG as she was driving. So, reluctantly, he sent the EKG as a photo from his phone. The cardiologist then called back, and said that she was a little concerned, but didn't think the patient needed to have a catheterization at this point. She was just going into another procedure, and asked the ED physician to text her the patient's name and medical record number. The ED physician again voiced his concerns, but the cardiologist again said that she was driving, and couldn't write anything down. So, once again, the information was reluctantly sent by text message.

The patient was admitted to the hospital, and the cardiologist said she would see him later that day. On his next shift, the ED physician heard that the patient went on to have a myocardial infarction (MI), as was

the concern. He was taken to the cardiac cath lab late in the day, had some arrhythmias and eventually received an intracoronary stent, having spent a brief period of time on an intra-aortic balloon pump.

About 6 months later the ED physician was contacted by the hospital counsel, who told him a medical malpractice claim had been filed. One of the contentions was that there was a Health Insurance Portability and Accountability Act (HIPAA) violation in that the patients protected health information (PHI) had been sent by a non-secured mechanism and the counsel wanted to know if that was indeed the case. The ED physician responded that the PHI had indeed been sent in that way. He had concerns at the time and had stated them twice, but the consultant's exigent circumstances had made it necessary to transmit the information as she requested.

Medical Approach

As communication capability improves, there are clear benefits of data sharing with immediacy and accuracy of the information transferred. The ability to have a visual representation of the data is sometimes invaluable. However, that being said, it is still necessary to be cautious about the transmission of unprotected health information.

The American College of Emergency Physicians (ACEP) developed an Emergency Department Information Systems (EDIS) White Paper Resolution 22 (07), defining electronic health record systems designed specifically to manage data and workflow in support of ED patient care and operations.[1] The EDIS should facilitate the delivery of patient care, conform to relevant data interoperability standards, and comply with applicable privacy and security constructs to ensure secure availability of relevant health-care information (Table 84.1).

Table 84.1 Electronic health record

1. Facilitate delivery of patient care
2. Conform to interoperability standards
3. Comply with privacy and security standards
4. Secure availability of relevant data

Reference: ACEP: Rothenhaus et al.[1]

Table 84.2 Correlates of protected health information data breach

Correlates	Significance % (95% CI)
1. Electronic media	67.4% (64.4–79.4%)
2. Theft	58.2% (55.0–61.3%)
3. Laptop computers, electronic devices	37.2% (29.7–35.7%)
4. States (CA, FL, IL, NY, TX)	34.1% (31.2–37.2%)
5. External vendors	28.8% (25.9–31.7%)

Reference: Liu et al.[2]

A systematic study of data breaches of PHI was performed by Liu by analyzing the online database of the US Department of Health and Human Services.[2] They targeted data breaches of unencrypted PHI, or individually identifiable information reported by covered entities, such as health plans or clinicians. When the data breaches affect 500 or more individuals, the report must include the name of the state of the entity breached, the number of records affected, the type and source of the breach, and the involvement of any external vendors (Table 84.2). Examples of unintended breaches include theft of unsecured laptops, dissemination of data in emails, and improper disposal of patient records.

There were 949 breaches affecting 29 million records between 2010 and 2013. There were six breaches that involved over a million records each, and breaches occurred in every state, the District of Columbia, and Puerto Rico. Five states – California, Texas, Florida, New York, and Illinois – accounted for 34.1% (95% CI, 31.2–37.2%) of all breaches. Most breaches occurred via electronic media (67.4%, 95% CI, 64.4–79.4%), frequently involving laptop computers or portable electronic devices (37.2%, 95% CI, 29.7–35.7%), involving theft (58.2%, 95% CI, 55.0–61.3%), and external vendors (28.8%, 95% CI, 25.9–31.7%). The number of breaches from hacking and unauthorized access or disclosure increased during the study period from 12.1% to 27.2% ($P = 0.003$).

The information technology requirements in this rapidly changing health-care environment are significant. Overhage et al. studied clinical information sharing between institutions, in which computerized information from another institution was shared with ED physicians.[3] There was no difference in workflow or information access, but a trend to a decreased cost per patient encounter with information sharing. However, standard precautions should be protocolized to protect inappropriate PHI release.

The confidentiality of medical records shared over the Internet was pioneered by the Boston Electronic Medical Record Collaborative.[4] They described an explicit protocol that makes it possible to electronically identify patients and providers, secure permission for the release in records, and track the information once it is reported. They stress a "scrubbed" data transfer process for additional safety.

The advent of email has raised concerns over patient confidentiality. Certainly, the use of email as a method of communication to optimize patient care has matured.[5] Most institutions have converted from email to an integrated, protected messaging system for patient–physician communication to ensure compliance.

There are physician concerns and precautions with email consultation. The radiology community was especially cautious as they were early adopters of the online patient communication process.[6] Medicolegal liability applies if there is a physician–patient relationship. First, it is assumed email contact concerning specific patient care establishes that relationship. Second, if there is electronic communication, it should ideally be within a closed and protected system. Third, if by necessity there is unsecured communication, it should be archived. Fourth, the provision of advice should be constrained by conventional evidence-based standards. Fifth, the provider should be aware of the patient's location and jurisdiction, and how that might affect their liability (Table 84.3).

One concern is how an internet-based educational program might reveal patient information. Weadock et al. evaluated 200 presentations from a general web-based search, in which 72% (143) featured images, image links, or notes.[7] They reported that 36% (52) contained PHI, and 24% (31) revealed the patient's name. Presentations located at US sites made up 66% (132) of the total. There were 71% (86) that contained

Table 84.3 Email communication and liability

1.	Email contact establishes physician–patient relationship
2.	Closed and protected system
3.	Archive communication
4.	Evidence-based standards advice
5.	Patient jurisdiction liability

Reference: Smith and Berlin.[6]

radiologic images, with 49% (34) containing PHI and 22% (19) showing the patient's name.

Legal Analysis

In *Board of Medical Quality Assurance* v. *Gherardini*, a state medical board requested the complete medical records of five patients in the investigation of a licensed physician.[8] The hospital refused to surrender the records, and the medical board sought and obtained a superior court order to compel. The hospital did not dispute the right to regulate the licensee physician, but here the patient's rights are under scrutiny. The Court of Appeals of California, Fourth District reversed the order to compel and remanded for further consideration. They acknowledged the individual's right to privacy is not absolute, and it may be outweighed by supervening public concerns. However, they felt the declaration set forth no showing of relevance or materiality of these medical records as they applied to this physician.

In *Law* v. *Zuckerman*, the patient had a surgical procedure, alleged complications, and brought suit.[9] The plaintiff requested an order precluding ex-parte discussion with another physician, a fact witness for the defendant. The trial court disagreed with the plaintiff's interpretation of HIPAA regulations, in that ex-parte conversation with a treating physician of the adverse party is prohibited. However, they issued an order permitting both sides to have ex-parte discussion with the physician. They then felt the statute was correctly applied. The district court held the patient should have the ability to withhold permission and to effectively block disclosure. However, HIPAA was applicable to the pretrial disclosure of medical information, as it is apparent that the court order remedied any potential violation, and the plaintiff's motion to preclude discussion was denied.[10]

In *O'Connor* v. *Pierson*, a tenured public school teacher was recommended for a leave of absence after alleged workplace behavioral issues.[11] The school requested a medical assessment and release of records to decide fitness to return. The plaintiff removed to federal court and raised due-process claims to the board's conditions regarding medical information. The district court granted summary judgment for the board of education. The United States Court of Appeals, Second Circuit affirmed, vacated, and remanded in part. They held that the property-based substantive due-process right is derivative of the privacy-based claim. The plaintiff must prove that the demand for medical records was constitutionally arbitrary and that he was deprived of a property right, which was precluded by the fact that while on sick leave he was not truly deprived of his property.

In *Arons* v. *Jutkowitz*, *Webb* v. *New York Methodist Hospital*, and *Kish* v. *Graham*, diverse plaintiffs filed lawsuits alleging medical malpractice in cases that were joined for resolution.[12] The Court of Appeals of the State of New York questioned whether the attorney may interview the adverse party's treating physician when the adverse party has affirmatively placed their medical condition in controversy. The court held that the attorney is permitted to do so, although HIPAA imposes procedural requirements unique to the informal discovery of health-care professionals.[10]

Conclusion

It is now common for unsecured photos to be sent from mobile phones and other electronic devices to better communicate patient circumstances. Unsecured email communication has also been used to discuss patient care and course and may reveal PHI. Any facility that still uses these insecure methods to communicate health-care information should install up-to-date software to secure this data as an absolute and urgent necessity.

References

1. Rothenhaus T, Kamens D, Keaton BF, Nathanson L, Nielson J, McClay JC, et al. Emergency department information systems: primer for emergency physicians, nurses and IT professionals. *ACEP Resolution 22(07) Task Force White Paper*. April 15, 2009.

2. Liu V, Musen MA, Chou T. Data breaches of protected health information in the United States. *JAMA*. 2015;313(14):1471–1473. DOI:10.1001/jama.2015.2252.

3. Overhage JM, Dexter PR, Perkins SM, Cordell WH, McGoff J, McGrath R, McDonald CJ. A randomized, controlled trial of clinical information shared from another institution. *Ann Emerg Med.* 2002;39(1):14–23. DOI:10.1067/mem.2002.120794.

4. Rind DM, Kohane IS, Szolovits P, Safran C, Cheuh HC, Barnett GO. Maintaining the confidentiality of medical records shared over the internet and the world wide web. *Ann Intern Med.* 1997;127(2):138–141. DOI:10.7326/0003-4819-127-2-199707150-00008.

5. Spiotta VL. Legal concerns surrounding e-mail use in a medical practice. *JONAS Healthc Law Ethics Regul.* 2003;5(3):53–57.

6. Smith JJ, Berlin L. Malpractice issues in radiology: e-mail consultation. *AJR Am J Roentgenol.* 2001;179(5):1133–1136. DOI:10.2214/ajr.179.5.1791133.

7. Weadock WJ, Londy FJ, Ellis JH, Goldman EB. Do radiology and other health care presentations posted on the internet contain accessible protected health information? *Radiology.* 2008;249(1):285–293. DOI:10.1148/radiol.2491080222.

8. Board of Medical Quality Assurance, 93 Cal. App.3d 669 (1979).

9. *Law* v. *Zuckerman MD*, 307 F. Supp.2d 705 (2004).

10. Health Insurance Portability and Accountability Act of 1996 (HIPAA), Title XI, Pub. L. 104–191, 110 Stat. 1936 (August 21, 1996), codified as 42 U.S.C. 1301 et seq.

11. *O'Connor* v. *Pierson*, 426 F.3d 187 (2005).

12. *Arons* v. *Jutkowitz, Webb* v. *New York Methodist Hospital, Kish, Jerge* v. *Graham*, 9 N.Y. 3d 393 (2007).

Psychiatric Care

Case

The police brought the patient to the emergency department (ED). He was aggressive, agitated, and intoxicated. That day he had started to make some family threats. He had made previous visits to the facility, and seemed to quiet down once he came to the ED. He had the standard psychiatric screening profile performed to ensure there were no medical issues. Laboratory testing was essentially normal but his blood alcohol was 0.25 mg/dL, so he was clinically intoxicated, with an alcohol level three times the normal upper limit for driving. The patient stayed in the ED for the evening and seemed to sober up, but the staff had concerns the next morning as he was still waiting for a bed to become available. The physician spoke to his family, asking about the availability of lethal means and recommending them to remove any sort of weapons from the house. Psychiatry was consulted during the evening, and the psychiatrist visited him in the morning.

After the evaluation, the psychiatrist said the patient was ready for discharge. Once again, the ED physician stressed the patient's presentation was a little different, as he seemed a little more violent or agitated than usual. It was thought he would benefit from a hospital stay, and all parties agreed. The search for a bed went on for the next 24 hours but still none was available. He remained in the ED with a sitter. Late the next evening, he was finally accommodated with a transfer bed at a facility a few miles away.

He was subsequently discharged after a 3-day stay and then apparently involved in some other law-enforcement issue. At this point, he was arrested, and brought back to the ED for evaluation. The family argued he should have been kept longer the last time. They were reminded that on this occasion he was admitted, referred to psychiatry, and competed

an inpatient stay under their care. The issue did not involve the ED.

Medical Approach

Psychiatric care in the ED is often complicated by a number of psychosocial factors including life and financial stressors, drug or alcohol abuse, and lack of care resources. In this particular case, the patient was evaluated appropriately and admitted to a psychiatric service, but unfortunately the recidivism rate is so high that he re-presented in a relatively short timeframe.

Assessment of the acute psychiatric patient in the ED involves analysis of multiple areas of risk (Table 85.1).[1] First, the new onset of a psychiatric disorder requires a careful and comprehensive analysis. Second, the assessment for medical clearance in an acute psychiatric presentation is a diagnosis of exclusion. Third, the assessment of the risk of suicidality is an area of significant focus. Fourth, a proper assessment must be completed before the patient departs the ED prematurely.

Another area of significant medicolegal concern is that of the agitated patient in the ED.[2] First, there is the continuum of informed consent and competence. Second, the use of chemical or physical restraint must be carefully planned and implemented. Third, there is a clear duty to protect the patient and the public. Fourth, appropriate patient boundaries should be

Table 85.1 Assessment of acute psychiatric patients in the ED

1. New-onset psychiatric disorders
2. Medical clearance
3. Suicide risk
4. Premature departure

Reference: Good et al.[1]

Table 85.2 Medicolegal concerns with the agitated patient

1.	Informed consent and competence continuum
2.	Chemical or physical restraint
3.	Protect the patient and the public
4.	Respect boundaries to avoid battery allegation
5.	Compelled care requirement
6.	Duty to warn while respecting confidentiality

Reference: Thomas and Moore.[2]

Table 85.3 Involuntary commitment procedure

1.	Detailed statement of reasons
2.	Closest relative identification
3.	Relationship with respondent
4.	Witness to help prove the facts
5.	Examination and admission within 72 hours

Reference: Illinois Compiled Statutes.[7]

respected to avoid a complaint of battery. Fifth, the requirements for compelled care should be defined to avoid a false imprisonment allegation. Sixth, there is an established duty to warn others of significant danger, even while respecting patient confidentiality (Table 85.2).

Mental health professionals have a clear duty to protect the public, and to warn against potential violent behavior of patients. The premise of patient confidentiality has roots dating back to the Hippocratic oath, but the seminal "duty to warn" case – *Tarasoff* v. *Regents of the University of California* – affected this balance.[3,4] This case triggered the "duty to warn" or "duty to protect" statutes passed in almost all states. The mandatory version has the provider liable for not reporting, as well as immunity, while the permissive version allows one to report, but does not compel it.

The majority of states (58%, 30), including the District of Columbia and Puerto Rico, have a mandatory duty to protect or warn, and 33% (17) of states have a permissive duty. The rest have an alternative requirement.[5] There are four states without a duty to warn (Nevada, Maine, North Carolina, and North Dakota), while Georgia allows discretionary disclosure. Another nuance is that Arizona, Delaware, and Illinois have established different profession-specific duties.

Legal Analysis

In *Arthur* v. *Lutheran General Hospital*, the patient presented to the ED with recurrent chest pain and shortness of breath, but allegedly became agitated and threatening concerning a previous disability determination[6] He received a psychological evaluation as part of the treatment plan. He allegedly made threats to others during the interview, and transfer to a psychiatric facility was recommended after his medical admission. Although he signed a voluntary commitment

on his initial admission, he balked on the mental health admission and involuntary commitment was required. He filed a claim for false imprisonment and the trial court awarded summary judgment to the defendant facility.

To begin the process of involuntary commitment, any person 18 years of age or older may present a petition to the director of a mental health facility, naming a respondent whose "immediate hospitalization is necessary for the protection of such a person or others from physical harm." [7] The petition must include: (1) a detailed statement of reasons, including a description of any acts or significant threats supporting, and the time and place of their occurrence; (2) name and address of closest relatives; (3) relationship with respondent; and (4) a witness who can help to prove the facts. The petition should be accompanied by a certificate executed by a physician, qualified examiner, or clinical psychologist stating that involuntary commitment and immediate hospitalization is required. The respondent should have been personally examined not more than 72 hours prior to the admission (Table 85.3).[7] In this case, the interval between examination and hospitalization was 96 hours. The Appellate Court of Illinois, First District affirmed the denial of summary judgment to the complainant, reversed that of the facility, and remanded to the trial court for further consideration.

Another area of critical focus in the ED is suicidal ideation. In *Sheron* v. *Lutheran Medical Center*, the plaintiff's husband was transported to the ED after ingesting a large quantity of prescription sleeping pills allegedly with stated suicidal intent.[8] After his medical condition was stabilized, he was evaluated by a mental health service clinician. They felt he was not "imminently dangerous" and could be discharged and seen the following day by a "mental health professional." The ED physician followed the psychiatric professional's recommendation and discharged the patient, who took his own life the next day. The trial court rendered a jury verdict and financial damages for the plaintiff. The facility appealed, attempting to shift liability to the ED physician, on a theory that the physician had sole admission or discharge capability. They alleged the jury instruction was misleading regarding ultimate liability for discharge. The hospital suggests the instruction should include the following wording:

> When a doctor diagnoses, treats or operates on a patient in a hospital, he is in command of these functions, and the hospital and its employees subserve him in his ministrations to the patient. He has the sole and the final control in the matter of diagnosis, treatment and surgery. Possessed of this authority, a doctor's actions are his responsibility.

The Colorado Court of Appeals affirmed, although the trial court reduced the award in relation to a contributory negligence of the patient himself.

In *Moses* v. *Providence Hospital and Medical Centers*, the patient presented to the ED with headaches, vomiting, hallucinations, and delusions.[9] His partner reported threatening behavior which she said made her fearful for her safety. The patient was admitted from the ED and was evaluated by an internist, a neurologist, and a psychiatrist. It was reported by his partner that he had tried to board a plane with a hunting knife, and she said he had told her "he had bought caskets." Although he was to have been admitted to a psychiatric facility, allegedly he was ultimately discharged home as medically stable. He subsequently murdered his partner 10 days after discharge. The plaintiff representing the estate of the deceased brought suit alleging the hospital violated the Emergency Medical Treatment and Labor Act (EMTALA) and committed other common-law negligence actions.[10] The trial court granted the summary judgment motion of the defendant, dismissing the plaintiff's claims. The United States Court of Appeals, Sixth Circuit reversed and remanded for further proceedings with respect to the hospital, but affirmed with respect to the psychiatrist. They held that EMTALA was not designed or intended to establish guidelines for patient care or to provide a suit for

medical negligence or malpractice. However, the hospital was required to admit and adequately stabilize the patient prior to discharge. To all appearances, the responsible physicians felt the patient was stable, and gave no indication of failure to improve or worsening.

Conclusion

From the ED perspective, it is crucial to recognize there is a "duty to warn" especially in cases in which the patient is a danger to society as well as themselves. Health-care professionals are obliged to warn in cases of significant threat, but must still protect the patient's rights and confidentiality as much as possible.

References

1. Good B, Walsh RM, Alexander G, Moore G. Assessment of the acute psychiatric patient in the emergency department: legal cases and caveats. *West J Emerg Med.* 2014;15(3):312–317. DOI:10.5811/westjem.2013.8.18378.

2. Thomas J, Moore G. Medical-legal issues in the agitated patient: cases and caveats. *West J Emerg Med.* 2013;14(5):559–565. DOI:10.5811/westjem.2013.4.16132.

3. *Tarasoff* v. *The Reagents of the University of California*, 17 Cal.3d 425 (1976).

4. Edelstein L. *The Hippocratic Oath: Text, Translation and Interpretation*, 2nd edition (Baltimore, MD: Johns Hopkins University Press, 1996).

5. National Conference of State Legislatures (NCSL). Mental Health Professionals Duty to Protect/Warn. January 2013.

6. *Arthur* v. *Lutheran General Hospital, Inc.*, 692 N.E.2d 1238 (Ill. App., 1998).

7. Illinois Compiled Statutes (ILCS): Mental Health and Developmental Disabilities. (405 ILCS 5/3–601(a,b), 602).

8. *Sheron* v. *Lutheran Medical Center*, 18 P.3d 796 (2000).

9. *Moses* v. *Providence Hospital and Medical Centers, Inc.*, 571 F.3d 573 (2009).

10. EMTALA, 42 U.S.C. §1395 dd.

Referral

Case

The patient presented to the emergency department (ED) with some facial numbness that had occurred 2 days ago. She had no current symptoms, but had called her primary care physician (PCP) and the PCP's office had referred her to the ED for evaluation. She had no difficulties with her motor function, no current sensation abnormalities, and no difficulties with speech or understanding, just a little left facial numbness that had gone away.

The ED physician performed a standard workup for a transient ischemic attack (TIA), ordering laboratory screening and a non-contrast head CT scan. The patient had a previous iodine allergy, which precluded any contrast studies, and it was late evening so MRI scanning was not available. The workup was essentially normal in all respects. The ED physician contacted her PCP, who suggested he would be glad to see her in his office and would then schedule an outpatient MRI. In the interim, she would be discharged on aspirin for secondary prevention of future cerebrovascular events.

In addition, the ED physician included the name of the on-call neurologist for follow-up. He did not contact the consultant again as it was late evening and the patient's symptoms had dissipated at this point. He stressed to the patient the importance of follow-up with her PCP and arranging the specialty physician referral to complete her discharge care plan.

About 6 months later the risk management department contacted the ED physician to say the patient had failed to show up for her follow-up appointment and subsequently had a stroke the week after her ED visit. One of the allegations in the complaint was that contact should have been made with neurology directly. The ED physician pointed out that he had included the neurologist information in her discharge instructions, but had not called neurology since the

PCP suggested that he would handle the follow-up issue and schedule the MRI.

Medical Approach

The standard contention in most medical malpractice allegations is that one is obliged to consult some specialty physician, as an absolute requirement in the emergency setting. Specialty consultation from the ED can sometimes be a very nebulous concept, contingent on availability depending on time of day, urgency of the complaint, or consultant staff availability. Often the ED physician generates a diagnosis and treatment plan in conjunction with the PCP that also involves an outpatient specialty referral.

Consultation and referral allow the traditional exchange of medical expertise between physicians, which benefits the patient.[1] The referral process has undergone a transition from a physician-based to a system-based process. However, it has direct effects on physician practice, which may include the potential for adverse financial impact, conflict of interest, or ethical dilemmas related to referral patterns. Most importantly, the physician may assume medicolegal liability either for not referring for additional care or for referring if an untoward outcome occurs.

Profiling the referral practice of individual practitioners allows a better understanding of the process. Forrest et al. evaluated 141 family physicians with 34,519 office visits, accompanied by 2534 referrals for consultation.[2] They found approximately 1 of 20 patients, or 5.1% of office visits, led to a referral to another physician for speciality care. The majority of referrals (68%) were made after physician evaluation, 18% after phone conversation, 11% by staff consulting with the physician, and 3% by staff. These PCPs sought specialist advice on diagnosis or treatment in half (52.1%) the referrals, asking their help with medical management in 25.9%, surgical management in

37.8%, and patient request in 13.6%. The most common referral was for surgery (45.4%), medical specialists (31.0%), non-physician clinicians (12.1%), obstetrician-gynecologists (4.6%), mental health professionals (4.2%), other practitioners (2.0%), and generalists (0.8%).

There can be marked variation in referral strategies, with referrals in business hours more predictable than after-hours emergency referrals.[3] There was a wide variation in family physician referral rates with a five-fold variation between the bottom and top quartiles. Referrals are often associated with off-hour (11 p.m. to 7 a.m.) evaluation.

Legal Analysis

In *Davis* v. *Dr. Weiskopf, Hagman*, the patient presented to the ED with knee pain and had radiography performed. The radiologist reported a concern of bony neoplasm to the ED physician.[4] The ED physician consulted the orthopedist for outpatient follow-up, but did not inform the patient of the diagnosis. The patient presented to the specialist's office for follow-up, but was rescheduled without being seen by the physician. The patient phoned ahead and was late for his second visit, but allegedly was not seen, nor referred to another physician or advised of the serious nature of his condition. The trial court determined that no physician–client relationship existed with the consultant, so no malpractice claim could arise. The Illinois Appellate Court, Second District reversed and remanded for further consideration. They held that a duty did indeed exist between a practicing physician, who accepted a referral and, having been advised the patient was suffering from severe illness, declined to treat him or refer him to another physician, to his damage.

In *Jett* v. *Penner*, the patient presented to the ED having fallen and injured his thumb. He was diagnosed with a metacarpal fracture. He was discharged with immobilization, analgesics, activity restriction, and a referral to orthopedics, "early this week" for a recheck appointment.[5] He was returned to a state of incarceration, followed by the physician there, maintained in splint with pain control, and saw orthopedics almost 8 weeks later as "routine." During subsequent follow-up, the injury was described as "well healed," an "old fracture," or "old fracture deformity." The plaintiff filed suit alleging (1) indifference to his serious medical needs in violation of his Eighth Amendment constitutional

rights and (2) violation of California Government Code §845.6 by failure to ensure prompt orthopedic follow-up.[6] The district court order adopted the magistrate judge's finding to award a summary judgment motion for the defendant. The United States Court of Appeals, Ninth Circuit reversed the summary judgment ruling, holding the plaintiff provided sufficient evidence of a valid medical referral, adverse consequences, and apparent indifference.

In *Shipley* v. *Williams*, a patient presented to the ED after abdominal surgery at the behest of her surgeon for evaluation by the ED physician.[7] The ED evaluation revealed an elevated white blood cell count, hypotension, and tachycardia and a discussion with her surgeon suggested an outpatient discharge plan. Allegedly, the surgeon did not have office hours the next day, and the patient was referred to her PCP for a "non-surgical" problem. She returned to the ED and was admitted in a critical condition with sepsis. The plaintiff filed suit against the ED physician, the operative surgeon, and the hospital. The trial court awarded summary judgment motions leaving her surgeon as the remaining defendant. The Supreme Court of Tennessee heard the appeal based on the "locality rule" for expert medical witnesses, in which the testimony is required to be compatible with the care provided in that community.[8] They held that the trial court's disqualification and exclusion of the claimant's expert witnesses was an error. They also reinstated the summary judgment motion in part of the surgeon on the failure to admit the claim of the appeal court. However, the defendant physician did not affirmatively negate, or suggest she could not prove elements of the plaintiff's claim. The burden of evidence production therefore did not shift to the plaintiff, vacating the trial court's summary judgment motion remanding for a new trial. This opinion was based on the testimony of the defense experts who were now reinstated to opine on this case, supporting the "locality rule" for expert witness testimony.

Conclusion

Ideally, in addition to just offering the consultant's contact information, the safest approach is to make consultative contact by phone to discuss the case. This ensures the consultant physician is available and desires to follow up with the patient and has an obligation for this issue if on call. Patient compliance, which is an important part of the diagnosis and treatment plan, often requires this additional intervention to ensure a valid referral.

References

1. Schaffer WA, Holloman FC. Consultation and referral between physicians in new medical practice environments. *Ann Intern Med*. 1985;103(4):600–605. DOI:10.7426/0003-4819-103-4-600.

2. Forrest CB, Nutting PA, Starfield B, Von Schrader S. Family physicians' referral decisions: results from the ASPN referral study. *J Fam Pract*. 2002;51(3):215–222.

3. Rossdale M, Kemple T, Payne S, Calnan M, Greenwood R. An observational study of variation in GPs' out-of-hours emergency referrals. *Br J Gen Pract*. 2007;57(535):152–154.

4. *Davis* v. *Weiskopf, Hagman*, 108 Ill. App. 3d 505 (1982).

5. *Jett* v. *Penner*, 439 F.3d 1091 (2006).

6. California Government Code §846.6: Police and Correctional Activities.

7. *Shipley* v. *Williams*, 350 S.W.3d 527 (2011).

8. Tennessee Code Annotated §29-26-115 (2000 & Supp 2010).

Chapter 87

Religion

Case

The paramedics brought the 75-year-old patient into the emergency department (ED). He had been the restrained driver in a motor vehicle accident. The patient had chest trauma, and what appeared to be a pelvic fracture and right femur fracture as well. This was designated Level II trauma. The remainder of the exam found no head injury, and no cause of intra-abdominal blood loss. However, the patient's hemoglobin level was low, only 8 g/dL, and he was scheduled to go to the operating room for fixation of the pelvis and femur fractures. The orthopedic resident asked that the ED staff consent the patient for blood transfusion, as they were in a hurry. During the consent procedure it became apparent the patient had a religious objection to blood transfusion. His daughter, who had now arrived in the ED, said her father was committed to this religious principle. He was awake and could corroborate this information even though he had been given a narcotic for pain. He appeared competent, with the capacity to decline blood transfusion, even if required to save his life.

Up to this point the patient had been maintained on a nasal cannula oxygen delivery system, but was now switched to a high-flow non-rebreathing face mask. After a brief time it was recognized that he would need to be intubated as he would require operative intervention. The physician then provided the patient with higher-flow oxygen to induce a hyperoxic state, with the bleeding resulting in lower blood counts. The patient was administered hetastarch and dextran in addition to fluids. The patient and family consented and accepted a dose of epoetin alfa (Epogen) to stimulate his bone marrow, but declined an experimental blood product as well.

The operating surgeon revisited the issue with the patient while he was still in the ED and suggested that a lethal outcome was indeed possible. The patient again declined a blood transfusion as he was committed to his religious principles. His family agreed and corroborated this, pointing out that until this point the patient had been healthy and made his own decisions.

Medical Approach

Patients' religious beliefs are often an important part of their medical care. Many patients object to blood transfusion. Other patients may refuse various chemotherapy treatments in deference to the hope of religious intervention. Religious accommodation may also be directed toward health-care personnel and the circumstances and environment in which the patient will be cared for. It is important to remember that cultural background and religious beliefs assist a significant proportion of patients in their understanding and coping with the disease process. Offering them that religious or cultural resources during their outpatient visit or hospital stay can often help to facilitate the recovery process.

It is helpful to understand patient preferences with regard to their religious beliefs. MacLean et al. presented a multi-center evaluation of 456 patients, in which one-third wanted to be asked about their religious beliefs and two-thirds felt their physician should be aware of their beliefs.[1] Patient agreement with physician spiritual interaction increased strongly with illness severity. There was 19% patient agreement with physician prayer in a routine office visit, 29% agreement in a hospital setting, and 50% agreement in a near-death scenario ($P < 0.001$). However, patient interest in spiritual or religious interaction declined when the intensity increased from simple discussion of spiritual issues (33%) to physician silent prayer (28%) to physician prayer with the patient (19%) ($P < 0.001$). Yet 10% of the patients would trade discussion time spent on medical issues for that discussing spiritual or religious issues.

Nurses play a huge part in assisting patients with their spiritual care needs. However, this has been adversely impacted by increasing workloads, documentation, and technology requirements. During their hospital stay patients may become anxious due to the fear of the unknown, uncertain future, and complications of their illness.[2] The ED is an area where patients may be particularly vulnerable. While technological advances improve the nurse's ability to objectively measure responses to care, the necessity of holistic health care with a spiritual component should not be forgotten.

The physician is often at the interface between religious beliefs and controversial clinical practice. Curlin et al. conducted a cross-sectional survey in which the patient requested a procedure that the physician had a moral or religious objection.[3] These procedures include administering terminal sedation to dying patients, providing abortion for failed contraception, and prescribing birth control to adolescents without parental consent. Of the 63% (1144/1820) of physicians who responded to the survey, the majority (86%) felt the physician was obligated to present all available options, 71% would refer the patient to a physician who would not object to the procedure, and 63% felt it was ethically permissible to discuss moral objections with the patient. Those physicians who were male, religious, or with personal objections to the procedures in question were less likely to believe that doctors must disclose information about other options, or refer them to others for the procedures (OR 0.3–0.5). Clearly, the focus should shift to the patient and away from the provider.

Perhaps the area of most importance to the emergency medicine professional is the care of Jehovah's Witness patients. Typically, Jehovah's Witnesses have a clear advance directive refusing blood transfusion, carried on their person as a wallet card: "Refusal to Accept Blood Products."[4] Today this record is often carried electronically. The information may also be conveyed by family or may be indicated by their registration details. The most difficult scenario is an unconscious patient known to be a Jehovah's Witness. Informed consent for the blood refusal should be sought and the "no transfusion" request should then be honored. If there is no documented blood transfusion refusal form, no previous medical record information, and no family member who communicates a transfusion prohibition request, then the standard risk/benefit analysis applies to blood transfusion.

Table 87.1 Individual vs. societal rights

Individual rights	Societal rights
1. Bodily control	Preservation of life
2. Privacy	Prevention of suicide
3. Medical decision-making	Protection of innocent third parties
4. Religious freedom	Maintenance of ethical integrity

Reference: Woolley.[5]

The ED physician is often left to balance individual rights, such as bodily control, right to privacy, right to medical decision-making, and right to religious freedom, which outweigh societal rights, such as preservation of life, prevention of suicide, protection of innocent third parties, and maintenance of ethical integrity of the medical profession (Table 87.1).[5] The Watchtower Society provides governance and establishes a decision-making pathway for adult Jehovah's Witnesses. The Medical Document card is signed, renewed annually, and witnessed by family members for adults. Clear immunity is offered for providers that follow these guidelines. For children and adolescents, decision-making is subject to judicial oversight if there is an area of controversy.

The area in which religious conviction is most controversial is parents not endorsing standard medical treatment for their child. Asser and Swan evaluated a cohort of 172 children who died between 1975 and 1995, in which faith healing was substituted for conventional medical care.[6] The majority of patients (81.4%, 140) had estimated survival of over 90%, 10.5% (18) had expected survival of over 50%, while 5.2% (9) were expected to have some benefit, and 1.8% (3) were not expected to have any treatment benefit. The exclusive use of faith healing to the exclusion of conventional medical care warrants public concern and often judicial intervention.

The "end-of-life" period can be an area of potential conflict between religious conviction and clinical judgment. Brett and Jersild defined the concept of religious justification for insistence of aggressive medical care near the end of life.[7] The reasons invoked include first, there is hope for a miracle at this point in care. Second, there is a refusal to give up on faith in God as health worsens. Third, the patient has a conviction that every moment of life is a gift from God and is worth preserving at any cost. Fourth, the patient may believe suffering has a redemptive value (Table 87.2).

Table 87.2 End-of-life religious conviction

1. Hope for a miracle
2. Refusal to abandon their faith in God
3. Life is worth preserving at any cost
4. Suffering may have redemptive value

Reference: Brett and Jersild.[7]

Clinicians are not obligated to provide care they feel to be medically inappropriate or inhumane, regardless of the patient's religious beliefs. With the assistance of clergy or the hospital chaplain, clinicians should discuss alternative religious interpretations with the patient and family. The group should attempt to reach a consensus on the implementation of life-sustaining therapy.

Legal Analysis

The caselaw is focused on the area of blood transfusion, which has undergone its own maturation. In *John F. Kennedy Memorial Hospital* v. *Heston*, the patient, a Jehovah's Witness, was involved in a motor vehicle accident. She required an emergency splenectomy for shock and it was felt she would die without a blood transfusion.[8] The unmarried patient and her family were firmly opposed to transfusion. The patient stated she did not want transfusion, although she was in an unstable state. Her mother stated her daughter declined the transfusion and signed a waiver for the facility alleviating their responsibility. The hospital sought a guardian to authorize transfusion, which was administered, surgery was performed, and the patient survived. The trial court declined to vacate the order, and the defendants (patient and family) appealed. The Supreme Court of New Jersey felt the case was moot since the patient had recovered and the likelihood of her return to that hospital was so remote that the declaratory judgment, or issued advisory opinion between parties, was unnecessary. The judgment was affirmed as the state's interest in preserving life is paramount.

These cases are even more emotive if an unborn child is involved. In *Jefferson* v. *Griffin*, the hospital petitioned the superior court for an order authorizing cesarean section and blood transfusion if necessary in a patient who was 39 weeks pregnant and refused consent for the transfusion.[9] The petition was filed, the defendant did not respond, and expert opinion was that neither she nor her child could survive a natural

delivery due to her complete placenta previa. The question raised was whether the unborn child has any legal right to court protection. The Supreme Court of Georgia found the state's interest in the unborn child outweighed the intrusion into the life of parents, and the motion for stay was declined.

In *Malette* v. *Shulman*, the patient was severely injured in a motor vehicle accident and presented to the ED in an unconscious state.[10] The ED physician ordered a blood transfusion, but a nurse found a card identifying the patient as a Jehovah's Witness and requesting no blood transfusion because of her religious convictions. As the nurse had a moral objection, the physician administered the transfusion himself, and did not follow the patient's daughter's instruction to discontinue. The physician felt he was obligated to provide this lifesaving intervention. The patient recovered and filed suit, where the trial judge ordered monetary damages for battery. The Ontario Court of Appeals denied the attendant appeal, as no evidence was presented to deny the validity of the transfusion prohibition card. The patient's right of self-control must prevail.

In *Matter of Dubreuil*, the patient was admitted through the ED at an advanced stage of pregnancy, signing a conventional consent form including blood transfusion.[11] She required a cesarean section to which she consented, but she did not consent to the blood transfusion because of her religious convictions as a Jehovah's Witness. The patient's condition precipitously declined but she still refused blood administration. The facility contacted her estranged husband (they were married but separated), who consented for her. The trial court held the patient could be compelled to receive medical treatment so that her death would not result in the abandonment of her children. The Supreme Court of Florida was asked for discretionary review and quashed the district court decision. They held that no evidence was offered to confirm the abandonment claim.

Perhaps the most emotive area involves pediatric patients. In *Newmark* v. *Williams/DCPS*, the patient was a child with advanced cancer, whose parents adhered to the Christian Science doctrine.[12] As members of the First Church of Christ, Scientist they rejected conventional medical treatment, choosing a course of spiritual aid and prayer. The parents filed suit citing Delaware statutory protections from abuse charges, exempting those who treat their children, "solely by spiritual means."[13] They also felt that removing the child from their custody violated their First Amendment constitutional right to freely exercise their religion.[14] The family court rejected both of these arguments and awarded custody to the Delaware Division of Child Protective Services (DCPS). The trial court issued an immediate stay and appeal was heard by the Supreme Court of Delaware. They held the child was neither abused nor neglected, and returned him to his parents. The DCPS was not able to sustain the heavy burden of demonstrating the benefit of a toxic chemotherapy regimen associated with a survival rate of less than 40%.

Conclusion

If the patient's refusal to give consent to a procedure may directly result in their death, a final appeal should be made. This appeal should involve the patient, family members, the primary care physician, specialty physicians, and other counselors. However, if the patient is a competent adult their request must be accommodated, even if the outcome is fatal. It is more complicated when these issues are made in the pediatric realm, by a minor or a parent. This requires a separate discussion.

References

1. MacLean CD, Susi B, Phifer N, Schultz L, Bynum D, Franco M, et al. Practice preference for physician discussion and practice of spirituality. *J Gen Int Med*. 2003;18(1):38–43. DOI:10.1046/j.1525–2003.20403.x.

2. McBrien B. Emergency nurses' provision of spiritual care: a literature review. *Br J Nurs*. 2010;19(12):768–773.

3. Curlin FA, Lawrence RE, Chin MH, Lantos JD. Religion, conscience and controversial clinical practices. *N Engl J Med*. 2007;356(6):593–600. DOI:10.1056/N ENGL J MEDsa065316.

4. Migden DR, Braen GR. The Jehovah's Witness blood refusal card: ethical and medicolegal considerations for emergency physicians. *Acad Emerg Med*. 1998;5(8):815–824. DOI:10.1111/acem.1998.5.issue-8/issuetoc.

5. Woolley S. Jehovah's Witnesses in the emergency department: what are their rights? *Emerg Med J*. 2005;22(12):869–871. DOI:10.1136/emj.2004.023382.

6. Asser SM, Swan R. Child fatalities from religion-motivated medical neglect. *Pediatrics*. 1998;101(4):625–629.

7. Brett AS, Jersild P. Inappropriate treatment near the end of life: conflict between religious convictions and clinical judgment. *Arch Int Med*. 2003;163(14):1645–1649. DOI:10.1001/archinte.163.14.1645.

8. *John F. Kennedy Memorial Hospital* v. *Heston*, 279 A.2d 670 (N.J. 1971).

9. *Jefferson* v. *Griffin Hospital Authority*, 274 S.E.2d 457 (1981).

10. *Malette* v. *Shulman*, 72 O.R. (2d) 417 (1990).

11. In Matter of Dubriel, 603 So. 2d 538 (1992).

12. *Newmark* v. *Williams/DCPS*, 588 A.2d 1108 (1991).

13. Delaware Code 10 §901 (11): Definitions Abuse, 16 §907: Neglect.

14. U.S. Const. Amend. I.

Research

Case

The patient presented to the emergency department (ED) in cardiac arrest. The paramedics had performed the usual prehospital interventions including cardiopulmonary resuscitation (CPR), intubation, and resuscitation drug administration. The facility was a tertiary care center with an experimental resuscitation intervention that could potentially be administered to the patient. The pretrial protocol had Institutional Review Board (IRB) approval with the capability of consent offered retrospectively, or because of its emergency nature it could be instituted by the investigator. There was a precedent for performing clinical resuscitation research, such as this intervention, under the doctrine of implied consent or a deferred informed consent protocol.

The patient was initially resuscitated and sent to the intensive care unit (ICU) but died the next day. Later in the week, the ED was informed the ethics committee had received an inquiry through the Patient Safety Committee, questioning the validity of the consent for this emergency cardiac arrest investigational trial. The ED physician stated that she was not a primary investigator, but was aware of the protocol as it had been discussed at a faculty meeting. The physician had only implemented a pre-established protocol and had no responsibility for its design. When asked if she administered the medication, she answered yes. When asked if she had obtained prospective informed consent from the patient, the physician answered that she obviously could not, since this was a cardiac arrest trial. She suggested the ethics committee should talk to the primary investigator and research staff.

Medical Approach

Emergency cardiac arrest research investigations are a necessary part of our emergency medicine clinical practice. We should participate as much as possible to improve the quality of care provided. Research does not, however, obviate the need for some type of consent. Typically, there is an IRB application and approval for a pathway that could include some form of consent. The doctrine of implied consent states that any patient in an emergency would want an intervention that had the potential to improve their outcome. Another option is the doctrine of proxy consent, in which the physician then actually has the informed discussion with family. If they choose to participate the data will be included, and if not, it will be excluded. Either way this requires a significant level of education for staff and other providers involved in the care so there is a better understanding of the risks and benefits of any of these interventions.

The issue of informed consent has always been problematic in emergency medicine research. Representatives from the Society for Academic Emergency Medicine and the American Heart Association were charged with developing a consensus statement with other stakeholders from the Office for Protection from Research Risks and the Food and Drug Administration (FDA).[1] They concluded that in some circumstances it is not feasible to obtain prospective or proxy consent for enrollment to an emergency research protocol. They felt patients may be vulnerable to research risks, but also to potentially beneficial therapy when no known effective therapy exists for a life-threatening illness. They offered recommendations when the critical nature of illness or injury, or the need to rapidly apply an investigational therapy, precludes prospective consent.

The "waiver of informed consent" pathway for acute care research was debated by the research and regulatory communities with limited public input and finalized in 1996. Smithline and Gerstle evaluated a sample of 212 patients presenting to an academic tertiary care ED.[2] The majority (73%) of patients approved of this waiver if the absolute risks were minimal, while

50% approved if the risk was incrementally greater than minimal. The only demographic correlates identified were educational and certain aspects of health status. However, there was a patient cohort that did not want to be enrolled regardless of the degree of risk or the availability of a family member to speak on their behalf. Waiver of consent poses an ethical dilemma, balancing individual rights against societal needs.

This issue has been addressed in the trauma population as well, balancing potential exploitation of a vulnerable population with deprivation of the benefits of advanced experimental trauma care. Morrison et al. performed a literature review in the 10-year period following passage of the FDA Common Rule 21 C.F.R. 50.24 and identified 21 published emergency research studies conducted under the waiver of informed consent.[3] The paradox of trauma resuscitation research in a population that is unconscious or with decreased decision-making capacity makes the idea of prospective informed consent difficult. The FDA memorialized this exception in 1995 as the "Common Rule" exception to the informed consent requirement in emergency medicine.[4] Problematic terms hindering implementation were language requiring "community consultation" and that existing treatments were "unproven or unsatisfactory." Researchers also cited difficulty with federal regulations and cumbersome internal review board processes as significant barriers to conducting trials.

The attitudes of ED patients and visitors regarding the "emergency exception" from informed consent in resuscitation research were surveyed by McClure et al. in face-to-face interviews in two academic trauma centers.[5] They evaluated 530 patients with an 82% response rate, with a demographic of mean age 41 years (range 18–95), 46% female, and 64% white. Most (88%) patients believed research subjects should be informed prior to enrollment, but 49% believed enrollment without prior consent would be acceptable, and 70% (369) would not object to enrollment in an emergency situation. Almost half (49%, 258) of the respondents stated they would attend a community meeting. These meetings were more likely to be attended by those with less education than those with college degrees (OR 0.53, 95% CI 0.33–0.85, $P = 0.008$). Another significant group (42%) would prefer to hear about "exception from informed consent" studies offered in their community via TV or radio. Only 5% were aware of any current applicable research studies in their area. Most participants disagreed with foregoing prospective informed consent for research participation, but many would be willing to participate in the "emergency exception" protocol.

The obvious question arises, "Do patients with acute medical conditions have the capacity to provide informed consent for emergency medicine research?" The premise is that, because of stress or illness, patients in emergency medicine may be temporarily cognitively impaired thereby rendering them incapable of participating in the informed consent process. Smithline et al. conducted a prospective study in which 25 patients were administered cognitive testing during standard ED care for an acute myocardial infarction.[6] They used the Weschler Adult Intelligence Scale – Revised (WAIS-R) for cognitive testing, with a score of less than 5 being abnormal, and a 10 cm visual analog scale was used to rate pain and nausea.[7,8]

The ED physicians felt that 8% (2) of the patients did not have capacity for consent. However, 20% (5) scored less than 5 on all WAIS-R subtests (κ = 0.5) and 32% (8) on at least one (κ = 0.3) Likewise, the initial to final subtest scores improved by discharge: median digit span (improved from 7 to 8), comprehension (5 to 7), and similarities (6 to 8). It is crucial to be aware that the patient's cognitive processing ability may be impaired, even though this may be difficult to recognize at times.

Legal Analysis

One of the early cases exploring the theory of lack of informed consent was *Mink* v. *University of Chicago*.[9] Here, 1000 women were given diethylstilbestrol to prevent miscarriage, as part of a double-blind study conducted by a university and a pharmaceutical company between 1950 and 1952. Allegedly, the patients were not informed of the experiment, nor of the medication that was administered. The patients alleged their children were at higher risk of cancer because of this intervention, and they were informed of this in 1975–1976. They claimed theories of liability to include: (1) battery by conducting an experiment without knowledge or consent; (2) product liability as a "defective and dangerous" drug; (3) breach of duty to inform of harm. The defendants moved to dismiss for failure to state a claim, and the district court denied the motion for the first cause of action, but granted for the second and third. The lack of consent allegation was a question of fact better left to the jury. The courts have authorized two theories of liability, including first an intentional tort, specifically assault and battery, in which a non-emergency treatment was performed without patient consent. The second is based on negligence theory, in which the physician is required to advise the patient of risks and benefits of an intervention to obtain informed consent.

In *Moore* v. *Regents of the University of California*, a patient with leukemia underwent a medically indicated splenectomy, but had tissue samples diverted for research without consent or approval.[10] These research activities, "were not intended to have any relation to … his medical care." The issue addressed was whether the use of the patient's cells for potentially lucrative research was violative of his rights. The superior court sustained all the defendants' demurrers to the third amended complaint, and reversed by the court of appeal. The Supreme Court of California held that the complaint states a valid cause of action for the beach of disclosure obligations, but not for property conversion. They held that:

> A physician who is seeking patient consent, to satisfy their fiduciary requirement, must disclose personal interests unrelated to the patient's health, whether research or economic, that may affect their medical judgment.

In *Grimes* v. *Kennedy Krieger Institute*, a prestigious research institute was studying a lead abatement program, which involved minor children.[11] An issue of concern was a research group and IRB that felt the potential accumulation of lead in the blood of otherwise healthy children was covered by parent consent. The trial court ruled for a motion on summary judgment for the defendant, holding the research entity did not have a duty to warn minor volunteer participants or guardians concerning potential harm. The Court of Appeals of Maryland reversed and remanded for further consideration. They held that a duty to warn of potentially foreseeable harm, and other obligations of special arrangement between subject and researcher, warranted further review of the evidence.

Conclusion

It is crucial to always maintain a high level of scrutiny with regard to the integrity of research studies. This requires a proper IRB, often focusing on the ethical analysis of the research on patients and their subsequent care. More recently, the focus has transitioned to analysis of potential financial conflict of interest for individuals, institutions, and industry.

References

1. Biros M, Lewis RJ, Olson CM, Runge JW, Cummins RO, Fost N. Informed consent in emergency research: consensus statement from the coalition conference of acute resuscitation and critical care researchers. *JAMA*. 1995;273(16):1283–1287. DOI:10.1001/jama.1995.03520400053044.

2. Smithline HA, Gerstle ML. Waiver of informed consent: a survey of emergency medicine patients. *Am J Emerg Med*. 1998;16(1):90–91. DOI:10.1016/S0735-6757(98)90074-2.

3. Morrison CA, Horsitz IB, Carrick MM. Ethical and legal issues on emergency research: barriers to conducting prospective randomized trials in an emergency setting. *J Surg Res*. 2009;157(1):115–122. DOI:10.1016/j.jss.2009.03.051.

4. 21 C.F.R. 50.24: Title 21: Protection of Human Subjects.

5. McClure KB, Delorio NM, Gunnels MD, Oschner MJ, Biros MH, Schmidt TA. Attitudes of emergency department patients and visitors regarding emergency exception from informed consent in resuscitation research, community consultation, and public notification. *Acad Emerg Med*. 2003;10(4):352–359.

6. Smithline HA, Mader TJ, Crenshaw BJ. Do patients with acute medical conditions have the capacity to give informed consent for emergency medicine research? *Acad Emerg Med*. 1999;6(8):776–780. DOI:10.1111/j.1553-2712.1999.tb01205.x.

7. Weschler D. *The Measurement of Adult Intelligence* (Baltimore, MD: Williams & Wilkins, 1939), p. 229.

8. Crichton N. Visual analog scale (VAS). J Clin Nurs. 2001;10(5):706.

9. *Mink* v. *University of Chicago*, 460 F. Supp. 713 (1978).

10. *Moore* v. *Regents of the University of California*, 793 P.2d 479 (1990).

11. *Grimes* v. *Kennedy Krieger Institute*, 782 A.2d 807 (2001).

Restraint

Chapter 89

Case

An agitated patient presented to the emergency department (ED). The nurse said, "We need to see this one pretty quick, she's being aggressive with the staff and says that she wants to kill herself." The physician quickly went to evaluate the patient and she was indeed very agitated. Security asked for her belongings for safekeeping, after the nurse asked her to get undressed. She then attacked the security staff and had to be physically restrained. The ED staff initially tried soft restraints, but she quickly broke through them and had to have more restrictive restraints applied to her wrists and ankles by security. The ED physician then administered a chemical rapid tranquilization regimen as well.

The nurse reminded the physician to put the order in for passive or active restraints, which he did, to comply with current guidelines. The patient was then evaluated by the psychiatry personnel for exacerbation of her chronic psychiatric conditions and suicidal ideation. The physical restraints were sequentially trialed for removal, and the patient's nutrition and other comfort ensured. She eventually calmed down and was admitted to the psychiatric facility.

An extra-regulatory review the next month raised questions concerning the restraint procedure, the order, and proper compliance with the restraint protocol. It was suggested that the protocol had been instituted appropriately: the ED physician had written the order for restraints to be used, and the restraints had been removed as required.

Medical Approach

The use of restraints, both physical and chemical, can often be required in the ED population. Typically, this relates to psychiatric illness and threats against patients themselves or others. There is a specific protocol that should be followed for patient safety,

having to do with both chemical restraint and physical restraint, requiring a proper order. The staff must have the capability to check the patient's well-being status frequently, as well as addressing their primary needs for nutrition, their ability to use the bathroom, and other standard medical needs during their stay in the ED.

The use of force and involuntary restraint is an area of close scrutiny in the ED. Lavoie reported on a cohort of 3637 ED patients, in which 8.5% (314) required involuntary treatment orders.[1] The majority (57%) of orders were for observation and detention, restraint in 26%, seclusion in 9%, and seclusion plus constraint in 7%. Most patients arrived with police or family or were self-referred, while 46% presented via emergency medical services (EMS). The most common time of presentation was on the second shift, from afternoon to midnight. Most patients requiring detention and seclusion received a psychiatric diagnosis and disposition, while 100% of the restrained patients were given a medical or surgical diagnosis, and 50% required a medical or surgical hospital admission.

We must recognize that the ED population often requires intervention for drug or alcohol intoxication or violent behavior distinct from psychiatric illness. This is a worldwide phenomenon, as reported by Cannon et al. who evaluated 116 Australasian EDs.[2] They estimated there were 3.3 episodes of patient restraint per 1000 ED presentations. The most common indications for physical restraint were violence or threat of violence (52%), psychosis (32%), and acute brain syndrome (10%). The contraindications include medical instability, risk of harm to staff, and alternatives to restraint. Manual restraint is frequently used as a prelude to chemical (87%), or less frequently mechanical restraint (69%). Seclusion training is only used in a minority (23%) of departments.

Chemical restraint utilizes major tranquilizers, most commonly haloperidol (93%), followed by

Table 89.1 Recommendations for use of physical restraints

1. Baseline cardiovascular evaluation
2. Consider risk factors
3. One-on-one clinical observation

Reference: Mohr et al.[3]

benzodiazepines such as midazolam (82%) and diazepam (59%). This combination of major tranquilizer and benzodiazepine is used in 97% of cases. Formal training is most commonly undertaken for chemical restraint, utilized in 33% of the departments surveyed. At that point in time, less than half of the EDs had written policies and in this study cohort only 11% audited their use of restraints.

The adverse effects of physical restraint are well known, and Mohr et al. performed a comprehensive assessment of the correlates to injury and death.[3] They made recommendations concerning the use of physical restraints. First, clinicians should obtain baseline cardiovascular evaluation to define any significant preexisting cardiac conditions. Second, clinicians should consider risk factors when restraints are used. Third, one-on-one observation should be the clinical standard when the patient is restrained (Table 89.1)

Many etiologies and contributing factors are hypothesized to cause the association of restraints and patient death. The most likely cause is restraint asphyxia, involving the effects of prone position combined with drugs or alcohol. Other explanations include death by aspiration, thoracic blunt trauma, combined effects of psychotropic drugs, rhabdomyolysis, thrombosis, and adverse psychological effects.

The correlation of factors associated with the sudden death of individuals requiring restraint for excited delirium has been reported by Stratton et al.[4] They evaluated the reports of 214 patients, in which 8.4% (18) suffered sudden death compared to 91.6% (196) who survived. These excited delirium patients were restrained at wrists and ankles, with the restraints attached behind their back. All cases of sudden death were found to be associated with a struggle by the victim, forced restraint, labored or agonal breathing, and cessation of the struggle resulting in cardiopulmonary arrest. Other associated factors include the use of a stimulant drug (78%), chronic disease (56%), and obesity (56%) in the mortality group. Interestingly, the initial rhythm of ventricular tachycardia was only

found in 8.6% (1/13) of patients and ventricular fibrillation found in none. The study offers some potential factors that could be tracked by EMS providers to avoid such transport catastrophes.

The complication profile of patient restraint in the ED has been reported by Zun in a study cohort of 298 patients collected over a 1-year period.[5] The mean age was 36.5 years (range 14–89 years) and they were predominantly male (68%). Patients were restrained for a mean of 4.8 (0.2–25.0) hours, in which 36% (106) had more than one indication for restraint with psychosis being the most frequent (33%) discharge diagnosis. They were most frequently restrained on a cart in the supine position (86%), with two restraints (59%) and 27.5% had chemical restraint added. Complications occurred in 7% (20) of patients, with getting out of the restraints the most common in half the cases followed by vomiting, injuring others, spitting, injury to self, and increased agitation. The study concluded there was a low rate of minor complications in these events.

Legal Analysis

In *Wyatt* v. *Stickney*, a class action suit was filed on behalf of patients involuntarily confined for mental health treatment in a psychiatric hospital.[6] The district court decreed that involuntarily committed patients:

> "unquestionably have a constitutional right to receive such individual treatment as will give each of them a realistic opportunity to be cured or to improve his or her mental condition."

More importantly, patients have the right to be free from unnecessary or excessive medication; and free from physical restraint and isolation.

> "Except for emergency situations, in which it is likely that patients could harm themselves or others and in which less restrictive means of restraint are not feasible, patients may be physically restrained or placed in isolation only on a Qualified Mental Health Professional's written order which explains the rationale for such an action."

The order requires personal evaluation and examination at least once an hour and requires renewal every 24 hours. The patient must be examined and their physical condition (if compromised) and psychiatric condition charted every hour, must have bathroom privileges every hour and must be bathed every 12 hours.

In *Baber* v. *Hospital Corporation of America*, a patient presented to the ED with nausea and agitation.

She also thought she might be pregnant.[7] She was tremulous, did not have orderly thought processes, had stopped taking her psychiatric medication, and was drinking heavily. The ED physician noted that she refused to remain on the stretcher and could not be verbally restrained. Her brother had not assisted to keep her from pacing throughout, and restraints would have increased her agitation. While waiting for her testing, she began to pace and was administered a major tranquilizer, thiamine, and magnesium. Afterwards she had a seizure and fell, striking her head and causing a laceration. The physician allegedly felt the seizure was due to her psychiatric condition and medication effect, arranged a transfer to a psychiatric facility, did not perform a scan, and chose a clinical observation route. She had another seizure, required cardiopulmonary resuscitation (CPR), was found to have a skull fracture and subdural hematoma, and died the next day. The brother filed a claim citing an Emergency Medical Treatment and Labor Act (EMTALA) theory, stating the physician and facility failed to perform an effective medical screening exam, or knew his sister had an emergency medical condition.[8] The district court granted summary judgment in favor of the defendants, and the United States Court of Appeals, Fourth Circuit affirmed, finding no error. They held the patient may have been misdiagnosed, but there was no evidence the facility failed to provide appropriate screening or treatment. The issue of medical negligence could be resolved at a later date if pursued outside the EMTALA claim.

In *Heastie* v. *Roberts*, a patient with borderline function was found intoxicated and was transported to a Level I trauma center ED.[9] He was alleged to be belligerent and combative and was considered to be a potential harm to himself or others. The restraint and seclusion protocol was activated by the charge nurse, where he would be secured to the cart and isolated from other patients. The patient was placed in the "cast room" as the regular seclusion room was in use. He was checked at 15-minute intervals but not again after 9 p.m., while the nurse attended to another patient. The patient was yelling, asking for a urinal, which was delivered. The fire alarm went off at 9:30 p.m. The patient's room was engulfed in flames, the restraints were cut, but the patient was severely burned, requiring resuscitation and transfer. A lighter was found afterwards in the room, with a defense presumption that the fire was started by the patient. The patient brought suit for negligence, and jury trial

verdict was returned in favor of the defendants. The appellate court reversed and remanded for a new trial on the grounds that the circuit court erred in dismissing a negligence count asserted by the plaintiff under the res ipsa loquitur doctrine.[10] The judgment of the appellate court affirmed in part, reversed in part, and remanded for further proceedings. The res ipsa negligence claim stated: (1) fires don't routinely start in patient's rooms; (2) the patient was not able to protect himself; (3) all interventions were under the control of the defendant. The Supreme Court of Illinois held that on retrial the plaintiff's cause of action should be limited to those subject to this appeal – the res ipsa claim and the negligence associated with not finding the lighter that allegedly was in his possession.

Conclusion

The use of patient restraints is one of the most highly monitored and regulated areas of medical practice. Each institution should issue clear guidelines for its implementation, maintenance, and discontinuation, and provide protocols and continuing education for the use of passive and active patient restraints.

References

1. Lavoie FW. Consent, involuntary treatment and the use of force in an urban emergency department. *Ann Emerg Med.* 1992;21(1):25–32. DOI:10.1016//S0196-0644(05)82232-2.

2. Cannon ME, Sptivulis P, McCarthy J. Restraint practices in Australasian emergency departments. *Aust N Z J Psychiatry.* 2001;35(4):464–467.

3. Mohr WK, Petti TA, Mohr BD. Adverse effects associated with physical restraint. *Can J Psychiatry.* 2003;48(5):330–337.

4. Stratton SJ, Rogers C, Brickett K, Gruzinski G. Factors associated with sudden death of individuals requiring restraint for excited delirium. *Am J Emerg Med.* 2001;19(3):187–191.

5. Zun LS. A Prospective study of the complication rate of use of patient restraint in the emergency department. *J Emerg Med.* 2003;24(2):119–124.

6. *Wyatt* v. *Stickney*, 344 F. Supp. 373 (1972).

7. *Baber* v. *Hospital Corporation of America*, 977 F.2d 872 (1992).

8. EMTALA 42 USCA §1395dd (a).

9. *Heastie* v. *Roberts*, 877 N.E.2d 1064 (2007).

10. Res Ipsa Loquitur. law.cornell.edu. Accessed March 16, 2016.

Chapter 90

Resuscitation

Case

A call came in to the medical command phone in the emergency department (ED). Emergency medical services (EMS) had been summoned to the scene to evaluate a patient who was "found down." The EMS radio gave the ED physician all the information that was necessary to provide medical command. The patient was an 89-year-old woman last seen by her family the evening before. She was found in cardiac arrest and was noted to be in asystole and unresponsive.

The paramedics were not sure if they should start resuscitative efforts. It seemed the patient had been down for some time, and they were not sure what to do. The physician asked them if the patient met any of the criteria for field termination of resuscitative efforts. They said they didn't think so, although she was asystolic, or without a heartbeat. The physician recommended they go ahead and transport, but if she met field criteria for death determination she could be pronounced there at home. The physician finished a busy shift and the patient was not brought to the ED.

The physician received a call from the EMS quality coordinator, who questioned if the patient needed to be resuscitated in the field. It was suggested the provider should have asked if there were clear criteria for death certification in the field, such as rigor mortis, dependent lividity, or catastrophic injury incompatible with life, such as decapitation. The physician had asked the crew to use their judgment about whether those criteria were met or not.

Medical Approach

There has clearly been progressive thinking about end-of-life care, recognizing that not every patient needs to undergo resuscitative efforts. Clearly at the end of life with asystole as the dominant rhythm, plus other factors suggesting this has been a prolonged event, resuscitation is not necessarily appropriate.

The conventional death certification criteria should be instituted for unequivocal presentation of death. Family input is crucial at this time so that the patient's last wishes may be honored, whether it be for resuscitation or not.

The medicolegal aspects of cardiopulmonary resuscitation (CPR) and emergency cardiac care (ECC) were defined in 1979 at the National Conference on CPR and ECC.[1] The following crucial aspects of resuscitation care were defined. First, focus on the decision-making, primarily the decision to initiate, withhold, and terminate CPR. Second, focus on the quality of performance once the decision to initiate is made. Third, guidelines for death determination should be clear, consistent, easy to implement, and not appear arbitrary. Fourth, the underpinning of the decision is the concept of doing the most "good" for the patient and family (Table 90.1).

The American Heart Association comments on several legal and ethical issues associated with provision of CPR.[2] First, they assure layperson liability protection, in which "Good Samaritan" laws exist in all 50 states. They grant limited immunity to lay rescuers when: (1) they perform a "good-faith" effort to save a life, as long as they are trying to help; (2) their actions are reasonable and not gross misconduct; (3) the rescuer receives no compensation; (4) they do not require formal CPR training; (5) for the general public, if CPR is not part of your job duty, there is no legal responsibility, but likely a moral responsibility to attempt

Table 90.1 Medicolegal aspects of CPR

1.	Decision-making to initiate, withhold, or terminate
2.	Quality of performance
3.	Clear guidelines for death determination
4.	Doing "good" for patient and family

Reference: McIntyre[1]

Table 90.2 "Good Samaritan" liability protection for CPR

1.	Limited liability for lay rescuers
2.	Actions are reasonable, without misconduct
3.	Rescuer receives no compensation
4.	No formal CPR training required
5.	No CPR job responsibility, no legal requirement
6.	CPR job responsibility, duty exists

Reference: American Heart Association[2]

Table 90.3 When to stop lay-rescuer CPR

1.	The patient begins to move
2.	An AED arrives
3.	Trained help takes over
4.	Too exhausted to continue
5.	Not safe to continue
6.	Trained help asks you to stop
7.	Obvious signs of death

Reference: American Heart Association[2]

Table 90.4 "Do not resuscitate" (DNR) profile

	Profile	Comparison
	n = 136	Mean
1.	Age	65 ± 15.9 years
2.	Organ systems	2.5 ± 1.2
3.	Hospitalization	22.7 ± 25.6 days
		Proportion (%)
4.	Medical futility	88 (120)
5.	Unable to participate	56 (76)
6.	Comatose	23 (31)
7.	Deaths	59 (80)

Reference: Lo et al.[5]

to assist; (6) if performing CPR is part of your job responsibility, there is a duty to perform (Table 90.2).

Second, they address the issue of when to stop lay-rescuer CPR once begun. It is recommended to stop CPR when: (1) the victim starts to move; (2) an automated external defibrillator (AED) arrives; (3) trained help arrives and takes over; (4) you are too exhausted to continue; (5) there is danger in continuing the CPR process; as an example, CPR on an active airplane flight requires you stop on approach and then resume upon landing; (6) trained help asks you to stop; (7) obvious signs of death have become apparent (Table 90.3).

Third, it is important to recognize when patients do not desire to have CPR performed. Many states have Do Not Attempt Resuscitation programs. The patient may have a wallet card, medical jewelry, or electronic information to that effect and a search should be made for these.

Fourth, the person's right to make end-of-life decisions was codified in the Patient Self Determination Act of 1990.[3] The simplest form of writing is a living will, in which the patient instructs physicians and caregivers on their care choices if the patient becomes terminally ill. The advance directive is the expression of the patient's hopes, wishes, and preferences in regard to end-of-life care. The document may include conversation, living wills, and durable power of attorney. The most recent reiteration is the Physician Orders for Life-Sustaining Treatment (POLST) form, which allows very specific and detailed directives concerning all aspects of the health-care continuum, not just resuscitation.[4]

Fifth, complexity is often encountered in an out-of-hospital cardiac arrest, where EMS providers are compelled to begin CPR. Their intervention is required unless there are obvious signs of death. A command physician can provide a countermanding verbal order, or the patient's physician may provide a written order with the patient. There are EMS-No CPR orders that are implemented in the field, assuring patients they can summon 911 for care assistance and comfort, without compelling the EMS to provide CPR against the patient's wishes.

The use of the Do Not Resuscitate (DNR) classification was profiled by Lo et. al studying 3282 medical inpatients, in which 4.1% (136) were DNR.[5] The patients were elderly, with more than one organ system involved, staying 3 weeks in the hospital, with futile care, unable to participate in decision-making, comatose, and dying during their stay (Table 90.4). The death rate was significantly higher than in the patients whose DNR status was not considered (4.4%, 137/3146, $P < 0.001$). Most importantly, further medical treatment was felt to be futile in most cases (88%, 120/136).

The obvious next question is whether an ED resuscitation is justified when emergency medical resuscitation has failed. Gray et al. evaluated 185 arrest patients presenting to the ED: only 9% (16) of patients were successfully resuscitated and admitted to the hospital.[6] The only correlation with better outcome was a brief duration of arrest. No patient survived to discharge and all but one was comatose. The mean hospital stay was 12.6 days (range 1–132), with 2.3 days (1–11) in the intensive care unit (ICU). They concluded that ongoing resuscitative efforts after failed prehospital resuscitation were unlikely to be successful.

ED physicians are often on the forefront of ethical dilemmas regarding resuscitation. Marco et al. polled 1252 respondents on their opinions concerning the initiation and termination of CPR.[7] Most (78%) providers acknowledge the legal advance directives regarding resuscitation, a few (7%) follow unofficial documents, and even fewer (6%) respond to verbal reports. The majority (62%) made resuscitation decisions because of fear of litigation or criticism, and attempted resuscitation (55%) despite expectations of futility. Most respondents (78%) feel that ideally, legal concerns should not influence resuscitation practice, but the vast majority (94%) recognize that legal issues universally influence practice.

Certainly, we recognize that ethical issues associated with resuscitation practice have evolved over time. Marco et al. revisited their earlier study and evaluated the change in emergency physician CPR practice from 1995 to 2007 evaluating 928 respondents anonymously with an 18% response rate.[8] The proportion of providers that honor legal advance directives has increased from 78% to 86%, an 8% increase (95%, CI 5–11%). However, very few honor verbal reports (12%) or unofficial documents (7%). The majority (56%) have attempted resuscitations that they felt to be futile. They reported factors that were important in their decision-making as including the presence of advance directives (78%), witnessed arrest (77%), extent of downtime (73%), family wishes (40%), presenting rhythm (38%), patient age (28%), and pre-arrest state of health (Table 90.5).

Legal Analysis

In *Estate of Leach* v. *Shapiro*, the patient suffered a respiratory-cardiac arrest, and was resuscitated but remained in a persistent vegetative state.[9] The family alleged she was placed on life support after resuscitation without their consent. The plaintiffs sought damages for the time she spent on life support. The trial court foreclosed additional evidence and granted the defendant's summary judgment motion. The Court of Appeals of Ohio, Summit County reversed and remanded for further consideration. They recognized that doctors must be free to exercise their best medical judgment in

Table 90.5 Resuscitation: decision factors

	Factor	Incidence (%)
1.	Advance directives	78
2.	Witnessed arrest	77
3.	Extent of downtime	73
4.	Family wishes	40
5.	Presenting rhythm	38
6.	Age	28
7.	State of health	25

Reference: Marco et al.[8]

treating a life-threatening emergency.[10] However, the plaintiff has the right to plead their version of the facts to the trial court in an attempt to obtain relief.

In *Lowry* v. *Henry Mayo Newhall Memorial Hospital*, the patient was admitted after a motor vehicle accident, and subsequently suffered cardiac arrest.[11] The "Code Blue" team responded and provided resuscitative efforts for 35 minutes, to which the patient did not respond. The family filed an amended complaint alleging medical malpractice by the physician who responded with the code team. The family alleged a deviation of care from the American Heart Association Guidelines for Advanced Cardiac Life Support, in which atropine was administered instead of epinephrine.[12] If this had been done, they claimed the chance for survival would have been "dramatically increased." The defendant responded her only contact had been as part of the code team, the patient's pupils were fixed and dilated on arrival, but the team began resuscitative efforts to be sure. The trial court granted summary judgment to the defendant based on the immunity offered to hospital-based rescue teams pursuant to the California Health and Safety Code §1317.[13] The plaintiff appealed, theorizing that this immunity only applied to volunteers, or "Good Samaritans," and not to paid professional providers, The Court of Appeals of California, Second District, Division Seven affirmed, holding that the immunity statute did indeed apply to "non-volunteer, non–Good Samaritan" members of the hospital code response team. They also held there was no triable issue of fact, in that the defendant clearly acted in good faith in an attempt to resuscitate the patient.

In *Bryan* v. *University of Virginia*, the patient was transferred to a tertiary care referral center with respiratory distress.[14] Her husband and children allegedly informed the facility that they were at all times to "take all necessary measures to keep her alive and trust in God's wisdom." The family alleged there was a violation of the Emergency Medical Treatment and Labor Act (EMTALA), as the hospital was alleged to have refused the family instruction and entered a DNR order. The patient was not stabilized and died 1 week later.[15] The trial court dismissed the complaint, alleging this statute applied to the transfer process, and there was no obligation once the patient was admitted. The case was dismissed on the merits, as the patient died 1 week after admission, and there was no tort action filed, which did potentially apply to the facts of the case. The family appealed, alleging "stabilization" was required no matter the duration of therapy required. The United States Court of Appeals (USCA), Fourth Circuit affirmed the trial court decision, reading that an indefinite stabilization process was neither plausible nor feasible. Once again, they remarked that the conduct may have violated other laws, but they were not included in the pleading so there would be no comment.

In *Toguchi* v. *Chung*, the patient was incarcerated with a lengthy mental health history and extensive history of illicit drug use.[16] The patient was taken to a lockdown unit and treated with multiple sequential medication treatments as his behavior became more confused and irrational. The patient had an arrest event from which he could not be resuscitated, and toxicology revealed multiple toxic drug levels. The family brought suit utilizing a 42 U.S.C. §1983 action alleging indifference to the patient's medical needs.[17] The trial court found there was no triable issue of material fact, and that the plaintiff's death was not due to provider indifference to his medical condition. The USCA, Ninth Circuit affirmed the trial court decision for the defense, noting "deliberate indifference" is a high legal standard. The showing of medical malpractice or negligence is insufficient to establish a constitutional deprivation under the Eighth Amendment.[18] "Mere medical malpractice does not constitute cruel and unusual punishment."[19]

Conclusion

Resuscitation is an area that is often a complex and highly emotive area for patient, family, and provider. Clear areas of responsibility, response protocols, and care guidelines help to minimize individual variation and subsequent risk exposure.

References

1. McIntyre KM. Medicolegal aspects of cardiopulmonary resuscitation (CPR) and emergency care (ECC). *JAMA*. 1980;244(5):511–512. DOI:10.1001/jama.1980.03310050075017.

2. American Heart Association. Advanced Cardiac Life Support: *CPR: Legal and Ethical Issues*. 2006:1–4.

3. Patient Self-Determination Act of 1990: H.R. 4449.

4. Jesus JE, Geiderman JM, Venkat A, Limehouse WE Jr, Derse AR, Larkin GL, Henrichs CW 3rd, ACEP Ethics Committee. Physician orders for life-sustaining treatment, and emergency medicine: ethical considerations, legal issues, and emerging trends. *Ann Emerg Med*. 2014;64(2):140–144. DOI:10.1016/j.annemergmed.2014.03.014.

5. Lo B, Saika G, Strull W, Thomas E, Showstack J. "Do not resuscitate" decisions: a prospective study at three teaching hospitals. *Arch Int Med*. 1985;145(6):1115–1117. DOI:10.1001/archinte.1985.00360060183028.

6. Gray WA, Capone RJ, Most AS. Unsuccessful emergency medical resuscitation – are continued efforts in the emergency department justified? *N Engl J Med*. 1991;325(20):1393–1398.

7. Marco CA, Bessman ES, Schoenfeld CN, Kelen GD. ethical issues of cardiopulmonary resuscitation: current practice among emergency physicians. *Acad Emerg Med*. 1997;4(9):898–904. DOI:10.1111/j.1553-2712.1997.tb03816.x.

8. Marco CA, Bessman ES, Kelen GD. Ethical issues of cardiopulmonary resuscitation: comparison of emergency physician practices from 1995 to 2007. *Acad Emerg Med*. 2009;16(3):270–273. DOI:10.1111/j.1553-2712.2008.00348.x.

9. *Estate of Leach* v. *Shapiro*, 13 Ohio App. 3d 393 (1984).

10. 61 American Jurisprudence 2d (1981) 314, Physicians, Surgeons, etc., Section 185.

11. *Lowry* v. *Henry Mayo Newhall Memorial Hospital*, 185 Cal. App.3d 188 (1986).

12. Cummins RO (ed.), ACLS: Principles and Practice (Dallas, TX: ACLS, 2003).

13. California Health and Safety Code: HSC §1371.

14. *Bryan* v. *University of Virginia*, 95 F.3d 349 (1996).

15. EMTALA 42 USCA §1395dd (a).

16. *Toguchi* v. *Chung*, 391 F.3d 1051 (2004).

17. 42 U.S.C. §1983 – Civil Action for Deprivation of Rights (1983).

18. U.S. Const. Amend. VIII.

19. *Hallett* v. *Morgan*, 296 F.3d 732 (2002).

Service Contract

Case

The physician group had been at the facility for years, providing a contracted service for patient care. Over time, there had been some personnel changes, involving transfer of ownership. Some normal attrition in the practice also occurred, where physicians in the group moved away or changed practice emphasis and focus.

The hospital administration then asked for contract proposals to perform the service and there was significant interest in the activity. In the final analysis it appeared that a change should be made. The concern was that although the physician group had performed admirably for years, there had been changes in the practice affecting their performance. The contract was awarded to another group.

Immediate concerns were raised by the physician group, suggesting the contract request for proposal (RFP) process was unfair and they would prefer things to remain as they were. The hospital decided to go ahead with the change, and offered all the physicians the option of keeping their current position but within a new work environment.

Medical Approach

These circumstances have become more common, with hospitals now subcontracting 50–60% of the physician-based service offered by the facility. Sometimes the subcontractor is a single physician or local multiple-location practice group; in other cases there may be a state, regional, or national presence with a larger management group.

The impact of external market forces is inevitable, causing significant change as we progress from clinical integration to an accountable care model. The challenges include a predominance of small group practices, dominant fee-for-service reimbursement methods, weaknesses of the traditional hospital medical staff structure, and the need to partner with commercial insurance companies.[1] The initial coordination was between providers and the hospital facilities. This was soon followed by hospital-wide to system-wide integration. Finally, the health-care system partners with the insurance company to form a commercial accountable care organization. This program will attempt to optimize care quality, patient safety, and cost-effectiveness. The commercial success of the contract requires implementation of strategies to avoid unnecessary admissions, avoid emergency department (ED) visits, expand primary care access, reduce readmissions, and enhance quality and patient safety (Table 91.1).

Hospital administration should be mindful of its own responsibilities, when it comes to rapid and frequent physician group turnover.[2] Often systemic or institutional factors are in operation, in addition to provider issues. The physician group should: first attempt to alleviate the impact of contract changes with proper awareness and planning; second, ensure that institutional goals and objectives are clearly understood by physicians and administration beforehand; third, recognize that transitions are always stressful and be on guard for staff morale problems; fourth, avoid contract transition at peak patient flow periods such as midwinter, or other inopportune times such as holiday periods; fifth, provide existing staff with adequate notice of the change, typically at least 6 months (Table 91.2).

Table 91.1 Accountable care organization

1. Avoid unnecessary admissions
2. Avoid ED visits
3. Expand primary care access
4. Reduce readmissions
5. Enhance quality and patient safety

Reference: Shields[1]

Table 91.2 Physician service contract transition

1. Proper awareness and planning can minimize impact
2. Ensure goals are understood beforehand
3. Transition always stressful, monitor morale
4. Avoid peak flow periods
5. Provide adequate notice, typically 6 months

Reference: ED Management[2]

Table 91.3 Successful contract management

1. Contract uncertainty should never come as a surprise
2. Communicate regularly with key audiences
3. Keep an "ear to the ground" for issues
4. Regular meetings with senior administration
5. Avoid relying on reactionary meetings
6. Seat on medical executive committee
7. Participate in community and family activities
8. Professional working relationship with nurse director

Reference: ED Management[3]

Contract change is often a contentious time between health-care providers and administration, and a power struggle may ensue.[3] First, the prospect of contract uncertainty should never come as a surprise to the physician administrator. Second, one should communicate regularly with key audiences within the hospital. Third, always keep an ear to the ground to anticipate real or potential issues. Fourth, establish regular routine meetings with senior administration. Fifth, avoid the habit of reactionary meetings only in times of conflict. Sixth, the group should attempt to obtain a seat on the hospital medical executive or governance committee. Seventh, participate in community activities with hospital leadership, including family-oriented activities. Eighth, a professional working relationship with the nurse director is essential for success (Table 91.3)

Uncertainty regarding employment contracts is a great stressor for practicing physicians. McNamara et al. performed an anonymous survey of 1035 ED physicians who were threatened with adverse contract actions concerning quality of care or financial issues, with a 37.6% (389) response rate.[4] The majority (86%) of the group were board certified, and over half had been in practice for over 16 years. From the provider group that answered, 62% (197/317) reported their employer could terminate their contract without due process and 76% (216/284) reported administration could remove them from the clinical schedule. Another 20% reported a possible or real threat to their employment if they raised quality of care concerns. They also noted financial pressures related to admission, discharge, and transfer of patients. These issues should be tracked and monitored carefully.

Legal Analysis

The first issue to define is classification as an independent contractor or a contracted physician.

In *Mduba* v. *Benedictine Hospital*, the patient presented to the ED after a motor vehicle accident (MVA) and was examined by the ED physician at 9:15 p.m.[5] At 9:40 p.m. she was evaluated by her own physician, who attempted to draw a blood sample for type and cross-matching at 10:15 p.m., but was unsuccessful. She had blood drawn by anesthesia at 10:45 p.m. and was taken to the operating room at 11 p.m. Blood was administered at 12:10 a.m., and she died at 1:45 a.m. The plaintiff filed suit against the hospital, contending the failure to obtain an early blood transfusion was a significant contributing factor resulting in the patient's death. The trial court dismissed the complaint, holding that the ED physician was under contract with the defendant hospital operating the ED and was an independent contractor and not an employee, so the hospital could not be held liable. However, the Appellate Division of the Supreme Court of New York, Third Department reversed and ordered a new trial. They held that, despite the wording of his contract with the hospital, the ED physician was in all actuality an employee with a guaranteed salary floor, clerical support, and fees set forth in the contract. They concluded the hospital held itself out to the public to provide emergency treatment, had a duty to perform those services, and was potentially liable for those furnished to provide that care. However, they did not have respondeat superior liability for all physicians providing care on their premises.

In *Thompson* v. *Nason Hospital*, the patient presented to the ED after an MVA, and the ED staff was advised the patient was taking warfarin (Coumadin).[6] The patient's personal physician was passing through the ED and was asked by nursing to assume care of the patient. Her physician orchestrated care, consulting other physicians and admitting her to the intensive care unit (ICU). The patient was subsequently transferred and was found to have a subdural hematoma and significant neurologic impairment. Plaintiff filed suit and the trial court honored the summary judgment motion of the physician and the hospital. The superior court appeal reversed the initial judgment in that there were genuine issues of material fact, precluding a summary judgment motion. The Supreme Court of Pennsylvania addressed the issue of corporate liability for hospitals. Under the doctrine of corporate liability or negligence, the hospital would be liable if it failed to uphold the proper standard of care owed the patient. This is a non-delegable duty that does not have to rely on demonstrating negligence of the third party. The court held this to be a viable doctrine and enough questions were raised that the summary judgment of the trial court should not have been granted.

In *Gilbert* v. *Sycamore Municipal Hospital*, the patient presented to the ED after lifting weights and was evaluated by a member of his physician's group practice.[7] The patient had no prior heart disease, had negative testing, was discharged, and succumbed to an autopsy-proven myocardial infarction (MI). The ED was considered a hospital function, not managed by a particular group: it employed the nurses, provided a call roster, and reviewed the care provided. The plaintiff filed suit and settled with the physician, and proceeded against the hospital. The circuit court granted summary judgment in favor of the hospital, as they were not vicariously liable because the physician in question was neither an agent nor an employee. The Supreme Court of Illinois reversed and remanded for further proceedings. They held that the "doctrine of apparent authority" applied, in which the hospital can be held vicariously liable for the negligent acts of a physician providing care at that hospital, regardless of whether the physician is an independent contractor, unless the patient knows, or should have known, that the physician is an independent contractor. The elements include: (1) the hospital or its agent acted in a manner that would lead a reasonable person to conclude that the individual who was alleged to be negligent was an employee or agent; (2) when the acts of the agent create the appearance of authority, the plaintiff must prove the hospital had knowledge of and acquiesced to them; and (3) the plaintiff acted in reliance upon the conduct of the hospital or its agent, consistent with ordinary care and prudence.[8]

Another area of litigation is contracted services. In *Jefferson Parish Hospital* v. *Hyde*, a board-certified anesthesiologist applied for medical staff privileges and was approved by the credentials committee and the medical ethics committee.[9] The hospital board denied the application, as they were party to a contract with another physician business entity providing exclusive service. The issue at hand is the validity of an exclusive contract between the hospital and physician group, and whether it restrains competition in violation of the Sherman Act §1.[10] Certain types of contractual arrangements are deemed unreasonable as a matter of law. The key to the analysis is an invalid tying agreement, in which two products are sold together to force the consumer to purchase an unwanted product. The Supreme Court of the United States held that the judgment of the United States Courts of Appeal (USCA), Fifth Circuit should be reversed and case remanded for the respondent's remaining claims. These arrangements must survive scrutiny under the rule of reason, in which the consumer does not suffer undue economic harm, and the provider is not excluded from a significant proportion of the marketplace.

In *Capital Imaging Associates* v. *Mohawk Valley Medical Associates*, a private radiology group brought an antitrust action against a health maintenance organization (HMO) and independent physician practice association (IPA) currently providing a radiology service to the enrollees.[11] The trial court granted the defendant's summary judgment motion focused on the "vertical" relationships between the HMO and the physicians' association. The USCA, Second Circuit affirmed the judgment of the district court, although they stressed the importance of considering the "horizontal" aspects of provider relationships, not considered initially. They focused on three components of the Sherman Act §1 analysis to evaluate the horizontal restraint of competition effects toward competing radiology physicians.[10] First, they evaluated the capacity of the IPA members to conspire. The court concluded they indeed had the capacity to shield the member provider group from external competition. Second, the analysis targeted the presence of actual conspiracy, and the court held there was at least circumstantial evidence there was exclusion, as an office in the service area was denied. Third, there is a "rule of reason" analysis of whether an unreasonable restraint of trade existed. Here, the plaintiff was unable to substantiate the case that the behavior of the IPA resulted in a change in their fee structure or patient harm.

In *Frost Street Medical Associates* v. *San Diego Internal Medicine Group*, the hospitalist physicians alleged an RFP process was flawed and unfair competition in a contract change.[12] They alleged they were unfairly excluded from a process compelling "unassigned" patients admitted through the ED to a designated group. The group ultimately awarded the contract was headed by the former facility chief of staff, and there were cross-allegations of care issues among the competitors. The plaintiff alleged the respondents were in violation of the Cartwright Act[13] and the Unfair Competition Act[14] through their intentional interference with its prospective business advantage. They alleged the RFP process was a pretext to favor the other group. The defendant contended the controlling caselaw precedent was *Centeno v. Roseville Community Hospital*.[15] Here, the operative test for whether a managerial decision by a hospital, made in a quasi-legislative capacity, must be set aside by the court requires a particularly high standard. For the hospital decision to be overturned by the court, the decision must have been "substantively irrational, unlawful, contrary to established public policy, or procedurally unfair." The defendant moves for summary judgment, or summary adjudication of issues, which the trial court decided in their favor. The Court of Appeals of California, Fourth District, on de novo review, concluded that the trial court correctly analyzed the undisputed facts on both sides of the argument and applied the appropriate test for evaluating a quasi-legislative policy decision (*Major*),[16] concurring with the trial court. It would not be appropriate to reverse the judgments to allow a trier of fact to effectively rationally second-guess hospital managerial decisions, and these rulings were legally correct.

Conclusion

There is clear legal precedent to suggest hospital facilities have a wide scope in their management of decision-making, according to judicial decisions, and typically have the capacity to make this change without concern or question.

References

1. Shields M. From clinical integration to accountable care. *Ann Health Law*. 2011;20(2):151–164.

2. Quick turnover of physician groups raises red flags for ED managers. *ED Manag*. 2005;17(4):37–39.

3. ED physicians group ousted, sues – power struggle with CEO blamed. *ED Manage*. 2007;19(7):73–75.

4. McNamara RM, Beier K, Blumstein H, Weiss LD, Wood J. A survey of emergency physicians regarding due process, financial pressures and the ability to advocate for patients. *J Emerg Med*. 2013;45(1):111–116.e3. DOI:10.1016/j.jemergmed.2012.12.019.

5. *Mduba* v. *Benedictine Hospital*, 52 A.D.2d 450 (1976).

6. *Thompson* v. *Nason Hospital*, 527 Pa. 330 (1991).

7. *Gilbert* v. *Sycamore Municipal Hospital*, 622 N.E.2d 788 (1993).

8. *Pamperin* v. *Trinity Memorial*, 144 Wis. 2d 188 (1988) at 855–56.

9. *Jefferson Parish Hospital* v. *Hyde*, 466 U.S. 2 (1984).

10. Sherman Act, 15 U.S.C. §§1–7 (1890).

11. *Capital Imaging* v. *Mohawk Valley Medical*, 996 F.2d 537 (1993).

12. *Frost Street Medical* v. *San Diego Internal Medicine*, September 18, 2014. Not Certified for Publication.

13. California Business and Professional Code §16700 et seq. Cartwright Act.

14. California Business and Professional Code §17200 et seq. Unfair Competition Law.

15. Centeno v Roseville Community Hospital, 107 Cal. App.3d 62 (1979).

16. *Major* v. *Memorial Hospitals Assn.*, 71 Cal. App.4th 1380 (1999).

92

Sexual Assault

Case

The nurse asked the emergency department (ED) physician to see the patient, who was still crying and had complained of an alleged assault involving a former significant other. There was no physical evidence of injury, but this was allegedly a non-consensual sexual event. The provider examined the patient and got the remainder of the history from the nursing report. He explained he would do a comprehensive assault exam, with the nurse performing part of the evaluation and the physician doing the rest. The physician asked the patient if she needed some time, and asked the nurse to get started with her portion of the evidence collection. The physician was summoned when that portion of the exam was finished and completed the remainder of the physical exam, obtaining all the appropriate cultures and specimens. These were placed into a forensic evaluation kit and the nurse was asked to seal and store this safely when she was done. The patient was told that "we were sorry about the event" and that there would be a law-enforcement intervention as well as some additional counseling, which she appreciated. She had safe transport home and a place to stay, and she was discharged from the ED with conventional instructions and infectious disease prophylaxis.

The ED physician was then called in as a fact witness for the criminal trial that occurred 2 years later. Apparently, there had been some issue with the chain of custody of the sexual assault kit. There was a challenge to the integrity of the kit, and the physician was required to validate its preparation as part of the collection process. It seemed there had been an issue with subsequent law-enforcement processing, but the provider was able to testify successfully regarding his actions.

Medical Approach

An alleged sexual assault case is often one of the more complex and difficult ED evaluations for all involved. The medical, psychosocial, forensic, and legal issues are all of concern and it is crucially important that a standardized process be in place to protect the patient's confidentiality in any evidence that is collected.

Sexual violence is a significant part of the violence directed against women, and accounts for 7% of all violent crime.[1] Typically, it involves a misuse of power by the perpetrator. Sexual abuse may involve professional sexual misconduct, sexual harassment, rape, or abuse of minors.

Analysis of the demographic profile of sexual assault patients is helpful in the recognition process. Avegno et al. evaluated 1172 ED patients presenting for alleged sexual assault, 692 of whom were women with a mean age of 27 years.[2] Over half (54%) of patients noted drug or alcohol involvement during the event, while 53% knew their attacker. Threats of force were common (72.4%), physical evidence of injury was present in over half (51.7%), and multiple assailants were unusual (18.1%). Multivariate analysis found race, age, threats, and substance use during the event were independent risk factors for evident trauma on physical exam. The most common profile was overwhelmingly female, relatively young, often knowing the perpetrator, likely to feel threatened, and showing signs of physical trauma.

Another robust demographic profile was offered by Riggs et al., who profiled 1067 patients with a mean age of 25 years (range 1–85), 96% (1036) female and 4% (41) male.[3] The assailant was a stranger in only 39% (409/1094) and multiple assailants involved in only 20% (208/1044) of cases. Force was used in a predominant number of cases (80%, 817/1027), but a weapon was only present in 27% (275/1014). The nature of the sexual assault was vaginal intercourse in 83% (851/1023) female victims, oral assault in 25% (271/1053), and anal penetration in 17% (178/1058). Assessment of general appearance found general body trauma was noted in 67% (621/927), genital trauma was noted in 53% (388/736), and in 20% (147/1712) no visible trauma was found. Although sperm was only found in 13% (93/716) of ED wet mount examinations, evidence of semen was found by the forensic crime laboratory in 48% (296/612) of cases. They concluded the typical profile involved general body trauma, often a known assailant, and DNA evidence found by the forensic lab.

Another interesting analysis performed by Feldhaus et al. reported on the lifetime sexual assault prevalence in an ED population of 442 women with an 81% (360) response rate.[4] The lifetime prevalence of sexual assault was 39% (139), and 70% (97) were older than 15 years at the time of the event. The assailant was an acquaintance, friend, or family member in 52% (49) of cases, a stranger in 30% (28), and a partner in 18% (17). The notification pattern found that less than half (46%, 46) reported to the police, 43% (42) sought medical care and 25% (23) contacted a social service agency. Those who were assaulted by a stranger were more likely to file a police report (79% vs. 18%, $P < 0.001$) or receive medical care (70% vs. 29%, $P < 0.01$). The lifetime prevalence of sexual assault in this population was significant, and the victims were less likely to report or seek care if the assailant was known to them.

Often the focus of the ED evaluation is on the physical stigmata of injury. Sugar et al. reported on a group of 819 female sexual assault victims in which 52% had general body injury, 41% were without bodily injury, and 20% had genital–anal trauma.[5] The presence of general trauma was associated with being hit or kicked (OR 7.7, 95% CI 5.1–11.7), attempted strangulation (OR 4.2, 95% CI 2.5–7.2), stranger assault (OR 2.4, 95%, CI 1.7–3.4), and oral–anal penetration (OR 95% CI 1.2–2.3). Specific genital–anal injury was more frequent in those who were younger than 20 or older than 49 years ($P < 0.05$), virginal (OR 2.7, 95% CI 1.4–5.4), examined within 24 hours of the event (OR 1.7, 95% CI 1.2–2.4), and after anal assault (OR 1.7, 95%, CI, 1.1–2.6). They concluded that general bodily injury is more common and related to situational factors, while genital–anal injury is more related to age, virginal status, or time of examination.

The recommended standard of evaluation involves the use of a Sexual Assault Nurse Examiner (SANE) program providing specially trained forensic nurses, providing first-response crisis care to rape survivors.[6] First, this program promotes the psychological recovery of survivors. Second, it provides consistent and comprehensive post-assault medical care including emergency contraception and STD prophylaxis. Third, complete and accurate collection and documentation of the forensic evidence of the crime. Fourth, improving the prosecution of sexual assault cases by providing better forensic analysis and expert testimony. Fifth, effecting community change by bringing multiple service providers together to provide a comprehensive care system for sexual violence (Table 92.1).

Most sexual assaults reported to law enforcement were never referred to prosecutors, or were not charged by the prosecutor's office (80–89%).[7] There was not a significant site-dependent change in prosecution rates after implementation of a SANE program, although positive trends were noted in aggregated data.

A more comprehensive analysis was performed by Ciancone et al., in which 66% (61) of 92 SANE programs responded, with 55% (32) of 58 operating for less than 5 years.[8] The initial exam was performed in the ED in 52% (30) of programs after written consent (97%, 57), typically headed by registered nurses with a median of 80 hours of education required. The interventions offered included pregnancy testing in 97% (56), pregnancy prophylaxis in 97% (57), and sexually transmitted disease (STD) prophylaxis in 90% (53). The median time for evaluation and evidence collection was 3 hours (range 1–8 hours). Evidence collection utilized the Wood's lamp in 86% (51), photographs in 78% (46), and colposcopic exam in 71% (42) of cases. Interestingly, few programs had prosecutorial results available to the staff. However, Rambow et al. performed a separate study of 182 female ED patients

Table 92.1 Sexual assault nurse examiner (SANE) program: benefits

1. Psychological recovery of survivors
2. Comprehensive post-assault care
3. Forensic evidence collection
4. Expert testimony
5. Community focus

Reference: Campbell et al.[6]

evaluating legal implications.[9] They noted a 9% rate of genital trauma, but only 29% complaining of pain or bleeding. They identified only 29% (53/182) of cases that had the potential for successful prosecution with both victim willing to testify and the assailant identified. From this group, one-third (34%) were successfully prosecuted, or only 9.9% for the overall group.

The prosecution of sexual assault cases often correlates with the forensic evidence identified. Gray-Eurom et al. reported on forensic exams on 801 sexual assault victims, predominantly female (97%).[10] The suspect was identified in less than half of cases (44%, 355), and arrests made in one-third (34%, 271). In 31% of cases there was not enough evidence to arrest after detention. Where the suspect was arrested (56%, 153), the majority were found guilty (58%, 89), 18% were still pending or sealed, and 1.3% (2) were subsequently found not guilty. There was evidence of trauma in 57% (202) of examinations and evidence of sperm found in 31% (110) of cases. Logistic regression found that a patient younger than 18 years, presence of trauma, and use of a weapon correlated with successful prosecution.

Lastly, McGregor et al. attempted to correlate the forensic evidence with successful sexual assault prosecution.[11] They reported on 462 cases, in which charges were filed in 32.7% (151) and a conviction obtained in 11.0% (51) of cases. Genital injury was noted in 41.8% (193) and sperm–semen positive forensic results obtained in 38.2% (100) of 262 samples tested. A gradient was noted relating injury severity score and subsequent charges filed. They ranged from mild injury (OR 2.85, 95% CI 1.09–7.45), through moderate injury (OR 4.00, 95% CI 1.63–9.84), to severe injury (OR 12.29, 95% CI 3.04–49.65). As well, the injury severity score defined as severe was the only variable correlated with actual conviction (OR 6.51, 95% CI 1.31–32.32). Documentation of the sexual assault service examiner evidence logged in the police filing also correlated with charges being filed (OR 3.45, 95% CI 1.82–6.56) (Table 92.2). They concluded that both extent of injury and the presence of forensic evidence are correlated with both filing of charges and conviction.

The ED is the cornerstone of care for the sexual assault victim, with successful prosecution contingent on proper evidence collection. In July 2000, the New York State Health Commission and Department of Criminal Justice imposed a substantial fine on Coney Island Hospital, and required them to hire a

Table 92.2 Sexual assault correlates with legal proceedings

Issue	Correlation
	OR, 95% CI
Charges filed	
Injury	
1. Mild	2.85, 1.09–7.45
2. Moderate	4.00, 1.63–9.84
3. Severe	12.29, 3.04–49.65
4. Forensic evidence documentation	3.45, 1.82–6.56
Conviction	
5. Severe injury	6.51, 1.31–32.32

Reference: McGregor et al.[11]

consultant to improve their practice.[12] They cited many deficiencies including a victim waiting over 3 hours for consultation, an inadequate sexual assault kit, improper or no collection of critical evidence, inappropriate doses of emergency contraception, lack of proper credentialing of the ED resident staff, and an inadequate follow-up plan for victims. The hospital was required to submit a plan of correction as it was held in violation of the New York Public Health Law: Article 28 Hospitals.[13]

Legal Analysis

In *State of North Carolina* v. *O'Hanlan*, the defendant was charged with multiple crimes including sexual assault.[14] The jury found the defendant guilty of all charges. The defendant alleged 46 different areas of appeal, including an error allowing testimony of the medical providers who performed the sexual assault evaluation. The rule governing expert witnesses states that:

> If scientific, technical or other specialized knowledge will assist the trier of fact to understand the evidence or to determine a fact in issue, a witness qualified as an expert by knowledge, skill, experience, training, or education, may testify thereto in the form of an opinion.[15]

The Court of Appeals of North Carolina held that the treating physician at the hospital is permitted to give the background reasons and basis for diagnosis and overruled the defendant's assignment of error as there was no evidence of prejudice.

In *State of Nebraska* v. *Vaught*, the defendant was convicted in district court of child sexual assault.[16]

The defendant objected that ED physician who treated and diagnosed the victim had testified that the victim had identified the defendant as the perpetrator of the assault. The district court ruling was upheld by the Nebraska Court of Appeals. The Supreme Court of Nebraska heard the defendant's appeal, again attempting to exclude the ED physician testimony under a hearsay rule. The ED physician testified that she examined the child, who was mature enough to understand the process and identified the perpetrator as part of the routine medical evaluation process. Statements are not excluded under the hearsay rule even though the declarant is available as a witness when they are made for the purposes of medical diagnosis or treatment and describing medical history, past or present symptoms, pain, sensations, or the inception or general character of the cause or external source insofar as reasonably pertinent to diagnosis or treatment.[17] The court denied the defendant appeal and upheld the initial conviction.

In *Ohio* v. *Stahl*, the defendant appealed the Court of Appeals, Ninth District decision that held that statements to a nurse practitioner during a medical examination at a specialty sexual assault unit identifying the accused were non-testimonial and admissible.[18] The Supreme Court of Ohio held that processes and procedures that are part of a routine medical evaluation are non-testimonial, referencing the Sixth Amendment Due Process Confrontation clause and admissible.[19] They held that the nurse practitioner's statement was not a testimonial statement meaning: (1) a statement made under circumstances that would lead an objective witness to reasonably expect that a statement would be used at a later trial and (2) a statement directed toward prosecutorial agents who would use it with an eye toward trial.

Conclusion

Ideally, a system should use a SANE program, or at least a nurse with suitable training in evidence collection and supportive interventions for the patient. Physicians are required to be meticulous in their evidence collection, including figures, photographs, diagrams, and any other corroborating evidence in their assessment, to allow the best chance of success for subsequent law-enforcement intervention.

References

1. Delahunta EA, Baram D. Sexual Assault. *Clin Obstet Gynecol.* 1997;40(3):648–660.

2. Avegno J, Mills TJ, Mills LD. Sexual assault victims in the emergency department: analysis by demographic and event characteristics. *J Emerg Med.* 2009;37(3):328–334. DOI:10.1016/j.jemermed.2007.10.025.

3. Riggs N, Houry D, Long G, Markovchick V, Feldhaus KM. Analysis of 1,076 cases of sexual assault. *Ann Emerg Med.* 2000;35(4):358–362. DOI:10.1016/S0196-0644(00)70054-0.

4. Feldhaus KM, Houry D, Kaminsky R. Lifetime sexual assault prevalence rates and reporting practices in an emergency department population. *Ann Emerg Med.* 2000;36(1):23–27. DOI:10.1067/mem.2000.1007660.

5. Sugar NF, Fine DN, Eckert LO. Physical injury after sexual assault: findings of a large case series. *Am J Obstet Gynecol.* 2004;190(1):71–76. DOI:10.1016/S0002-9378(03)00912-8.

6. Campbell R, Patterson D, Lichty LF. The effectiveness of sexual assault nurse examiner (SANE) programs: a review of psychological, medical, legal and community outcomes. *Trauma Violence Abuse.* 2005;6(4):313–329. DOI:1177/1524838005280328.

7. Campbell R, Bybee D, Townsend SM, Shaw J, Karim N, Markowitz J. The impact of sexual assault nurse examiner programs on criminal justice case outcomes. *Violence Again Women.* 2014;20(5):607–625. DOI:10.1177/1077801214536286.

8. Ciancone AC, Wilson C, Collette R, Gerson LW. Sexual assault nurse examiner programs in the United States. *Ann Emerg Med.* 2000;35(4):353–357. DOI:10.1026/S0196-0644(00)70053-9.

9. Rambow B, Adkinson C, Frost TH, Peterson GF. Female sexual assault: medical and legal implications. *Ann Emerg Med.* 1992;21(6):727–731. DOI:10.1016//S0196-0644(05)82788-X.

10. Gray-Eurom KG, Seaberg DC, Wears RL. The prosecution of sexual assault cases: correlation with forensic evidence. *Ann Emerg Med.* 2002;39(1):39–46. DOI:10.1067/mem.2002.118013.

11. McGregor MJ, DuMont J, Myhr TL. Sexual assault forensic medical examination: is evidence related to successful prosecution? *Ann Emerg Med.* 2002;39(6):639–647. DOI:10.1067/mem.2002.123694.

12. New York State Department of Health. Press Release: Health Department Fines Coney Island Hospital $46,000 for Deficiencies in Sex Assault Case. July 2000.

13. New York Public Health Law. Article 28: Hospitals.

14. *North Carolina* v. *O'Hanlan*, 570 S.E.2d 751 (2002).

15. North Carolina General Statutes §8C-1, Rule 702 (2001).

16. *State of Nebraska* v. *Vaught*, 268 Neb. 316 (2004).

17. Nebraska Revised Statutes. §27–803(3) (Cum. Supp.2002).

18. *Ohio* v. *Stahl*, 111 Ohio St. 3d 186 (2006).

19. U.S. Const. Amend. VI.

Chapter 93

Social Media

Case

The trauma pager went off again and a patient came in to the emergency department (ED) with a penetrating wound. Everyone around cringed as they saw a substantial wooden stake impaled in the patient's thigh. He had been transported with the impaled object in place: it was about 3 feet long and the thickness of a baseball bat, piercing the vascular region of the medial thigh. Although he had been given appropriate analgesics he was in obvious pain.

Someone in the ED commented, "Boy, that is unbelievable," and some staff even felt a little nauseous when they looked at it. The patient's distal vascular system was intact and a quick CT scan was ordered to define the anatomy and the nature of the injury. As the patient was leaving the ED a few of the residents quickly snapped photos on their phones and were comparing notes. The patient went to the operating room, had the object successfully removed, and went on to recover in the hospital.

The next day a concern was raised because in this small community a family member had expressed concerns that photos of their relative taken during this event appeared on a social media site. The pictures looked to have been taken in the ED, and an inquiry found that was indeed the case. The photos and stories on social media were quickly taken down and additional resident education about appropriate use of social media was instituted.

Medical Approach

The advent of electronic information sharing has allowed exponential improvements in the health-care delivery process. However, the explosion of social media, social networking, and dozens of public sites where photos and text can be shared, warrants the utmost caution in the health-care arena today.

How patients search for online information has been reviewed by Morahan-Martin.[1] Worldwide, approximately 4.5% of all web searches are for health-related information, but the quality of information retrieved is questionable. The issues appeared to be related to the use of short search terms, often misspelled, and seldom going beyond the first page of search results. The public is interested in reliable information and will avoid overly commercialized sites, but they do not search for other indicators of credibility. A partnership between patient and provider to facilitate the educational process is most helpful.

The issue of unsecured email between patients and physicians has been settled. Recupero described the experience of psychiatrists and their patients.[2] They specifically examined the scenario of some physicians responding to unsolicited emails, to suggest diagnosis or offer advice. The existence of communication may be enough to establish a patient–physician relationship. There are difficult ethics-related decisions regarding unsolicited email for the public, current patients, and third parties, such as family members.

The scenario above envisages health-care providers taking pictures in the hospital setting. Bhangoo et al. solicited 150 EDs in the United Kingdom for clinical photography protocols with a 78% (117) response rate.[3] The majority (45.2%, 53) take clinical photographs with no existent policy, 18% (21) have a written policy, 5.9% (7) take assault or domestic violence images, where only slightly over half (4) document consent. All photographs are taken for clinical or teaching purposes, and 27.3% (32) without a policy attach the photograph to the clinical record.

The issues of consent, archiving, and confidentiality are especially important with the advent of digital image handling and manipulation. The concepts of electronic information sharing are constantly evolving. The term "social media" refers to web-based tools

Table 93.1 Social media outlets

	Type	Sites	
1.	Social networking	MySpace	
		Facebook	
		Twitter	
		GooglePlus	
		Snapchat	
2.	Professional networking	LinkedIn	
		Doximity	
3.	Media sharing	YouTube	
		Instagram	
		Flickr	
4.	Content production		
		Blogs	Tumblr
			Blogger
		Microblogs	Twitter
5.	Knowledge aggregation	Wikipedia	
6.	Virtual reality/gaming	Second Life	

Reference: Ventola.[4]

that allow communication, collaboration, information, and content sharing between individuals and groups in real time.[4] Although the term social networking may be used synonymously, it implies a more active process of interacting with others, rather than simple information or content sharing. Social media sites are growing exponentially and include social networking, media sharing, content production, web log or blogs, microblogs, wikis, gaming, and virtual reality sites (Table 93.1).

The impact of social networking sites on patient care in the ED is ever increasing. For example, the use of Facebook is ubiquitous among both patients and health-care providers, and concerns have been expressed. The use of Facebook in the ED setting can have beneficial effects on the patient encounter as well assisting in diagnosis or intervention. Bennett et al. describe a juvenile patient who presented to the ED with a concern for suicidal ideation.[5] The case was assisted by her parents, who showed the staff Facebook posts referring to her intent, facilitating a diagnosis and subsequent care plan.

The use of social media can benefit patients, enhance professional networks, and advance understanding of public health issues. George et al. postulated the dangers of social media could be mitigated

by changing the functionality of privacy settings.[6] Sites such as Google+ and Facebook have added privacy and modified their grouping methodology so that there are definite boundaries between friends and work colleagues.

The American Medical Association has published guidelines on the maintenance of the physician's online presence,[7] and these recommendations have been expanded upon (Table 93.2). First, physicians should be aware of patient privacy and confidentiality standards, maintain them online, and refrain from posting identifiable patient information online. Second, physicians using social networking must use appropriate privacy settings to safeguard personal information and content. Third, it is crucial to recognize the privacy settings are not absolute, and assume anything posted on the internet as permanent. Fourth, physicians should routinely monitor their own internet presence to ensure its professional nature and accuracy; and that content about the physician posted by others is accurate. Fifth, any patient–physician interaction over the internet needs to respect the appropriate professional ethical boundaries and guidelines. Sixth, physicians should consider separating personal and professional content online to maintain appropriate professional boundaries. Seventh, physicians have a responsibility to discuss inappropriate content posted by colleagues so they can self-correct. Eighth, if the behavior is significantly violative of professional norms and there is no individual correction, it should be referred to appropriate authorities. Ninth, health-care workers

Table 93.2 Professionalism in the use of social media

1.	Be aware of online patient privacy and confidentiality standards
2.	Use appropriate privacy settings for online contents
3.	Recognize that privacy settings are not absolute
4.	Monitor your personal web presence for accuracy
5.	Patient–physician interaction online has same boundaries
6.	Separate personal and professional online content
7.	Discuss inappropriate online content with colleagues
8.	Refer significant or refractory violations
9.	Online content can affect reputation
10.	May have impact on later career of medical trainees
11.	Online content may undermine public trust

Reference: AMA Opinion 9.124 (adapted).[7]

should recognize that online actions and negative content posted may negatively affect their reputations among patients and colleagues. Tenth, these content choices may have later career impact for medical students and physicians in training. Eleventh, inappropriate online content may undermine the public trust in the profession as a whole.

The issue distills down to the appearance of protected health information (PHI) on social networking sites. Thompson et al. performed a cross-sectional analysis of all 2053 medical students and resident study participants at a single university program who had a Facebook profile.[8] Almost half (49.8%, 1023) had online profiles, and 1.2% (12) of profiles had photos of patient care posted. However, no identifiable patient likeness or information in text form was posted. These events were more common with medical students than residents, increased over time, and were clustered around medical mission trips. The photos typically included trainees interacting with identifiable patients, performing medical examinations and procedures. The obvious conclusion is education, orientation, and supervision.

The goal is the implementation of a social media strategy compliant with the Health Insurance Portability and Accountability Act (HIPAA), as offered by Hinmon.[9] First, one must understand the statute itself, allowing information sharing only within the health-care team and select identified groups. Second, limit the facility's liability by establishing clear policies and procedures. Third, train and educate the staff in proper policies and procedures. Fourth, avoid the temptation to practice medicine online without the appropriate authorizations and protocol. Fifth, regularly monitor your social media platforms (some would suggest daily) for irregularities. Sixth, prepare a rapid action team to intervene if a problem is found (Table 93.3).

Table 93.3 HIPAA-compliant social media strategy

1.	Understand HIPAA statute
2.	Establish clear policies and procedures
3.	Train and educate staff
4.	Avoid practicing medicine online
5.	Regularly monitor your social media platforms
6.	Rapid intervention if problem found

Reference: Hinmon.[9]

Another crucial question is who is responsible for social media comments. The Communications Decency Act of 1996, Section 230 states that, "No provider or user of an interactive computer service shall be treated as the publisher or speaker of any information provided by another information content provider."[10] This statute resulted in the protection of internet service providers and any other online services that publish third-party content. The next step in the analysis questions the facility's liability for posted content or comments. The facility is liable if there is disclosure of PHI, or inappropriate or unprofessional employee or affiliate comments. It is less likely to be liable for public forum postings that are dealt with professionally when encountered.

Legal Analysis

In *In The Matter of Thran*, the State of Rhode Island Department of Health and Board of Medical Licensure evaluated the case of an emergency physician who used Facebook in such a manner as to allegedly violate patient confidentiality.[11] The respondent did not use patient names and had no intention to reveal any confidential patient information. A patient was identified by an unauthorized third party, and the respondent deleted the account immediately. The respondent was the subject of a consent order held in violation of Rhode Island General Law 5–37–5 (19) revealing personally identifiable information of third parties.[12]

In *Puetz* v. *Spectrum Health Hospitals*, an ED physician was allegedly terminated for an ostensible HIPPA violation after a social media conversation.[13] The physician had a long-term facility relationship with administrative responsibilities, and other facility contributions that she felt were at issue. The physician did not post the photo, but allegedly added a question, which included potentially identifying initials, to the discussion stream. The court issued an order to show cause to the parties on issues related to intellectual property ownership, alleging a case of actual controversy. The district court concluded it lacked subject-matter jurisdiction over the plaintiff request for declaratory judgment and dismissed.

In *Yath* v. *Fairview Clinics*, a clinic employee saw an acquaintance there, allegedly read their medical file, and disclosed information to others. Someone forged a MySpace profile disclosing protected information to 60–80 "friends."[14] The district court granted summary judgment to the defendants on most claims.

The Court of Appeals of Minnesota upheld the district court judgments that: (1) declined to impose sanctions for spoliation, as there was no proof the destroyed computer files contained the internet postings; (2) held that the invasion of privacy claim failed because there was no "publicity"; (3) dismissed the negligent infliction of emotional distress claim for failing to meet the invasion threshold; (4) held that the clinic could not be held liable for unauthorized acts of employees; (5) held that "breach of a confidential relationship" is not a recognized cause of action. However, they reversed and remanded the decision to the district court, holding that HIPAA does not preempt Minnesota Statute 144.335, allowing a private cause of action for releasing health records.[15]

Conclusion

All staff should be educated about the impropriety of PHI appearing in a public venue even though the individuals are not clearly identified. In a small town or rural environment there is often little or no confidentiality with regard to health-care issues. Even in larger urban areas, photos or information posted online may assume a new importance because they are so widely circulated. Staff should be reminded that in no circumstances should any photos be taken without the patient's permission, and certainly not for circulation or posting to a social media website.

References

1. Morahan-Martin JM. How internet users find, evaluate and use online health information: a cross-cultural review. *Cyberpsychol Behav.* 2004;7(5):497–510. DOI:10.1089/CPG.2004.7.497.

2. Recupero PR. E-mail and the psychiatrist-patient relationship. *J Am Acad Psychiatry Law.* 2005;33(4):465–475.

3. Bhangoo P, Maconochle IK, Batrick N, Henry E. Clinicians taking pictures – a survey of current practice in emergency departments and proposed recommendations of best practice. *Emerg Med J.* 2005;22(11):761–765. DOI:10.1136/emj.2004.016972.

4. Ventola CL. Social media and health care professionals: benefits, risks and best practices. *PT.* 2014;39(7):491–499, 520.

5. Bennett A, Pourmand A, Shesser R, Sanchez J, Joyce J. Impacts of social networking sites on patient care in the emergency department. *Telemed J E Health.* 2014;20(1):1–3.

6. George DR, Rovniak LS, Kraschnewski JL. Dangers and opportunities for social media in medicine. *Clin Obstet Gynecol.* 2013;56(3):453–462. DOI:10.1097/GRF.0b013e318297dc38.

7. *Opinion 9.124 – Professionalism in the Use of Social Media* (Chicago, IL: American Medical Association, 2011).

8. Thompson LA, Black E, Duff WP, Black NP, Saliba H. Protected health information on social networking sites: ethical and legal considerations. *J Med Internet Res.* 2011;13(1):e8. DOI:10.2196/jmir.1590.

9. Hinmon D. Understand the rules for a HIPAA-compliant social media strategy. Blog, February 15, 2011.

10. 47 U.S.C. §230. Communications Decency Act of 1996.

11. In The Matter of Tranh, No. C10-156. April 13, 2011.

12. Rhode Island General Law, Chapter 5-37. Board of Medical Licensure and Discipline. §5-37-5.1. Unprofessional Conduct (2012).

13. *Puetz v. Spectrum Health Professionals*, USDC, Western District of Michigan, Southern Division. No. 1:14-cv-00275-GJQ. June 26, 2015.

14. *Yath v. Fairview Clinics*, 767 N.W.2d 34 (2009).

15. Minnesota Statutes, Chapter 144, §144.335. Access to Health Records.

Staff Privileges

Chapter

94

Case

He was an excellent physician – proficient, kind, and caring. He had cared for a large patient population that had been with this practice for years. He was a member of a number of hospital committees and was known as a strong contributor to the overall hospital mission. Within the last few months a new administrative team had started at the hospital, and the physician had made a number of statements concerning the hospital's new course and direction. Some of the new initiatives and plans were helpful and seemed to benefit the local population, and some were harder for the physicians to understand. This particular physician, who was a member of the hospital quality committee and medical executive board office, spoke out in opposition to the changes. His rationale was well founded and backed by evidence that the business decisions made regarding the hospital practice suggested another course. Finally, after years of argument back and forth, the physician's staff privileges were revoked, ostensibly for quality issues. Some cases were reviewed but there was no clear evidence of practice variation and he filed suit to regain his hospital privileges. Even though factors favored restoration of those privileges, they were not restored. The physician changed his practice location and went on to be successful there as well.

Medical Approach

It is important to realize staff privileges are indeed privileges, not rights, even when the evidence clearly supports ongoing privileges. The judiciary has given wide scope to hospitals and facilities to make their own decisions regarding staff privileging and they feel they are on the side of the hospital in individual disputes. Physicians should recognize they truly have no right to their staff privileges although there are other remedies that may apply such as discrimination, inappropriate termination, bias, and other legal theories.

The crucial question is the effect of medical or surgical skill, as judged by peers, on complication rates or patient outcome. Birkmeyer et al. evaluated the skill set of 20 bariatric surgeons, with a video-recorded procedure then reviewed by 10 peer-reviewed surgeons.[1] The mean technical skill rating was 2.6–4.8 across 10 surgeons rated 1 (low) to 5 (high). The highest complication rate (14.5 vs. 5.2%, $P < 0.001$) and higher mortality (0.26 vs. 0.05%, $P = 0.01$) was associated with the bottom quartile of surgical skill. In addition, the lowest skill quartile was associated with longer operations (137 vs. 98 minutes, $P < 0.001$), higher rates of reoperation (3.4 vs. 1.6%, $P = 0.01$), and readmission rates (6.3 vs. 2.7%, $P < 0.001$). They concluded that peer review was an effective strategy in defining surgical proficiency (Table 94.1).

A factor often cited in areas of controversy is the presence of workplace discrimination. Tolbert Coombs and King mailed questionnaires to 1930 practicing physicians evaluating exposure to discrimination with a 24% (445) response rate.[2] They identified four types of alleged discrimination affecting career advancement, punitive behaviors, practice barriers, and hiring barriers. The majority of the respondents (63%) felt they had experienced some type of discrimination. Demographic analysis found that 46% of respondents were women, 42% were from a racial or ethnic minority, and 40% were international medical school graduates. The majority (60%) felt discrimination against international graduates was significant and 27% thought there was bias against women as well. However, the low response rate to the questionnaire is acknowledged.

Table 94.1 Peer review analysis of surgical skill: lowest to highest quartile

	Outcome	Incidence %, $P < 0.001$
1.	Complication rates	14.5 vs. 5.2
2.	Mortality	0.26 vs. 0.05
3.	Operation length	137 vs. 98
4.	Reoperation	3.4 vs. 1.6
5.	Readmission	6.3 vs. 2.7

Reference: Birkmeyer et al.[1]

Legal Analysis

In *Alexander* v. *Rush North Shore*, a staff anesthesiologist was on call for the emergency department (ED) when an airway emergency occurred[3]. The anesthesiologist was allegedly contacted for assistance, did not present, and general surgery presented to perform a tracheostomy and stabilize the patient. A complaint was filed, and an inquiry was held. The plaintiff and other witnesses alleged various reasons why the on-call physician did not appear, including: (1) the ED physician did not ask; (2) the facility did not possess the appropriate equipment; (3) he questioned whether it was necessary for him to come in; (4) the fact that the fiberoptic procedure failed mandated a tracheostomy. The hospital convened various quality review panels, and informed the physician that his staff privileges were revoked. The plaintiff filed suit, alleging the revocation of staff privileges constituted unlawful discrimination in violation of the Civil Rights Act of 1964.[4] The defendant moved for summary judgment under the theories that: (1) the plaintiff was an independent contractor not an employee and precluded from filing a Title VII claim, and (2) the plaintiff could offer no evidence to support the discharge based on the pretext claim. The United States Court of Appeals (USCA), Seventh Circuit affirmed the trial court ruling for the defendants, holding there was ample opportunity for both parties to discuss the independent contractor–employment status before the summary judgment stage. They did offer guidance on the determination, citing *Ost* v. *West Suburban Travelers Limousine, Inc*, offering a five-factor test for employee status.[5] First, the extent of control and supervision including directions on scheduling and work performance. Second, the type of occupation and the nature of skill required, including whether skills are obtained

in the workplace. Third, who bears the responsibility for the costs of operation including equipment, supplies, fees, licenses, workplace, and maintenance of operations. Fourth, the method and form of payments and benefits. Fifth, the length of job commitment and performance expectations. They concluded that:

> If an employer has the right to control and direct the work of an individual, not only as to the result achieved, but also as to the details by which that result is achieved, an employer/employee relationship is likely to exist. *Ost*, 88 F.3d at 439 (quoting *Spirides* v. *Reinhardt*).[5,6]

In *Menkowitz* v. *Pottstown Memorial Medical Center*, the physician, a specialist surgeon, was diagnosed with attention deficit disorder but produced a written evaluation by a clinical psychologist demonstrating fitness in patient and staff interactions.[7] The physician was accused of various infractions of hospital policy, which he described as "a pattern of harassment and intimidation." His staff privileges were initially suspended, allegedly without a hearing, then for 6 months after committee discussion. Finally, a National Practitioner Data Bank (NPDB) Adverse Information Report was filed. The appellant filed claims under the Americans with Disabilities Act (ADA) and Section 504 of the Rehabilitation Act of 1973 (largely eclipsed by the former).[8,9] The district court held that the appellant failed to show that the hospital had suspended his staff privileges "solely for reasons of disability" and the claim was dismissed. The appellant raises an issue of first impression, whether Title III of the ADA prohibits disability discrimination against a medical doctor with "staff privileges" at a hospital.[8] The district court held that normal usage applies to "public accommodation" and for a hospital it would apply to patients or visitors, not the employees working there. The USCA, Third Circuit reversed the district court order on the federal claims and vacated the order, declining to exercise supplemental jurisdiction over the appellant's state-law claims. They held that the appellant set forth sufficient factual circumstances to permit an inference to be drawn that the medical staff privileges were suspended by reason of handicap. This extends the public space protection of Title III to physicians as well. They clarified that Section 504 of the Rehabilitation Act requires the appellant to provide factual evidence that the disability was the sole reason for action.

In *Freilich* v. *Upper Chesapeake Health*, a physician's staff privileges were terminated after an

Table 94.2 Minimum standards for credentialing

1. Analyzing filed claims
2. Define utilization, quality, and risk
3. Review of clinical skills
4. Follow hospital bylaws, policies, and procedures
5. Continuing education requirements
6. Mental health and physical status

Reference: Maryland Health Code §19–319.[13]

Table 94.3 Process for physician reappointment: "collect, verify, review, and document"

1. Claims filed against physician
2. Utilization, quality and risk data
3. Review of clinical skills
4. Adherence to hospital bylaws, policies and procedures
5. Continuing medical education requirements
6. Mental and physical health status
7. Attitude, cooperation, work with others

Reference: COMAR §10.07.01.24 (E).[14]

extensive review of a reappointment application.[10] The physician stated she advocated for patient rights and quality of care and opposed hospital outsourcing of oversight functions. Claims were filed under ADA, the Rehabilitation Act, and 42 U.S.C. §1983.[8,9,11] However, the focus was on a constitutional challenge to the statutes that grant qualified immunity to peer review participants, citing the federal Health Care Quality Improvement Act (HCQIA).[12] The challenge also included the Maryland statutes and regulations covering physician credentialing.[13,14] The HCQIA limits liability for damages for those who participate in the peer review process, which is accompanied by the appropriate due-process safeguards. The professional review action must be taken (1) "in the reasonable belief that the action was in the furtherance of quality health care," (2) "after a reasonable effort to obtain the facts of the matter," (3) "after adequate notice and hearing procedures are afforded," and (4) "in the reasonable belief that the action was warranted by the facts known after such reasonable effort to obtain facts."[15] The Maryland Code requires the Secretary of Health and Mental Hygiene to establish minimum standards for formal credentialing that must take place every 2 years.[13] They must review the physician's pattern of performance by: (1) analysis of filed claims; (2) data defining utilization, quality, and risk; (3) review of clinical skills; (4) adherence to hospital bylaws, policies and procedures; (5) compliance with continuing education requirements; and (6) mental health and physical status (Table 94.2). The Code of Maryland Regulations (COMAR) require each Maryland hospital to establish a process for physician reappointment.[13] The hospitals must "collect, verify, review and document" the physician's pattern of performance, including: (1) claims filed against the physician; (2) utilization, quality, and risk data; (3) review of clinical skills; (4) adherence to hospital bylaws, policies, and procedures; (5) compliance with continuing

medical education; (6) assessment of current mental and physical health status; (7) attitudes, cooperation, and the ability to work with others (Table 94.3). These processes are essentially identical and largely objective with the exception of the "attitude and cooperation" requirement, which is subjective and challenged most often in cases of controversy.

The district court dismissed the federal claims with prejudice, and the state-law claims without prejudice. The judgment was affirmed by the USCA, Fourth Circuit. They held that the federal court was not to supervise what amounts to a physician–hospital dispute or the expenditure of resources. They held that the hospital medical staff reappointment codes, statutes, and guidelines are indeed constitutional on their face.

In *Poliner* v. *Texas Health System*, a jury awarded an interventional cardiologist a $366 million settlement over a 29-day suspension while a peer review investigation proceeded concerning alleged patient care issues.[16] The hospital department-based peer review ultimately led to a 5-month suspension. The plaintiff sued the hospital and its peer review committee, alleging various federal and state law violations. The medical issue was related to an allegedly missed coronary occlusion during an interventional procedure, difficulty in reaching the provider afterwards, and the care of four other patients subsequently referred to the committee. The district court held that the suspension enjoyed immunity from monetary damages under the HCQIA, and granted partial summary judgment. However, they considered that the question of temporary restriction of privileges during the investigation was a matter for the jury. The jury found for the physician on the defamation claim with a $90 million award for mental anguish and injury to career, and $110 million in punitive damages. The

USCA, Fifth Circuit reversed the district court and rendered judgment for the defendants. The plaintiff failed to rebut the statutory presumption that the peer review actions were in compliance with accepted standards, and HCQIA offered immunity to peer review members.

However, in *Adkins* v. *P. Christie*, the question of validity of evidentiary "medical peer-review privilege" is called into question.[17] This privilege attempts to protect from discovery and disclosure physician records containing performance reviews from their peers in connection with their hospital-based practice. The physician felt he was under extraordinary scrutiny as a new staff physician, with the reviews increased in number and depth, allegedly due to discriminatory motives. The facility alleged difficulty with call, medical records completion, failure to follow admission protocol, and a patient care issue. The district court granted the defendant's summary judgment motion for failure to state a claim. The plaintiff appealed, requesting peer review records on all physicians who underwent the peer review process for a 7-year period. The defendants filed a protective order motion. The court ordered a limited disclosure of the unidentified reasons to generate peer review, and only for physicians in similar circumstances. The USCA, Eleventh Circuit joined the Fourth and Seventh Circuits in declining to recognize the privilege for the documents proper relating to medical peer review in federal discrimination cases. They held that the district court improperly limited the scope of discovery, prematurely granting a summary judgment motion for the defendant, reversed and remanded. They concluded that "the social goal of eliminating employment discrimination" overrides the policy concern over peer review privileging.

Conclusion

The controversy over staff privileges often comes down to the following points: (1) staff privileges are not a protected right; (2) the facility has wide scope in decision-making; (3) some semblance of due process is required; (4) the official peer review process offers immunity to the participants but some aspects of the actual work product may be scrutinized.

References

1. Birkmeyer JD, Finks JF, O'Reilly A, Oerline M, Carlin AM, Nunn AR, et al. for Michigan Bariatric Surgery Collaborative. Surgical skill and complication rates after surgery. *N Engl J Med*. 2013;369(15):1434–1442. DOI:10.1056/NEJMsa1300625.

2. Tolbert Coombs AA, King RK. Workplace discrimination: experiences of practicing physicians. *J Nat Med Assoc*. 2005;97(4):467–477.

3. *Alexander* v. *Rush North Shore Medical Center*, 101 F.3d 487 (1996).

4. Civil Rights Act of 1964, Title VII, 42 U.S.C. §2000e et seq. (4).

5. *Ost* v. *West Suburban Travelers Limousine, Inc.*, 88 F.3d 440 (1996).

6. *Spirides* v. *Reinhardt*, 613 F.2d 826 (1979).

7. *Menkowitz* v. *Pottstown Memorial Medical Center*, 154 F.3d 113 (1998).

8. Americans with Disabilities Act (ADA), 42 U.S.C. §§12101–12213 (1994).

9. Rehabilitation Act of 1973, 29 U.S.C. §794 (1994): Section 504.

10. *Freilich* v. *Upper Chesapeake Health*, 418 Md. 586, 16 A.3d 977 (2011).

11. 42 U.S.C. §1983 – Civil Action for Deprivation of Rights (1983).

12. Healthcare Quality Improvement Act (HCQIA), 42 §11101 et seq.

13. Maryland Code, Health – General §19–319 (e) (2010).

14. Code of Maryland Regulations (COMAR) §10.07.01.24 (2011).

15. 42 U.S. Code §11112 – Standards for Professional Review Actions.

16. *Poliner* v. *Texas Health Systems*, 537 F.3d 368 (2008).

17. *Adkins* v. *P. Christie*, 488 F.3d 1324 (2007).

Chapter 95

Subpoena

Case

The medical staff office received a certified envelope addressed to the emergency department (ED) physician. The secretary said she thought it looked legal and asked if they should forward it to the legal office. It turned out to be a subpoena, requiring the physician to testify in a medical care matter. The physician requested that it be sent to the legal department, but she wanted a copy. Later that day during her shift in the ED she received a call from an attorney who introduced himself as the counsel requested to address the subpoena regarding some medical care that had been provided. The physician told him she was in the middle of her shift and couldn't talk to him; the requesting group would have to work through the hospital legal counsel. He replied that the physician was not the subject of a lawsuit. His client had been treated in the ED and was now involved in a workers' compensation matter. The attorney needed some information about his health condition. The physician agreed to speak to him for a few minutes. The attorney asked her some questions about the patient's care and his health condition. What diagnostic evaluation was performed? How did they think he was doing? When did they think he would be able to return to work? The physician said she was not in charge of defining long-term disability, but thought the patient would be recovered in a couple weeks after the on-the-job accident.

Later that day, the hospital attorney contacted the physician, and she described her interaction with the outside attorney. The hospital attorney expressed concern that this may have been something more than a worker's compensation matter. Often that sort of approach is a ruse to get information about the medical care provided. Sure enough, within a month, the hospital received a pleading alleging medical malpractice during the ED visit.

Medical Approach

It is important to recognize that every subpoena is a formal legal document that should be passed on to the hospital legal counsel. Anyone receiving a subpoena can be compelled to appear in court, so the document requires due diligence and cannot be ignored. It is also important to be aware that the reason for the request stated in the subpoena can sometimes be masked by a request to appear as a fact witness on another matter, whereas in fact the real target is information regarding an alleged medical malpractice event.

The confidentiality of patient-related information is the cornerstone of the patient–physician relationship;[1] the patient feels their confidential information should never be released without their consent. The interface between legal process and compelled production of evidence often rests with the subpoena process. A covered health-care provider or health plan may disclose protected health information (PHI) required by a judicial court order, or administrative tribunal, but may only disclose the information specifically described in that order.[2,3] However, if the subpoena is issued not by the judge, but by someone else such as a court clerk or attorney, the information can only be released if proper notification is made under the Privacy Rules. The Privacy Rules require that before the covered entity may respond to the subpoena, there must be evidence that reasonable efforts were made: (1) to notify the person who is the subject of the information about the request, so the individual had a chance to object and; (2) to seek a qualified protective order for the information from the court.[2,3]

The Health Insurance Portability and Accountability Act (HIPAA) supersedes most aspects of state disclosure regulations as described by Thornton (Table 95.1).[4,5]

First, there are changes in the notice provision required so the subpoena now becomes a two-step

Table 95.1 Compelled production of evidence

1.	Two-step notification and response
2.	Discovery liberal admission process
3.	"Minimum necessary" disclosure
4.	"Qualified protective order" single-use release

Reference: Thorton.[5]

Table 95.2 Forms of legal process

1.	Subpoena
2.	Subpoena duces tecum
3.	District attorney subpoena
4.	Federal subpoena
5.	Search warrant
6.	Court order
7.	Administrative subpoena or warrant

Reference: Iowa Medical Society.[7]

process. In California, for example, there is a 10-day notice of requirement and the provider has 15 days to respond.[6] However, HIPPA requires "satisfactory assurance" that the provider (1) be given written documentation from the party seeking release that it has attempted to notify the patient and (2) be provided with a written statement that either the patient did not object in a timely fashion, or the objection was involved in the favor of disclosure.

Second, the scope of discovery is typically wide – solicitation of medical records from the last 5–10 years, if relevant, and introduced into evidence by the patient as part of the controversy. California law states the criteria as "admissible in evidence or appears reasonably calculated to lead to the discovery of admissible evidence."[6]

Third, HIPAA imposes a "minimum necessary" requirement designed to limit the amount of medical information that may be disclosed in the litigation process. This has resulted in an extraordinary workload involving record review to identify the appropriate information to provide.

Fourth, the patient may consent to a "qualified protective order" that allows the information only to be used expressly for litigation. All information must be returned to the provider or destroyed when the case is complete.

Most importantly, providers should only comply with subpoenas that are HIPPA compliant, to avoid liability for disclosure. It is essential for physicians at least to be familiar with this aspect of the legal process.

There are different types of subpoenas. The term means literally "under penalty" and compels a person to appear and give testimony for either a deposition or a court proceeding (Table 95.2).[7] A subpoena is issued by a clerk of court, under the court's authority, without showing cause and subject to sanctions. A *subpoena duces tecum* compels you to "bring things with you," typically documents. It is not a court order, but is supported by court authority to mandate response. The

district attorney subpoena typically issued in criminal cases is usually the equivalent of a court order. A *federal court subpoena* is issued through the federal court system and is equivalent to a state court order.

A *search warrant* is used by law enforcement to conduct a search and seizure for information, based on probable cause, and is the equivalent of a court order. A *court order request for medical records* is issued after a hearing by both parties, determining merit to produce. Typically, both the court and the judge requesting are specified in the document. An *administrative subpoena or warrant* is issued under the authority of a state or federal agency that has investigative and enforcement authority, backed by the authority to compel production.

Frequently law enforcement personnel accompany patients or seek access to them while they are in the ED.[8] Although the ED and trauma bays are highly regulated areas, law enforcement personnel typically fall outside of the ethical and institutional guidelines of health-care institutions. The law enforcement presence is a potential area of conflict that can affect patient care, provider liability, and the effectiveness of law enforcement: patients are quick to notice the collaboration or lack thereof between hospital and law enforcement personnel. An important aspect of this relationship is the interface with law enforcement. The ED director should meet with the police chief and develop conjoint management protocols in advance of the interaction.[9] Second, they should establish orientation sessions so both groups of professionals know what to expect. Third, it is helpful to arrange ED tours for law enforcement personnel, to help them understand operations and confidentiality standards. Fourth, ED personnel should be exposed to standard law enforcement practice as well (Table 95.3).

Table 95.3 ED–law enforcement interface

1. Conjoint management protocols
2. Establish orientation sessions
3. ED tours for law enforcement
4. Law enforcement tours for ED

Reference: Selbst et al.[9]

Table 95.4 Subpoenaed physician testimony

1. Nature and extent of treatment relationship
2. Medical and laboratory support of opinion
3. Opinion incorporates all evidence
4. Persuasiveness of opinion
5. Consistency of opinion with record
6. Physician specialization

Reference: Butera.[13]

Legal Analysis

In *Greene* v. *Rogers*, the patient presented to the ED with chest pain, received an EKG and single cardiac enzyme, and was admitted to a general medical ward.[10] The plaintiff alleged misdiagnosis, inappropriate testing, and failure to admit to the critical care unit proximately caused her death. The trial court awarded summary judgment to the hospital, ruling that the ED physician was not an agent of the hospital. The appellant asserted the trial court erred in denying the appellant's new trial motion based on the hospital's representation of a witness who refused to testify at an out-of-state evidence deposition. They alleged the former nurse was instructed not to testify and hid her identity until trial. The Illinois Appellate Court affirmed the trial court dismissal. They held that a non-party witness may insist on a subpoena before testifying. They felt the appellant attorney could have subpoenaed but did not, after the hospital attorney informed the court that the nurse was represented and would not testify. Likewise, there was no evidence the testimony would have changed the course of the trial.

In *Yancey* v. *Apfel*, a patient applied for disability benefits based on a chronic rheumatological condition.[11] These benefits were denied by an administrative-law judge (ALJ), and at a second appeal a subpoena request was denied. The ALJ held that the other evidence was sufficient to fully adjudicate the case. The appellant theorized that the Fifth Amendment to the Constitution and notions of fundamental fairness should compel the issuance of the physician subpoena.[12] The United States Court of Appeals (USCA), Second District held that the administrative decision rested on adequate findings, and there was no basis that substantial evidence was lacking. They held that due process in an administrative proceeding does not require that a reporting physician be subpoenaed any time a claimant makes such a request.

In *Butera* v. *Apfel*, the patient sought treatment in an ED for severe back and hip pain, with preliminary screening indicating degenerative disease.[13] He was referred to orthopedic surgery for evaluation, revealing an acceptable exam, and MRI revealing a disk herniation. The patient's disability claim was denied, as well as request for physician subpoena. The USCA, Seventh Circuit concurred that the appellant failed to demonstrate that a subpoena was reasonably necessary for full presentation of the case.

The court weighs the value of compelled physician testimony to include: (1) nature and extent of treatment relationships; (2) degree to which the medical signs and laboratory findings support the opinion; (3) degree to which opinion takes into account all pertinent evidence; (4) persuasiveness of the opinion rendered; (5) consistency of opinion with record as a whole; (6) specialization of the physician (Table 95.4).[14]

In *United States* v. *Zamora*, the government charged the defendant for driving under the influence on government property. She claimed onset of asthma symptoms and was taken to the hospital for evaluation.[15] While there she received a blood alcohol test, and the government issued a subpoena for medical records. The hospital filed a motion challenging the requested disclosure based on HIPAA,[4] the Texas Health and Safety Code,[16] and Title 42 United States Code §290dd-2.[17] The government filed a motion to quash the denial, arguing that HIPAA allows disclosure without patient consent for legitimate law enforcement purposes, and the records were properly requested by the clerk of courts. Section 290dd-2 also allows disclosure of confidential substance abuse and mental health records by "an appropriate order of a court of competent jurisdiction granted after application

Table 95.5 Subpoena–provider interface

1.	Professionals for testimony
2.	Delivered through proxy
3.	Refer to hospital attorney
4.	Civil or criminal matter
5.	Summoned as fact witness
6.	No compensation
7.	Consider your own attorney
8.	Appear regardless of work schedule
9.	Contempt or fine for non-compliance

showing good cause."[17] The district court denied the hospital protective order to quash and the facility was ordered to produce the medical records.

Conclusion

Health-care professionals should always be cautious regarding subpoenas (Table 95.5). First, they are typically issued when testimony is required for a legal proceeding. Second, the document is often delivered through a proxy, typically the hospital attorney. Third, if a subpoena is not delivered through a proxy, it should be referred to risk management or the hospital attorney for processing. Fourth, you may be summoned to offer testimony in both civil and criminal matters. Fifth, you are usually summoned as a fact witness and not an expert witness. Sixth, there is often no fee or compensation reimbursement for medical fact testimony. Seventh, if you have concerns then consult the hospital attorney, although consider retaining an attorney personally if there are potential conflicts of interest. Eighth, realize that you can be compelled to appear regardless of your work schedule. Ninth, although it is unlikely, you can be compelled to appear and held in contempt or fined if you do not appear as mandated by the court.

References

1. Wiener BA, Wettstein RM. Confidentiality of patient-related information. *Arch Opthalmol.* 1994;112(8):1032–1036. DOI:10.1001/archopth.1994.01090200038018.

2. Health Information Privacy. Court orders and subpoenas. US Department of Health & Human Services. www.hhs.gov. Accessed November 20, 2015.

3. 45 C.F.R. 164.512 – Uses and Disclosures for Which an Authorization or Opportunity to Agree or Object Is Not Required.

4. Health Insurance Portability and Accountability Act of 1996 (HIPAA), Title XI, Pub. L. 104–191, 110 Stat. 1936 (August 21, 1996), codified as 42 U.S.C. 1301 et seq.

5. Thornton TE. HIPAA affects docs' response to subpoenas for medical data. *Managed Care.* June 2002.

6. California Civil Code §56.10–56.16.

7. HIPAA: Responding to Legal Process. Iowa Medical Society. September 2005.

8. Tahouni MR, Liscord E, Mowafi H. Managing law enforcement presence in the emergency department: highlighting the need for new policy recommendations. *J Emerg Med.* 2015;49(4):523–529. DOI:10.1016/j.jemergmed.2015.04.001.

9. Selbst SM, King C, Ludwig S, Schwartz GR, Barcliff C. Interfacing with police in the pediatric emergency department. *Pediatr Emerg Care.* 1992;8(3):152–156.

10. *Greene* v. *Rogers,* 498 N.E.2d 867 (1986).

11. *Yancey* v. *Apfel,* 145 F.3d 106 (1998).

12. U.S. Const. Amend. V.

13. *Butera* v. *Apfel,* 173 F.3d 104 (1999).

14. 20 C.F.R. §§404.1527 (d), 416.927: Evaluating Opinion Evidence.

15. *USA* v. *Zamora,* 408 F. Supp.2d 295 (2006).

16. Texas Health and Safety Code §81.103.

17. 42 U.S.C. §290dd-2: Confidentiality of Records.

Substance Abuse

Case

Recently there had been talk among some of the staff about one of the physicians. People said she was a wonderful physician, an excellent clinician, and caring toward the patients, but they thought she seemed to be slipping a little bit. They were concerned because it was public knowledge she had recently been through a divorce and a contentious custody battle.

It had started subtly with some patient complaints, which was very unusual for her. Then, she seemed irascible with some of the staff that she had been friendly with for years. There was absence from work as well and concerns were raised with hospital administration. At one point it was suggested she had come to work smelling a little of alcohol. When she was questioned, she said it was just hand sanitizer.

When she was confronted with the issue in an administrative setting, her initial response was denial. She left the premises and called off her next shift. After discussion with administration, a subsequent meeting was arranged. This time the planned intervention, involving a physician colleague she was friendly with, was successful. At this point she finally acknowledged the issue, agreed to self-report, and then enrolled in a treatment and counseling program.

Medical Approach

The prevalence of substance use in the physician population approximates that of the general population with various studies indicating an average of 10% (range 5–15%) of physicians who abuse drugs or alcohol. However, there are some specialty-based practice correlates to note. Hughes et al. reported on a national sample of 9600 physicians with a 59% response rate that required three mailings.[1] Physicians were less likely than their age and gender counterparts abstracted from the National Household Survey on Drug Abuse to use cigarettes and illicit substances

such as marijuana, cocaine, and heroin.[2] However, they were more likely to have used alcohol and prescription medications including minor opiates and benzodiazepine tranquilizers. The prescription medications were used for self-treatment, whereas illicit substances and alcohol were used in a "recreational" fashion.

The presence of psychiatric comorbidity is often intertwined with substance abuse as covariables. Brooke et al. evaluated 144 physicians who had received treatment for substance abuse.[3] There was no difference between general practitioners and hospital-based physicians in substance misuse or outcome. However, there were differences between more senior consultants and more junior staff. The consultants were older at the onset of problematic substance use (42.6 ± 8.6 years vs. 29.9 ± 9.8 years), experienced fewer career problems, and misused fewer substances. Psychiatric correlates most commonly include personality difficulties (52.8%, 76) and anxiety or depression (31.9%, 46). History of depression (36) was associated with perceived stress at work ($P = 0.014$) or at home ($P = 0.035$). Past neurotic disturbances (20) were associated with personality difficulties ($P = 0.035$), anxiety or depression ($P = 0.004$), and an earlier onset of problematic substance use (30.2 ± 8.3 vs. 36.5 ± 9.8 years, $P = 0.014$). They quantified a "disturbance score" demonstrating a reduction in age of onset of problematic substance use.

The misuse of alcohol and drugs among physicians can be associated with malpractice, absenteeism, and patient complaints. Alves et al. evaluated by questionnaire 198 physicians enrolled in an outpatient substance use treatment program.[4] Most subjects were male (87.8%) and married (60.1%) with a mean age of 39.4 ± 10.7 years. The majority (66%) had previously been in an inpatient treatment program. As well, the majority (69%) practiced as specialists – internal medicine, anesthesiology, and surgery.

Psychiatric comorbidity was diagnosed in 27.7% for DSM-IV Axis I and in 6% for Axis II diagnosis. The most frequent pattern of abuse involved both alcohol and drugs (36.8%), alcohol alone (34.3%), and use of drugs exclusively (28.3%). The mean interval between the onset of substance misuse and seeking treatment was 3.7 years, while 30% attempted a self-treatment approach. The majority of these physicians (84.5%) presented impact on their professional lives, while 8.5% had issues with an oversight medical council. The social and legal problems encountered include marital problems and divorce (52%), motor vehicle accidents (42%), unemployment (33%), and legal problems (19%). The impact is significant, so prevention and supportive intervention is ideal.

It has been suggested that emergency physicians may have a higher rate of substance use disorder (SUD). Rose et al. performed a 5-year longitudinal cohort study of 904 physicians diagnosed with SUD admitted to 16 physician health programs (PHP).[5] They compared a cohort of emergency physicians (7.2%, 56) to physicians of other specialties (92.8%, 724). Emergency physicians had a higher than expected rate of SUD (OR. 2.7, CI 2.1–3.5, $P < 0.001$). Roughly half of each group enrolled due to alcohol-related issues (49 vs. 50%) and one-third of each group enrolled for opioid use (38% vs. 34%). During the PHP monitoring period, there was positive drug testing in 13% of the emergency physicians and 22% of other physicians, a non-significant difference. After the 5-year monitoring period, 71% of the emergency physicians and 64% of the other physicians completed their PHP contract successfully and no longer required monitoring (OR 1.4, CI 0.8–2.6, $P = 0.31$). The proportion of emergency physicians that continued practice was as high as the other physician group (84% vs. 72%, OR 2.0, CI 1.0–41, $P = 0.06$). Although the emergency physicians had a higher incidence of SUD, the majority (84%) completed their program successfully and had returned to practice at 5 years. The emergency physicians had a higher rate of success on three outcome measures – relapse rate, successful completion of monitoring, and return to clinical practice – compared to the other physician cohort.

Legal Analysis

The implication of the "impaired physician" allegation may often manifest in the setting of malpractice litigation. In *Dudley* v. *Humana Hospital*, a patient had a total hip replacement performed, required a second surgery, and sued the physician and facility for alleged malpractice.[6] The plaintiff alleged the physician was impaired, allegedly due to a federal investigation regarding dispensing of prescription drugs. The trial court agreed this evidence was "more prejudicial than probative" and excluded it as irrelevant. The defendants were awarded directed verdicts, and appealed the investigation evidence exclusion. The Court of Appeals of Texas, Houston upheld the trial court decision as no evidence was introduced suggesting the physician gave any outward appearance of being impaired as it related to the surgical procedure.

In *Kirbens* v. *Wyoming State Board of Medicine*, the question arises whether state and federal statutes offer protection to an allegedly impaired physician facing disciplinary action for misconduct he attributed to his disability.[7] The physician was subject to a board complaint and temporary restriction of practice, due to disciplinary action, followed by indefinite suspension for alleged patient care issues at two facilities, pursuant to Wyoming state law.[8] He attended a Professional Assessment Program where his substance abuse screening was negative, but was recommended to enter a Physician in Crisis Program. The board revoked his medical license, and despite an alleged initial public release the final disposition was sealed from public disclosure. The Supreme Court of Wyoming affirmed the license revocation order. They held that departmental regulations and Title III of the Americans with Disabilities Act (ADA) provides that a "public accommodation is not required to permit an individual to participate in or benefit from goods, services, facilities, privileges, advantages and accommodations, if that individual poses a direct threat to the health and safety of others."[9] They define a "direct threat" as a significant risk to the health or safety of others that cannot be eliminated by a modification of policies, practices, or procedures or by the provision of auxiliary aids or services.

In *Albany Urology Clinic* v. *Cleveland*, certiorari was granted to consider the appellate court ruling that a patient was authorized to bring a claim against a physician for failure to disclose alleged drug use.[10] The patient sued for medical malpractice after a surgical intervention with complications, and the physician was obligated to disclose alleged drug use. The Georgia Informed Consent Doctrine states that six specified categories of information must be disclosed by health-care providers before specified surgical or diagnostic procedures.[11] The Supreme Court of Georgia held that neither common law, public policy, nor code requirements impose a duty on a physician or other professional to disclose personal life factors that might adversely affect occupational performance. The plaintiff cannot assert that, as an independent factor, this non-disclosure would establish a medical malpractice claim, but it could be used in support of a claim. They reversed the appellate court decision that this disclosure was required.

In *Griffiths* v. *Superior Court of Los Angeles County*, a physician with multiple driving under the influence (DUI) citations had medical license intervention.[12] The California Business and Professions Code §2239 provides that if a physician sustains two or more misdemeanor convictions, than a basis for unprofessional conduct exists.[13] There was no evidence that the physicians's office-based medical practice was adversely affected. The plaintiff filed a petition for a writ of mandamus, in which an inferior governmental official would be compelled to comply with an official duty or correct an abuse of discretion.[14] The appellate court held that a nexus, or logical connection, exists between convictions and a physician's fitness to practice medicine. Therefore imposing this §2239 discipline does not violate the due process of the Fifth and Fourteenth Amendments and the equal protection clause of the Fourteenth Amendment to the United States Constitution,[13,15,16] and establishes conclusive evidence of unprofessional conduct that may affect medical licensure.

Conclusion

There are work-related correlates to substance abuse that seem self-evident, including behavioral issues, work absence, performance issues, and relationship difficulties. The key is early intervention, action, and referral. The standard is referral to a program for impaired physicians so to enable recovery, work reentry, and reintegration. These programs typically require an ongoing monitoring program, often for years, but for many physicians this can be a lifelong issue requiring constant vigilance.

References

1. Hughes PH, Brandenberg N, Baldwin DC, Storr CL, Williams KM, Anthony JC, Sheehan DV. Prevalence of substance use among US physicians. *JAMA*. 1992;267(17):2333–2339.

2. National Institute on Drug Abuse. *National Household Survey on Drug Abuse: Population Estimates 1990* (Rockville, MD: US Dept of Health and Human Services, 1990).

3. Brooke D, Edwards G, Andrews T. Doctors and substance misuse: types of doctors, types of problems. *Addiction*. 1993;88(5):655–663.

4. Alves HN, Surjan JC, Nogueira-Martins LA, Marques AC, Ramos SP, Laranjeira RR. Clinical and demographical aspects of alcohol and drug dependent physicians. *Rev Assoc Meds Bras*. 2005;51(3):139–143.

5. Rose JS, Campbell M, Skipper G. Prognosis for emergency physicians with substance abuse recovery: 5-year outcome study. *West J Emerg Med*. 2014;15(1):20–25. DOI:10.5811/ westjem.2013.7.17871.

6. *Dudley* v. *Humana Hospital Corporation*, 817 S.W.2d 124 (1991).

7. *Kirbens* v. *Wyoming State Board of Medicine*, 992 P.2d 1056 (1999).

8. Wyoming Statutes Annotated §§33-26-402 (a) (xxii-xviii): Grounds for Suspension; Revocation; Restriction; Imposition of Conditions; Refusal to Renew or Other Disciplinary Action.

9. 28 C.F.R. 36.208 – Direct Threat.

10. *Albany Urology Clinic* v. *Cleveland*, 528 S.E.2d 777 (2000).

11. OCGA §31-9-6.1: Informed Consent Doctrine.

12. *Griffiths* v. *Superior Court of Los Angeles County*, 117 Cal. Rptr.2d 445 (2002).

13. California Business and Professions Code, Section 2239 (a).

14. Mandamus Definition. law.cornell.edu.

15. U.S Const. Amend. V.

16. U.S. Const. Amend. XIV.

Chapter 97

Suicide

Case

The patient had visited the emergency department (ED) before. She had significant multiple sclerosis and was debilitated by disease. The paramedics had transported her for a decrease in her ability to eat or drink, and she looked tired and certainly appeared clinically dehydrated. There was nothing else: she had no fever, no pain, and had been compliant with her medicine regimen. After the ED physician did an evaluation, he suggested they could give her some fluid to get her rehydrated and then get her admitted to the hospital.

She weakly said that she didn't want to be admitted and wanted to go home. A family member who was with her objected: "No, you have to come in to the hospital, you're not eating or drinking anything at home." The patient replied, "I don't want to eat or drink anything, I just want to go home, this is the end."

The provider did a quick assessment and realized the patient was competent and had an advance directive that precluded aggressive resuscitation, but there was no comment about nutrition and rehydration.

Her family ushered the physician out of the room again, suggesting the patient "didn't know what she wanted." The provider answered that according to his assessment she seemed competent and did not want to be rehydrated. He offered some additional assistance by calling her primary care physician, social service, and psychiatry and offering to call the hospital chaplain or to ask for an ethics consultation as possible approaches.

The patient repeated that she did not want to be admitted to the hospital, but again declined any resuscitative measures directed at giving her nutrition or rehydration. She was fine with the blood work, but didn't want anything else done. The provider discharged her home with additional care. The next month she re-presented to ED after allegedly taking too much pain medicine, saying she didn't want to go on, and was admitted for additional care.

Medical Approach

The patient's ability to determine their own care and course is paramount to what we do. We recognize that a patient can actively refuse nutrition and rehydration as long as they are competent. The health-care system accommodates that right of patient self-determination but this is often difficult for families to accept. Certainly, an intervention to assist the family dynamic in the understanding of this "right to die" concept should be attempted. The use of hospice and end-of-life palliative care consultants can assist in this process for both the patient and family understanding.

The National Study of US Emergency Department Visits for Attempted Suicide and Self-Inflicted Injury 1997–2001 reported on 412,000, or 0.4%, of all annual ED visits.[1] In the United States, the annual visit rate for attempted suicide was 1.5 (range 1.3–1.7) visits per 1000 of the population. The mean patient age was 31 years, and self-injury was most common among younger patients, age 15–19 years (OR 3.3, 95% CI 2.1–4.4). The ED visit rates were higher among female patients (1.7 vs. 1.3) and non-white patients (1.9 vs. 1.5). The most common methods of injury were poisoning (68%) and cutting or piercing (20%). One-third of patients were admitted to the hospital, with 31% of admissions going to the intensive care unit (ICU). The patient was ultimately diagnosed with a psychiatric condition in 55%, depressive disorder in 34%, and alcohol abuse in 16%. These ED visits for attempted suicide are most common in adolescents attempting self-poisoning, raising issues of psychiatric illness and substance abuse.

Trends in ED visits for suicide attempts were also profiled for 1992–2001, in which visits related to mental health increased by 27.5% from 17.1 to 23.6 per

1000 ($P < 0.001$) and suicide or self-injury by 47% (0.8 to 1.5) visits per 1000 US population ($P = 0.04$).[2] Suicide attempt visits increased in non-Hispanic whites, pediatric patients younger than 15 years of age, older patients of 59–69 years, in urban areas, and among the privately insured. Although there has been an increase in ED visits for suicide attempts, there has been a reciprocal decrease in post-attempt hospitalization.

The adolescent population is at particular risk for suicidal behavior. King et al. studied 298 adolescents, 13–17 years of age, in which 16% (48) screened positive for elevated suicide risk.[3] They used multiple screening tools including the Problem Oriented Screening Instrument for Teenagers (POSIT).[4] Of the 48 who screened positive, they found 98% reported severe suicidal ideation or recent suicide attempt (46% attempt and ideation, 42% ideation, 10% attempt), and 27% reported alcohol abuse or depression. In the subgroup positive for depression and alcohol abuse 90% reported severe suicidal ideation or recent attempt, and more impulsivity than other adolescents. The adolescents most at suicide risk included those with depression, alcohol abuse, and impulsivity.

The key to effective intervention with a potentially suicidal ED patient is anticipation and early intervention. Claassen et al. evaluated the prevalence of suicide risk in 1590 ED patients, in which 11.6% (185) had ideation and 2% (31) had a plan.[5] Almost all of those with suicidal ideation (97%) acknowledged symptoms typical of mood disorder, anxiety, or substance use disorder. Structured medical record review revealed 81% (25/31) of those patients planning suicide went undetected during their index visit. Thereafter, 13% (4/31) of this ideation group attempted suicide within 45 days of the ED visit.

Applying additional screening methodology, a cohort of 219 probable suicides was identified, in which 39% (85) had an ED visit in the previous year and 15% of these visits were due to non-fatal self-harm, often shortly (median 38 days) before the suicide event.[6] However, as many as a fifth of the patients were not in contact with local mental health services. It is crucial to recognize the ED is as common a presentation forum for these patients as mental health resources.

Solicitation of care in the ED prior to suicide in a cohort of 286 mental health patients was studied by Da Cruz et al.[7] They identified that 43% (124) of these individuals had attended the ED at least once in the

year prior to their death, and 28% (35) had attended the ED on more than three occasions. The more frequent ED users and those with a history of alcohol misuse had a history of early death following ED attendance. Since 40% of the patient group visited the ED in the year prior to their suicide, this venue offers a crucial opportunity to intercede to prevent self-harm.

Another possible bellwether for at-risk suicide patients is the monitoring of self-harm patients who present to the ED and depart without a psychiatric assessment. Hickey et al. evaluated 256 deliberate self-harm patients over a 2-year period, in which 58.9% (145) were discharged without a psychiatric assessment.[8] Those who were not assessed more often had a past history of self-harm, were in the 20–34-year age group, and exhibited difficult behavior in the ED. Timing correlates indicated that those that present between 9 a.m. and 5 p.m. were more likely to receive a psychiatric consultation than those presenting between 5 p.m. and 9 a.m. During the following year, more non-assessed patients were subject to self-harm and completed suicide than those assessed (37.5 vs. 18.2%). The focus on self-harm patients should include a psychiatric consult to address this issue.

Lastly, the definitive endpoint is to examine subsequent suicide mortality after an ED visit for suicidal behavior. Crandall et al. evaluated 218,304 patients comparing suicide attempt or ideation, self-harm, or overdose cohort compared to a control group and followed for 6 years.[9] There were 408 suicide deaths, with an incidence rate of 31.2 per 100,000. Suicide rates after an ED visit are higher in males, those with previous overdose visits, suicidal ideation, or self-harm (Table 97.1). The suicide rate is higher in ED patients than population-based estimates, offering a chance to intervene with awareness and screening programs.

Table 97.1 Suicide risk after ED visit for suicidal behavior

	Predictors	Correlation
		RR, 95% CI
1.	Male	3.6, 2.8–3.6
2.	ED overdose visit	5.7, 4.5–7.4
3.	Self-harm	5.8, 5.1–10.6
4.	Suicidal ideation	6.7, 5.0–9.1

Reference: Crandall et al.[9]

Legal Analysis

In *Tabor* v. *Doctors Memorial Hospital*, the patient presented to the ED with a suspected overdose and depression after a family stressor.[10] The decision was made to admit him voluntarily to a psychiatric facility for 72 hours. The patient went missing, being allegedly in the car smoking, but returned to the ED. He then encountered difficulty with an insurance co-payment. A physician waiver was possible, but a decision was made to discharge home with family observation. Although under parental observation, he slipped away and suffered an allegedly self-inflicted gunshot wound. A medical review panel found a breach of the standard of care, but this was not judged to be the cause of the patient outcome. A second jury trial also found for the physician and hospital. The family sued for failure to admit, and the trial court found for defendants. The Supreme Court of Louisiana granted certiorari to review the decision. They affirmed the decision for the defendant medical facility, but reversed the decision regarding the emergency physician and service group and reduced the financial award by 20% in light of a comparative fault theory involving family decision-making as well.

In *Baker* v. *Adventist Health*, the patient took his own life 2 days after release from a community hospital ED.[11] The small rural facility had no psychiatric resources, but a written policy that directed ED personnel to call the county mental health department for assistance. The patient was brought in by family requesting a "mental health evaluation" and symptoms included "apathy, unable to communicate, depressed." A call was made to the county resource, a crisis worker evaluated the patient and concluded he was not "a danger to himself or others," not meeting criteria for an involuntary hold.[12] He was discharged for follow-up the next day with the counseling center, but was found to have allegedly taken his own life 2 days later. The family filed suit under the Emergency Medical Treatment and Labor Act (EMTALA) and the California Health and Safety Code for failure to perform an adequate medical screen.[13,14] The trial court granted summary judgment for the defendants. The United States Court of Appeals, Ninth Circuit held that the attempt to seek redress for failure to perform adequate medical screening, ostensibly for lack of payment, was misdirected and affirmed the trial court judgment.

In *Kassen* v. *Hatley*, the patient was found walking on an expressway, taking additional prescribed medicine and threatening to harm herself, and was taken to a psychiatric emergency room.[15] There was allegedly a dispute with hospital staff over her medication. The ED offered a taxi ride home as a quid pro quo, security came to escort her, and according to court records she left the ED voluntarily. She allegedly stepped in front of freeway traffic a short time later and died as a result. The family filed a wrongful-death action. The nurse argued she was not liable because the Texas Civil Practice and Remedies Code provides an affirmative defense in the case of suicide.[16] The trial court granted summary judgment for the resident physician and Southwestern (the training program), while proceeding to trial against the nurse and Parkland (the treating facility), again with directed defense verdicts. The Supreme Court of Texas held that the question of official immunity was not properly established. They reversed the appellate court summary judgment for the nurse and the directed verdict for the physician and remanded to trial court for further proceedings. They concluded the plaintiff failed to allege an injury from a condition or use of property and reversed the appellate court judgment for the hospital defendants. The Texas Civil Practice and Remedies Code addresses the question of whether the patient's suicide was caused by the deprivation of her personal property in the setting of her medical records, the difficult patient file, the ED procedures manual, and the confiscated medication as evidence.[17] Both hospital facilities were entitled to prevail on their defense of sovereign immunity.

Conclusion

Suicide is perhaps the ultimate tragedy that can be encountered in the practice of health care, so an especially high level of scrutiny is required in the ED. An integrated care program involving mental health resources, community support networks, and family is required to establish an effective care and safety plan.

References

1. Doshi A, Boudreaux ED, Wang N, Pelletier AJ, Carmago CA. National study of US emergency department visits for attempted suicide and self-inflicted injury, 1997–2001. *Ann Emerg Med.* 2005;46(4):369–375. DOI:10.1016// j.annemergmed.2005.04.018.

2. Larkin GL, Smith RP, Beautrais AL. Trends in US emergency department visits for suicide attempts, 1992–2001. *Crisis.* 2008;29(2):73–80. DOI:10.1027/0227-5910.29.2.73.

3. King CA, O'Mara RM, Hayward CN, Cunningham RM. Adolescent suicide risk screening in the emergency department. *Acad Emerg Med.* 2009;16(11):1234–1241. DOI:1111/j.1553-2712.2009.00500.x.

4. Problem Oriented Screening Instrument for Teenagers (POSIT) (Bethesda, MD: National Institute of Drug Abuse, 1991).

5. Claassen CA, Larkin GL. Occult suicidality in an emergency department population. *Br J Psychiatry.* 2005;186(4):352–353. DOI:10.1192/bjp.186.4.352.

6. Gairin I, House A, Owens D. Attendance at the accident and emergency department in the year before suicide: retrospective study. *Br J Psychiatry.* 2003;183(1):28–33. DOI:10.1192/bjp.183.1.28.

7. Da Cruz D, Pearson A, Saini P, Miles C, While D, Swinson N, et al. Emergency department contact prior to suicide in mental health patients. *Emerg Med J.* 2011;28(6):467–471. DOI:10.1136/emj.2009.081869.

8. Hickey L, Hawton K, Fagg J, Weitzel H. Deliberate self-harm patients who leave the accident and emergency department without a psychiatric assessment: a neglected population at risk of suicide. *J Psychom Res.* 2001;50(2):87–93. DOI:10.1016/S0022-3999(00)00225-7.

9. Crandall C, Fullerton-Gleason L, Aguero R, LaValley J. Subsequent suicide mortality among emergency department patients seen for suicidal behavior. *Acad Emerg Med.* 2006;13(4):435–442. DOI:10.1197/j.aem.2005.11.072.

10. *Tabor* v. *Doctors Memorial Hospital*, 563 So. 2d 233 (1990).

11. *Baker* v. *Adventist Health*, 260 F.3d 987 (2001).

12. California Welfare and Institutions Code §5150.

13. EMTALA, 42 U.S.C. §1395 dd.

14. California Health and Safety Code §1317 (2011).

15. *Kassen* v. *Hatley*, 887 S.W.2d 4 (1994).

16. Texas Civil Practice and Remedies Code §93.001 (a) (2): Assumption of the Risk: Affirmative Defense.

17. Texas Civil Practice and Remedies Code §101.021 (2): Governmental Liability.

Telemedicine

Chapter

Case

The physician had practiced emergency medicine for a long time, and done his share of nights, weekends, and holidays. He was also concerned about the malpractice litigation risk in his current work environment, so decided to pursue a career in telemedicine instead. This allowed him to work from home with lower-acuity patients. He was quite satisfied with his new practice, which consisted mainly of minor emergencies, typically coughs and colds and miscellaneous aches. He occasionally prescribed antibiotics, and always referred the patient back to their primary care physician (PCP) for additional care.

About 6 months after he started this telemedicine practice, he was contacted by the legal counsel retained by the group who suggested there was an allegation of medical malpractice involving both the group and himself. The physician responded that these were lower-acuity cases, and he wondered how anything could go wrong in that environment. The attorney replied that the case was more complicated than it appeared. The telemedicine practice was a new medical endeavor and it was indeed a lower-risk specialty, but there was an allegation of individual medical malpractice that had to be defended.

Medical Approach

The telemedicine program is an exciting new area of acute care medicine allowing convenience for the patient and family, as well as a new work approach for both newly qualified and experienced practicing physicians. The typical scenario allows the physician to work from a home setting either in a consistent time block or intermittently over time.

The telemedicine marketplace is rapidly evolving, although there is significantly more experience in the international marketplace with time and distance

constraints. The globalization of health-care services allows technology to be exported from sophisticated environments to be imported by those with fewer resources.[1] Multilateral trade agreements and an effective communications network are key. The "importing" countries receive more rapid care delivery in a more cost-effective fashion as remote labor and technology are provided at lower cost in the offshore environment. In return, the "exporting" countries receive foreign exchange, financial benefit, and quality improvement.

The most common current use of telemedicine in the United States is for minor complaints. Mair reported on a minor injury telemedicine service providing oversight to 15 community hospital-based minor injury units.[2] They studied 112 patients referred to the emergency department (ED) by three minor injury units and observed several trends. The facility with the highest telemedicine use had the lowest ED transfer rate (2%). The facility that had all radiographs reviewed offsite referred the most (85%). They concluded that the advent of telemedicine would reduce the 80–85% rate of ED referral.

The use of telemedicine may also help to facilitate early hospital discharge. Early discharge plans are often met with concerns over safety, malpractice litigation, and patient or family anxiety.[3] The telemedicine approach allows communication from a remote monitoring center to a home-based computer transmitting audio, video, and vital signs data. The benefits include cost savings and more rapid convalescence at home.

Eron et al. described a plan in which patients with pneumonia, cellulitis, or urinary tract infection may be potentially treated at home depending on disease severity, comorbidities, and Karnofsky Performance Status.[4] The Karnofsky score, often used in oncology patients, assesses functional capability and ranges from 0 (death) to 100 (perfect health).[5] Patients treated with telemedicine manifest satisfactory clinical outcomes and appear to recover more rapidly than comparable hospitalized patients.

To evaluate the cost-saving benefits of telemedicine programs, McCue et al. studied a cohort of 290 correctional patients cared for within a telemedicine program.[6] They balanced the cost of operating the telemedicine system, transportation, litigation avoidance, and the quality of the medical care itself. There was a slight decrease in cost (3.6%), but greater access to medical care.

In a meta-analysis, Miller studied the effect of telemedicine on physician–patient communication.[7] Of the 38 studies identified, 55.2% (21) were post-encounter patient surveys, 29% (11) were analyses of behavior, and 16% (6) studied provider and community attitudes. The majority (55%, 21) of programs were based in the United States, with the remainder at international sites. The overall majority (80%) of respondents favored telemedicine with positive opinions. However, in a minority of categories sampled (7%, 2/28), specifically non-verbal behavior and lack of touch, opinion was negative. Verbal content analysis is the cornerstone of a quality improvement program to facilitate physician–patient communication.

The overall effectiveness of telemedicine has been evaluated by Ekeland et al. in a systematic review.[8] They evaluated 1593 telemedicine articles or abstracts and identified 12% (80) heterogeneous systematic reviews. They found 26% (21) of reviews demonstrated effectiveness, 22.5% (18) found evidence was promising but incomplete, and 51.2% (41) found evidence that was limited and inconsistent. New studies should focus on controlled interventions measuring economic analysis and patient benefits, and monitoring collaborative programs.

The implementation of any new technology requires management of all aspects of clinical risk. Telemedicine allows one to transfer clinical information and decision-making capability, to reduce clinical risk.[9] The telemedicine system must ensure that the clinical data and discussion are preserved for clinical audit and quality monitoring. The system also requires equipment that has adequate technical specifications and is sufficiently reliable, with secure information storage and adequate backup in the case of system failure.

The key to medicolegal management is the use of protocols, guidelines, and care standards. Loane reviewed three types of telemedicine guidelines: clinical, operational, and technical (Table 98.1).[10] The

Table 98.1 Telemedicine guidelines and standards

1.	Clinical	Teleradiology
		Telepsychiatry
		Home telenursing
		Minor injury telemedicine
		Surgical telemedicine
		Teledermatology
		Telepathology
2.	Operational	Email communications
		Internet access
		Videoconferencing
3.	Technical	American Telemedicine Association
		US Office for the Advancement of Telehealth
4.	Standards	International Telecommunications Union
		DICOM

Reference: Loane.[10]

clinical guidelines included those for teleradiology, telepsychiatry, home telenursing, minor injury telemedicine, surgical telemedicine, teledermatology, and telepathology. Operational guidelines identified include those for email communication, high-speed internet access, and videoconferencing. Technical guidelines included those from the American Telehealth Association and the US Office for the Advancement of Telehealth. The standards relevant to telemedicine practice included those of the International Telecommunications Union and the DICOM standard.

The rapidly changing telecommunications technology requires a proactive legal approach to ensure the patient's right to confidentiality and the security of medical records are not breached. There are seven interfaces of direct concern: informed consent, physician liability, non-physician liability, costs, practice parameters, physician–patient relationships, and ergonomics (Table 98.2).[11] The risk management or legal department should have early input into project design.

As with any new discipline there can be medicolegal challenges, and currently there is discussion concerning proper state-based licensing of practitioners challenging the ability to treat patients or prescribe across state lines. Although the majority of patients are not acutely unwell, standard concerns still apply.

Table 98.2 High-risk areas in telemedicine

1. Informed consent
2. Physician liability
3. Non-physician liability
4. Costs
5. Practice parameters
6. Physician–patient relationships
7. Ergonomics

Reference Lott[11]

This may include referral to the ED, the PCP, or a specialty physician for proper follow-up.

Legal and regulatory barriers to telemedicine have come to the fore. Telemedicine is defined as "the use of medical information exchanged from one site to another via electronic communications to improve patients' health status."[12] The benefits include making a better quality of care available at a decreased cost. However, in the United States the state-based medical regulatory process can complicate and inhibit this transaction. To be most effective, advanced telemedicine will require federal oversight of interstate commerce or international regulation of global encounters.

One of the most crucial issues in telemedicine is proper security for patient information. The key is to ensure the right information is associated with the right patient. The exponential increase in the number of electronic health-care document exchanges has increased the risk of document drop-out or address errors.[13] "Watermarking" or the embedding of security elements, such as a digital signature, within a document can be used to ensure reliability. Encryption provides a-priori protection, requiring processing for reviewing. Watermarking provides a-posteriori protection, allowing free document access but still verifying data integrity, maintaining the patient record link and the reader interpretation link. However, there can be questions of validity regarding the proof and its legal acceptability.

Legal Analysis

In *USA* v. *Quinones*, a retailer and a physician allegedly authorized controlled substance prescriptions after an online questionnaire was completed and credit card payment authorized.[14] The defendants were charged in a superseding indictment with conspiracy to distribute, and possess with intent to distribute, controlled substances in violation of 21 U.S.C. §§841–846.[15] All defendants but the physician moved to dismiss on the grounds the acts they were alleged to have committed are not proscribed by federal drug laws; and alternatively they are unconstitutionally vague. The United States District Court, E.D. New York denied the defendant's motion for dismissal, which was previously affirmed as proper. They relied on Puerto Rico's Telemedicine Act, which authorizes licensed physicians to provide medical services, including prescriptions via "advanced technology telecommunication means" to patients in "distant geographical areas."[16] In addition, "oral and written informed consent of the patient" is required before performing telemedicine services. Even assuming the website information constituted "written consent," no physician ever spoke with the patient. The court held that most reasonable people would feel the statute applied to situations like this without having to consider exceptions, citing "a statute or regulation is not required to specify every prohibited act." [17]

In *Hageseth* v. *Superior Court of San Mateo County*, the district attorney filed a criminal complaint alleging unlawful practice of medicine in California without a license.[18] The patient, a resident of California, purchased an online prescription from an overseas interactive website, after a domestic physician subcontractor in Colorado forwarded the patient questionnaire to the corporate headquarters in Florida with a prescription shipped from a Mississippi pharmacy. The petitioner claimed the alleged acts occurred outside the state and jurisdiction should be denied. The trial court felt the evidence was sufficient to survive the demurrer and denied the motion to dismiss. The issue of personal or territorial jurisdiction-based internet or "network-mediated" contacts are more rooted in civil than criminal proceedings under the "minimum contact" standards of *International Shoe Co.* v. *Washington*.[19] The forum state cannot assert personal jurisdiction over an out-of-state resident unless they have availed themselves of the privileges and benefits of conducting activities within the forum. The practice of telemedicine, or health-care delivery, diagnosis, consultation, treatment, transfer of medical data and education using interactive audio, video, or data communications, is specifically authorized by the Telemedicine Development Act of 1996.[20] The Medical Practice Act exempts from the unlawful practice of medicine a practitioner located outside the state, when in actual consultation, whether within the state or across state lines, with a licensed practitioner of the state, provided only that the out-of-state practitioner does not "appoint a place to meet patients (in the state), receive calls from patients within the limits of his state, give orders or have ultimate authority over the care or primary diagnosis of a patient who is located within the state." [21] The California Court of Appeals, First District held there is no persuasive reason why the petitioner's or other business partners' use of cyberspace should defeat the application of traditional legal principles to define extraterritorial jurisdiction. The petition to dismiss was denied, and the temporary stay dissolved.

In *MacDonald* v. *Schriro*, the patient was treated for a left knee injury, had a conservative course implemented, and then MRI to follow.[22] There was a subsequent telemedicine evaluation, during which the plaintiff was fully clothed and seated, with a treatment course including a knee brace and anti-inflammatory medications. The plaintiff alleged deliberate indifference to his medical condition filed as a 42 U.S.C. §1983 complaint implementing an Eighth Amendment claim of cruel and unusual punishment.[23] The United States Court of Appeals, D. Arizona denied the defendant's summary judgment motion, and proceeded to trial to evaluate whether deliberate indifference toward his health condition was indeed exhibited.

In *USA* v. *Maye*, the physician notified the New York Office of Professional Medical Conduct he would resume practice as a telemedicine consultant providing phone and online consultation to customers seeking medications over the internet.[24] He would establish bona fide physician–patient relationships as required, obtained medical histories, reviewed files and approved or denied prescription requests. The physician was convicted for allegedly distributing and dispensing controlled substances not in the usual course of medical practice. The district court went on to grant the government request for a preliminary order of forfeiture in a reduced amount.

Conclusion

The explosive growth of telemedicine is coming under greater medicolegal scrutiny each day. As this is a novel way of practicing medicine, primary education in the discipline is essential. It is also a nascent medicolegal risk area requiring a comprehensive risk mitigation strategy.

References

1. Alvarez MA, Chanda R, Smith RD. How is telemedicine perceived? A qualitative study of perspectives from the UK and India. *Global Health*. 2011;17:17. DOI:10.1186/1744-8603-7-17.

2. Mair F. More patients with minor injuries could be seen by telemedicine. *J Telemed Telecare*. 2008;14(3):132–134. DOI:10.1258/jtt.2008.003009.

3. Eron L. Telemedicine: the future of outpatient therapy? *Clin Infect Dis*. 2010;51(S2):S224–S230. DOI:10.1086/653524.

4. Eron L, King P, Marineau M, Yonehara C. Treating acute infections by telemedicine in the home. *Clin Infect Dis*. 2004;39(8):1175–1181. DOI.10.1086/424671.

5. Karnofsky DA, Abelmann WH, Craver LF, Burchenal JH. The use of nitrogen mustards in the palliative treatment of carcinoma, with particular reference to bronchogenic carcinoma. *Cancer*. 1948;1(4):634–656.

6. McCue MJ, Mazmznian PE, Hampton CL, Marks TK, Fisher EJ, Parpart F, et al. Cost-minimization analysis: a follow-up study of a telemedicine program. *Telemed J*. 1998;4(4):323–327. doi10.1089/tmj.1.1998.4.323.

7. Miller EA. Telemedicine and doctor-patient communication: an analytical survey of the literature. *J Telemed Telecare*. 2001;7(1):1–17. DOI:10.1258/1357633011936075.

8. Ekeland AG, Bowes A, Flottoro S. Effectiveness of telemedicine: a systematic review of reviews. *Med Inform*. 2010;79(11):736–771. DOI:10.1016/ijmedinf.2010.08.006.

9. Darkins A. The management of clinical risk in telemedicine applications. *J Telemed Telecare*. 1996;2(4):179–184. DOI:10.1258/1357633961930022.

10. Loane M. A review of guidelines and standards for telemedicine. *J Telemed Telecare*. 2002;8(2):63–71. DOI:10.1258/1357633021937479.

11. Lott CM. Legal interfaces in telemedicine technology. *Mil Med*. 1996;161(5):280–283.

12. Sao D, Gupta A, Gantz DA. Legal and regulatory barriers to telemedicine in the United States: public and private approaches toward health care reform. Chapter 20 in: *The Globalization of Health Care: Legal and Ethical Issues*, ed. I. Glenn Cohen (Oxford: Oxford University Press, 2013), pp. 359–380.

13. Coatrieux G, Quantin C, Allaert FA. Watermarking as a traceability standard. In: *Quality of Life Through Quality of Information*, ed. J. Mantas et al. (Amsterdam: IOS Press, 2012), pp. 761–765. DOI:3233/978-1-61499-101-4-761.

14. *United States* v. *Quinones*, 536 F. Supp.2d 267 (2008).

15. 21 U.S.C. §§841, 846. Prohibited Acts, Attempt and Conspiracy.

16. 20 L.P.R.A. §6001: Telemedicine Act.

17. *Perez* v. *Hoblock*, 368 F.3d 166, 175. 2d Cir. (2004).

18. *Hageseth* v. *Superior Court of San Mateo County*, 59 Cal. Rptr.3d 385 (2007).

19. *International Shoe Co.* v. *Washington*, 326 U.S. 310, 66 S Ct. 154, 90 L.Ed. 95 (1945).

20. California Business and Professions Code §2290.5, subd (a) (1) Telemedicine Development Act of 1996.

21. California Business and Professions Code §2060: Legal Medical Consultation with Doctors Outside California.

22. *MacDonald* v. *Schriro*, No. CV 04-1001-PHX-SMM (MHB). Arizona. July 17, 2008.

23. 42 U.S. Code §1983, Civil Action for Deprivation of Rights.

24. *USA* v. *Maye*, No. 08-CR-194S. New York. April 23, 2014.

Telephone Advice

Case

The call came in to the emergency department (ED) and was transferred to the triage nurse. It was a mother wanting some information about her child's health. The nurse listened politely and suggested the ED could not offer any medical advice and she should call her pediatrician, but the ED was available for evaluation at all times. The mother asked if the department was busy and the nurse told her it was always busy, but they would see patients who were in need and she should bring her daughter in if she thought it was warranted. As she was about to end the call, the mother asked one more question: "Do you know the dose of Tylenol that I might give her?" The nurse again cautioned she was prohibited from giving medical advice, but she had daughters of her own. She calculated the proper 10 mg/kg dose of Tylenol [acetaminophen, paracetamol] and gave the mother that information.

Six months later the hospital was in receipt of a lawsuit suggesting the child had indeed had meningitis but the mother was not advised to bring the child in and was allegedly instructed to give her Tylenol and see how she did at home. The ED director was questioned, asking if they had a protocol in place for the nurses to give telephone advice. The director replied they had clear guidelines on what is recommended in various scenarios.

Medical Approach

These cases at the intersection of protocol and caring are often difficult. Health-care providers – both nurses and physicians – have an inherent desire to try to give patients helpful advice. It has become clear over time that the medicolegal risk of telephone advice outweighs the benefits. So, in most institutions the recommended course includes: first, advise that you are not allowed to give telephone medical advice; second, the ED is available for immediate care. There should

be no comments on whether the ED is busy or not busy, or about the triage process, patients just need to know the ED is there and available for them; third, it is often suggested that the patient call their primary care physician (PCP) instead of presenting to the ED. This recommendation is typically not warranted in a situation like this, and poses another potential risk bordering on Emergency Medical Treatment and Labor Act (EMTALA) concerns (Table 99.1).

Management of telephone liability risk is a major area of concern in patient referral call lines. Bartlett described a screening call system in which the majority (28.5%) are pediatric patients, then internal medicine (24.6%), obstetric and gynecology (19.6%), and family medicine (19.4%).[1]

Analysis of medical malpractice related to a telephone nursing system was examined by Ernesater et al.[2] They analyzed 33 claims stemming from phone advice calls in which 39% (13) of the patients died, and 36% (12) were admitted to the intensive care unit (ICU). They cited failure to listen to the caller as the most common issue (36%, 12), and discussion within the work group (39%, 13) the most common intervention. The most common symptoms were abdominal pain (33%, 11) and chest pain (18%, 6). Telenurses followed up in 18.6% of cases to ensure adequate patient understanding. Third-party health calls create an area of risk, and reevaluation is required in those with multiple repeat contacts.

Telephone triage programs are a common use of this technology. Barber et al. evaluated 133 physician referrals compared to 260 control patients to a pediatric emergency department.[3] They used a blinded Delphi rating system to review the referrals and if two of three pediatric emergency medicine physicians agreed, then it was an appropriate referral. (The Delphi methodology, borrowing its name from the Ancient Greek oracle, assumes that an informed group makes a better subjective assessment than an

Table 99.1 Telephone advice protocol

1.	Advise you are not permitted to give phone advice
2.	ED is available for immediate care
3.	Recommendation to contact primary care not required
4.	Insurance contact not required

unselected group.[4]) They found that referrals from the Pediatric Health Information Line (80.2%) had a higher appropriate referral rate compared to controls (60.5%, x^2 = 14.6369, OR 2.65, 95% CI 1.5759–4.5008). The study supports the use of a speciality referral line with 33% higher accuracy rate.

The provision of unsolicited advice from the ED is felt to be a high-risk area. The American College of Emergency Physicians (ACEP) has published a policy resource and education paper commenting on the matter.[5] The ED frequently receives unsolicited calls from the public, requesting detailed instruction or medical advice. Managed care networks make extensive use of the telephone referral process. Caselaw indicates that expectations for those receiving telephone-based medical advice will not be significantly less than those with on-site triage.

A prospective study of telephone calls for medical advice to an accident and emergency (A&E) department was performed by Singh et al.[6] They evaluated 154 calls over a 10-day period, averaging 15.4 calls per day. The public felt that the A&E department was the most logical area to contact. However, less than one-third (30%)[46] had attempted to seek advice from their general practitioner before calling A&E.

The standard for medicolegal analysis is a closed claims review of telephone physician–patient encounters. Katz et al. reported on 32 claims involving 40 defendants, in which the leading practitioners sued included internists, pediatricians, and obstetricians.[7] The cases were reviewed by a physician experienced in telephone medicine with the input of two additional risk management analysts. The majority (60%, 24) of cases were settled or awarded to the plaintiff, with an average indemnity of $518,932. The most common allegation was failed diagnosis (68%) and the most common injury was death (44%). The most common setting was a general internal medicine ambulatory practice. The leading errors were in documentation (88%), followed by faulty triage (84%). It is crucial to recognize telephone-related claims were costly and injuries were catastrophic.

Legal Analysis

In *St. John* v. *Pope*, the patient presented to the ED complaining of back pain and fever after back surgery with an elevated white blood cell count.[8] The ED physician allegedly diagnosed the patient with back pain and psychosis. The wife requested transfer to a facility closer to their home. Contact with the on-call physician, an internist, suggested the patient would be better served by a hospital that routinely handled neurologic or neurosurgical emergencies. The ED physician then contacted the physician at another facility, but the ED refused to accept the transfer. The wife did not want to admit to that facility and took the patient home against advice, where he suffered a bout of meningitis with sequelae. The issue raised in the filing was whether consulting the on-call physician by the ED physician by telephone created a physician–patient relationship based on that physician's recommendation to transfer to another facility. The trial court rendered a take-nothing summary judgment, in which there would be no financial reward even if there was merit, in favor of the physician. The appellate court reversed the trial court decision, holding the facility owed "a duty of ordinary care to the patient such that a reasonably prudent person would recognize that such acts would place the patient in danger." However, the Supreme Court of Texas reversed the appellate court decision, restoring the take-nothing verdict to the physician. The defendant established that no relationship was established by the call, so no duty was owed.

In *Weaver* v. *University of Michigan Board of Regents*, a pediatric patient with hydrocephalus had a shunt implanted and was followed up until the parents transferred care to a more local neurosurgeon and had two office visits.[9] The patient subsequently complained of visual issues and was seen by their pediatrician, who ordered a CT scan, and was seen by neurosurgery. The neurosurgeon allegedly concluded the shunt had become disconnected, but thought this did not constitute an emergency and suggested they should seek a "second opinion." They called a second neurosurgeon, booked an appointment in a month's time, then rescheduled earlier. At that appointment the second neurosurgeon felt emergency surgery was required, but unfortunately significant visual loss occurred. The family filed suit against the pediatrician, neurosurgeon, and hospital, followed by a settlement, and a grant of summary disposition to the remaining defendant. The Michigan Court of Appeals declined to recognize a physician–patient relationship from a single telephone call from a parent to schedule an appointment, when no medical advice was sought or obtained in that call.

In *Adams* v. *Christi Regional Medical Center*, the patient, who was pregnant, presented to the ED with significant abdominal pain.[10] The family contacted their PCP, a family practitioner, who had not seen their daughter, and who no longer provided obstetric care, although the family stated they had not received written notice of this. The family notified their PCP, and the history was allegedly variable regarding an ED referral, but she was offered an office appointment the next day. She worsened by midnight, was taken to the ED, and suffered a catastrophic event. Her PCP was contacted late the next afternoon, and support was withdrawn. The parents filed suit, settled hospital claims, and jury awarded trial verdict to the family as well against their PCP. Because the parents had already received the statutory financial limit the jury awarded no judgment for wrongful death damages. The parents appealed the judgment and the PCP cross-claimed on liability. The case was transferred to the Supreme Court of Kansas to assign the case properly.[11] That court held that the phone discussion with family about the patient's medical condition renewed the medical relationship, even though the PCP did not speak to the patient herself. The family alleged the cross-appellant did not submit an adequate record to establish the claimed error, and without an adequate record the claim fails.[12] The judgment on wrongful death damages was reversed, and the matter remanded to district court to enter a financial judgment against the PCP.

In *Medley* v. *Jewish Hospital*, the patient presented to the ED initially complaining of chest pain radiating to her back.[13] By the time an ED physician examined her, the documented complaint was abdominal pain and an episode of bloody diarrhea. The patient was admitted after a number of diagnostic tests, admitted to her internal medicine physician after telephone consult, and then transferred to the intensive care unit after a gastrointestinal consult by telephone as well. Because of a bed delay, the patient remained in the ED, the evaluating ED physician's shift ended, and the oncoming ED physician was not aware of the patient's presence. There was a radiology overread of the admission chest radiograph with a concern for aneurysm. There were conflicting reports in

the record of the transfer of this information between the numerous health-care providers. The Court of Appeals of Kentucky heard the appeal and cross-appeal of the defense verdict on the medical malpractice case alleging failure to diagnose aortic dissection, and affirmed. They commented that the oncoming ED physician owed no additional special duty since the patient did not have any clinical change while in the ED. Likewise, they dismissed additional claims based on the statute of limitations. Although it appears the radiographs were not visualized by some defendants, radiology reading logs were accessed by others. Phone communications between health care providers were considered part of the factual record.

Another area of focus is the use of telephone triage for health-care referrals. In *Thornton* v. *Shah*, the patient, who was pregnant, called the insurance after-hours nursing line, complaining of bleeding and contractions.[14] There were a number of calls over the next week to the referral line, involving the obstetrician, and the patient was apparently told to present to the ED when contractions were 10 minutes apart. There was a subsequent office visit, absent fetal heart tones, and an induced delivery with fetal demise. The plaintiff filed suit against the physician and subsequently the health maintenance organization (HMO), in which the first two counts addressed the physician's response to the call center. There was a factual dispute between the physician and nurses staffing the call center concerning notification of patient findings. The nurse described the telephone triage protocol, in which there was a section to note physician contact, the physician's decision to return the patient's call, and the nurse had the ability to render their own decision without contacting the physician. Further counts were directed against the HMO alleging a contract breach for not allowing physician access. The final count alleged negligent spoliation, as the call records were not retained for review. The circuit court dismissed all claims except the first two counts with prejudice. The Appellate Court of Illinois, First District affirmed the proper dismissal of these claims.

Conclusion

The "one more question" telephone scenario must be avoided. Even something as benign as advising a proper medication dose can be construed as offering medical care advice, resulting in the allegation of establishing a care relationship. Specific scripted protocols should provide clear guidelines to the staff on the proper response to phone inquiries.

References

1. Bartlett EE, Managing your telephone liability risks. *J Health Risk Manag*. 1995;15(3):30–36. DOI:10.1002/jhrm.5600150307.

2. Ernesater A, Winblad U, Engstrom M, Holmstrom IK. Malpractice claims regarding calls to Swedish telephone advice nursing: what went wrong and why? *J Telemed Telecare*. 2012;18(7):379–383. DOI:10.1258/jtt.2012.120416.

3. Barber JW, King WD, Monroe KW, Nichols MH. Evaluation of emergency department referrals by telephone triage. *Pediatrics*. 2000;105(4 Pt 1):819–821.

4. Brown BB. Delphi process: a methodology used for the elicitation of opinions of experts. An earlier paper published by RAND, Document No. P-3925, 1968, 15.

5. Proctor JH, Hirshberg AJ, Kazzi AA, Parker RB. Providing telephone advice from the emergency department. *Ann Emerg Med*. 2002;49(2):217–219. DOI:10.1067/mem.2002.126398.

6. Singh G, Barton D, Bodiwais GG. Accident & emergency department's response to patients' inquiries by telephone. *J Roy Soc Med*. 1991;84(6):345–346. DOI:10.1177/014107689108400613.

7. Katz HP, Kaltsounis D, Halloran L, Mondor M. Patient safety and telephone medicine: some lessons from closed claim case review. *J Gen Int Med*. 2008;23(5):517–522. DOI:10.1007/s11606-007-0491-y.

8. *St John M.D.* v. *Pope*, 901 S.W.2d 420 (1995).

9. *Weaver* v. *University of Michigan Board of Regents*, 506 N.W.2d 264 (1993).

10. *Adams* v. *Christi Regional Medical Center*, 19 P.3d 132 (2001).

11. Kansas Statutes Annotated K.S.A. 20–3018 (c): Transfer of Cases.

12. *Adams* v. *Christi*, 180 S.W.3d 386 (Tex. App. 2005).

13. *Medley et al.* v. *Jewish Hospital Inc., et al.*, Nos. 2008-CA-001111-MR, 001192-MR, 001244-MR, October 9, 2009.

14. *Thornton* v. *Shah*, 777 N.E.2d 396 (2002).

Third-Party Duty

Case

The physicians had worked in the hospital's emergency department (ED) for a good number of years as hospital-based employees. However, recently the hospital system had been sold, resulting in a change in hospital management. The new owners felt that subcontracting the ED service to a third-party employed group would have financial benefits for the facility, as well as minimizing their medicolegal risk. This was the standardized process throughout their hospital system. The director discussed this with the partners in the group, pointing out the financial benefits. At this point the recommendation was to set up an independent corporation to provide professional services, and operations were largely unchanged.

Later that year, the hospital's retained corporate counsel was in receipt of a professional liability medical malpractice claim that threatened a seven-figure claim alleging medical malpractice. The legal process entailed that the physician group had initially filed a claim with an equal portion of the liability directed at the hospital. However, the hospital attempted to obtain a summary judgment motion excluding themselves from litigation as they had no third-party agency relationship with this professional service group, who bore the responsibility for ED operations. Since the hospital entirely subcontracted the service, the corporate counsel then stated that the plaintiff attempted to shift the entire medicolegal burden and financial demand to the ED physician group. He added that this move was typically not successful, as the hospital was perceived as being in charge of the facility's operation.

The attorney asked to see the physician staff's hospital identification badges. The director had brought his with him, but had left it in his car. Another physician's badge stated the name of the hospital with "Staff Physician" underneath. The attorney pointed out that this is just one of many factors that would be take

into consideration, but it would tend to support the contention that the physicians were indeed hospital employees. Later that week the badges were reissued identifying the holders as "Contracted Physicians"

Medical Approach

The provision of medical care often requires examination for third-party relationships in that an oversight organization is typically the hospital. They are often perceived as having the "deepest pockets" in the business relationship. The facilities are typically equally split between those that employ their physicians and those that use a subcontracted group. With a subcontracted group, the liabilities are felt to be put at arm's length and the theory is there is no agency relationship or responsibility for the hospital to cover the actions of the group providing professional service, except in the most egregious of circumstances. However, this is often not the public perception.

The "business" of medicine undergoes almost continuous change. There has been a drive for integration to capture market share. *Vertical integration* is the combination of the hierarchy of the entire sequential chain of health-care delivery service from system entry to exit.[1] *Horizontal integration* captures market share by acquiring the entire level of the same health-care resource in an area, such as all the physicians. The balance is controlling enough of the marketplace to matter, while still avoiding antitrust concerns.

The strategic integration of hospitals and physicians has often been suggested to improve care efficiency in the managed care model. An evaluation by Cuellar and Gertler demonstrated little effect on care efficiency, with a tendency to increase prices especially when the integrated care organization is exclusive, occurring in less competitive marketplaces.[2]

Lee evaluated hospital clinical integration based on data from a number of health-care system databases.[3]

This study tested the hypothesis that structural clinical integration is negatively related to average total charge and positively related to adverse patient outcomes. Significant associations were found between structural clinical integration and average total charge per admission, between average total charge per admission and surgical complication, and between surgical complication and in-hospital death. However, the study did not demonstrate the expected reduction in total charge per admission.

Another study utilized Donabedian's model for health-care outcomes research, analyzing three areas including structure, process, and outcomes to draw inferences on quality.[4] They concluded that highly integrated structures demonstrated no immediate financial benefit, and structural clinical integration had only an indirect effect on patient care outcomes.

Lake et al. studied recent developments in hospital–physician relationships in 12 randomly selected metropolitan areas, interviewing 895 respondents.[5] As the benefits of HMO enrollment and capitation plateaued, 65% of facilities still owned primary care practices. The ownership is more prevalent in concentrated marketplaces, but the majority (55%) of hospitals have decreased the size of these practices. They have returned to a strategy of pursuing specialists, seeking additional fee-for-service revenue. Some of the interest in the formation of integrated care delivery systems, emphasizing primary care and coordinating hospital and physician services, has waned as definable quality goals may not have materialized. There is a newer emphasis on hospital–specialist partnerships which may improve hospital finances and address quality issues in specific markets, but may increase health-care costs incurred by consumers.

The nature of the hospital–physician affiliation can be predictive of both financial expenditures and patient outcomes. Madison performed a multivariate regression analysis of hospital–physician affiliations, such as physician–hospital organizations or salaried employment, and treatment of Medicare patients with myocardial infarction.[6] The integrated salary model was associated with slightly higher procedure rates and higher patient expenditure. There was little evidence that the type of hospital–physician affiliation had any appreciable impact on patient treatment or outcome.

Hospital–physician relationships (HPR), such as gain sharing, bundled payments, and

Table 100.1 Strategies for hospital–physician collaboration

1.	Better physician financial conditions
2.	Change to internal operations
3.	Application of behavioral skills to management
4.	Change provider payment model
5.	Simultaneous change

Reference: Burns and Muller.[7]

pay-for-performance (P4P) can have tremendous impact on a hospital's financial success.[7] There is often only partial overlap of interests in achieving the meritable goals of improving quality and reducing cost. Currently, the relationship between clinical integration and financial benefit that has been studied is weak and inconsistent.

The success of the HPR is often contingent on several factors. First, providing better financial conditions or incentives for physicians. Second, changes to internal operations and systems. Third, the application of behavioral skills to the HPR management improves operation. Fourth, changes in the provider payment model can impact efficiency. Fifth, significant systematic change may need to be applied simultaneously to achieve success (Table 100.1).[7]

Legal Analysis

Most legal cases turn on the issue of hospital corporate liability. In *Elam* v. *College Park Hospital*, the plaintiff alleged medical malpractice after a surgical procedure, alleging the hospital was obligated to ensure physician quality.[8] The question addressed is whether the hospital is liable under a doctrine of corporate liability for the negligent conduct of independent physicians, who are members of the medical staff, but are neither employees nor agents of the hospital.[9] The Court of Appeals of California answered this question in the affirmative and reversed the trial court judgment. They found that no appellate decision of this state addressing precisely this application of corporate hospital liability, so the matter was treated as one of first impression. The premise accords with statutory authority recognizing hospital accountability or the quality of the medical care provided and the competency of the medical staff according to the state Health and Safety Code.[10] They held that the hospital generally owes a duty to ensure the competency of its medical staff, and to evaluate the quality of the medical care delivered on the premises.

In *Jackson* v. *Power*, a teenage patient had a significant fall and was airlifted to the hospital ED.[11] He was examined by an ED physician working in an independent contractor relationship. Tests and diagnostics were ordered, but allegedly the patient suffered significant renal vascular injury and subsequent renal failure. The family filed suit alleging negligence, attempting to hold the facility vicariously liable under three theories: (1) enterprise liability; (2) apparent authority; (3) a non-delegable duty. The superior court held the facility could not be held liable by an enterprise liability theory, but summary judgment motion was not granted as there was a factual dispute concerning the other theories. First, the "enterprise liability" theory finds liability whenever the enterprise of the employer would have benefited by the context of the act of the employee, "but for" the unfortunate injury that may have occurred.[12] Second, the "apparent" or "ostensible" agency provides that:

One who employs an independent contractor to perform services for another which are accepted in the reasonable belief that the services are rendered by the employer or by his servants, is subject to liability for physical harm caused by the negligence of the contractor in supplying such services, to the same extent as though the employer were supplying himself or by his servants.[13]

There are two relevant factors to find for ostensible agency: (1) whether the patient looks to the institution rather than the individual physician for care, and (2) whether the hospital "holds out" the physician as its employee.[14] Third, the "non-delegable duty" requires that if a hospital undertakes to operate an emergency medicine facility as an integral part of its health-care enterprise, public policy dictates that it is not allowed to insulate itself from liability by shunting it to another individual or entity. The Supreme Court of Alaska affirmed the trial court denial of summary judgment based on enterprise liability and apparent authority. However, they held the facility did have a non-delegable duty to provide non-negligent physician care in the ED. The trial court summary judgment for the defense was reversed and remanded, with a partial summary judgment verdict for vicarious liability in favor of the plaintiff.

In *Gilbert* v. *Sycamore Municipal Hospital*, the patient presented with chest pain while weightlifting, received testing which was normal, was discharged,

and subsequently died.[15] The ED was staffed by rotating "on-call" physicians as independent contractors, who had medical staff privileges and their own private practices. The question raised was whether the hospital could be held liable for the alleged negligence of a physician who was not a hospital employee. The circuit court granted summary judgment in favor of the hospital. The Supreme Court of Illinois reversed and remanded for further proceedings, holding the hospital vicariously liable under the doctrine of "apparent authority":

For a hospital to be liable, a plaintiff must show that: (1) the hospital, or its agent, acted in a manner that would lead a reasonable person to conclude that the individual who was alleged to be negligent was an employee or agent of the hospital; (2) where the acts of the agent create the appearance of authority, the plaintiff must also prove that the hospital had knowledge of and acquiesced in them; (3) plaintiff acted in reliance upon the conduct of the hospital or its agent, consistent with ordinary care and prudence.[16]

The court found there was a general issue of fact about the agency of the physician, and the patient's understanding of the process, and this should be decided by a fact finder.

In *Baptist Memorial Hospital* v. *Sampson*, the patient presented to the ED with a bite later identified to be from a brown recluse spider.[17] She was treated conservatively, discharged, and re-presented to another facility in septic shock. The plaintiff filed a medical negligence lawsuit, and the Supreme Court of Texas addressed the question of whether the hospital was vicariously liable for the ED physician. The hospital may not be responsible for the acts of an independent contractor without meeting the requisites of ostensible agency:

Apparent authority in Texas is based on estoppel. It may arise either from a principal knowingly permitting an agent to hold oneself out as having authority, or by a principal's actions which lack such ordinary care as to clothe an agent with the indicia of authority, thus leading a reasonably prudent person to believe that the agent has the authority they purport to exercise. A prerequisite to a proper finding of apparent authority is evidence of the conduct by the principal relied upon by the party asserting the estoppel defense which would lead a reasonably prudent person to believe an agent had authority to act.[18]

The Supreme Court of Texas reversed the judgment of the Court of Appeals and decided against financial recovery for the plaintiff. They held that no conduct of the hospital would lead a reasonable patient to believe that the treating emergency physicians were hospital employees.

In *Simmons* v. *Tuoemy Regional Medical Center*, the patient was involved in a moped accident, presented to the ED, allegedly confused, was discharged, re-presented to another facility with subdural hematoma, and died.[19] The daughter signed the treatment consent form that read:

> The physicians practicing in this emergency room are not employees of Tuoemy Regional Medical Center. They are independent physicians, as are all physicians practicing at this hospital.

This arrangement was replicated in the professional service contract between the group and facility, and the facility agreed to not: "exercise any control over the means, manner or methods by which any Physician supplied by carried out their duties." The family filed suit for negligent care, the trial court awarded summary judgment to the facility attributing significance to the notice and contract. The Court of Appeals of South Carolina heard the plaintiff appeal citing actual agency, apparent agency, and nondelegable duty. Traditionally, employers have avoided vicarious liability for the torts of their employees, which agency law has imposed through the doctrine of "respondeat superior," by utilizing an independent contractor arrangement.[20] However, "a person who delegates to an independent contractor an absolute duty owed to another person remains liable for the negligence of the independent contractor just as if they were an employee."[21,22]

There are at least five criteria that should be considered in determining the presence of a "master–servant" relationship. First, who has the power to select and engage the servant. Second, the payment of wages. Third, the power to discharge the worker. Fourth, the power to control the servant's conduct. Fifth, whether the work is a part of the regular business of the employee. The controlling factor appears to be controlling conduct, the right to control and direct the servant in the performance of work, and the manner in which the work is to be done.(Table 100.2).[23] The Simmons trial decision was reversed and remanded for further consideration. The court's opinion was that it was public policy, and not traditional rules of the law of agency or torts, which should underlie the decision to hold hospitals liable for malpractice which occurs in the ED.

Table 100.2 Criteria for "master–servant" relationship

1.	Power to select and engage
2.	Payment of wages
3.	Power to discharge
4.	Control of the worker's conduct
5.	Part of the regular business of employee

Reference: Keitz.[23]

In *Boren* v. *Weeks*, the patient was brought to the ED by her husband, who signed an extensive three-page consent form, although he stated, "he was not asked to read anything."[24] The consent form disavowed the existence of any employment or agency relationship with the emergency physicians. The patient presented with a fall, was diagnosed with contusions, discharged, and returned with worsening symptoms, was admitted and succumbed allegedly to a pulmonary embolism. The trial court denied the hospital's summary judgment motion as there is a dispute of material fact concerning vicarious liability. The appellate court reversed the trial court's decision, granting summary judgment to the hospital on all grounds. They held that, "efforts to disavow that the ED physicians were agents of the hospital were sufficient to preclude the plaintiff's claim based on apparent agency." The Supreme Court of Tennessee reversed the summary judgment and remanded for further consideration, as there are genuine issues of fact concerning vicarious liability under the apparent agency theory. They held that the patient and family relied on the hospital to provide emergency medical care, not relying on a particular physician. They accepted services with the belief the ED physicians were hospital employees, and could not say as a matter of law that the consent form provided adequate notice.

In summary, the hospital's duties have been classified into four general areas as cited in *Thompson* v. *Nason Hospital*.[25] First, the duty to use reasonable care in the maintenance of safe and adequate facilities and equipment.[26] Second, a duty to select and retain only competent physicians.[27] Third, a duty to oversee all persons who practice medicine within its walls related to patient care.[28] Fourth, a duty to formulate, adopt, and enforce adequate rules and policies to ensure quality patient care (Table 100.3).[29]

Table 100.3 Summary of hospital duties

1.	Maintenance of safe and adequate facilities and equipment
2.	Select and retain only competent physicians
3.	Oversee all persons practicing medicine within the walls
4.	Formulate, adopt, and enforce patient care policies to ensure quality

References: [25–29].

Conclusion

A number of factors must be considered in the analysis of the provider relationship, but the name of the group itself, the badge identification, who makes the schedule, and who collects and bills for services are often deciding factors in making a distinction between these two business models. The final decision has import in the medicolegal financial liability in alleged medical malpractice cases.

In the employed physician model, the hospital typically takes ultimate responsibility for the group's actions and liabilities. It is important to recognize whether it is the professional service group that maintains responsibility for care provided versus a shared responsibility plan, with the obvious financial repercussions of this decision.

References

1. Conrad DA, Dowling WL. Vertical integration in health service: theory and managerial implications. *Health Care Manag Rev* 1990;15:9–22.

2. Cuellar AE. Gertler PJ. Strategic integration of hospitals and physicians. *J Health Econ*. 2006;25(1):1–28. DOI:10.1016/j.jhealeco.2005.04.009.

3. Lee K. Effects of hospitals' structural clinical integration on efficiency and patient outcome. *Health Serv Manag Res*. 2002;15(4):234–244. DOI:10.1258/095148402320589037.

4. Donabedian A. The quality of care: how can it be assessed? *JAMA*. 1988;260(12):1743–1748. DOI:10.1001/jama.1988.0341012008903.

5. Lake T, Devers K, Brewster L, Casalino L. Something old, something new: recent developments in hospital–physician relationships. *Health Serv Res*. 2003;38(1 Pt 2):471–488. DOI:10.1111/1475-6773.00125.

6. Madison K. Hospital–physician affiliations and patient treatments, expenditures and outcomes. *Health Serv Res*. 2004;39(2):257–278. DOI:10.1111/j.1475–6773.200400227.x.

7. Burns LR, Muller RW. Hospital–physician collaboration: landscape of economic integration and impact on clinical integration. *Milbank Q*. 2008;86(3):375–434. DOI.10:1111/j.1468-0009.2008.00527.x.

8. *Elam* v. *College Park Hospital*, 132 Cal. App.3d 332 (1982).

9. Shensky ES. Corporate negligence in medical malpractice. *National Law Review*, February 5, 2017.

10. California Health and Safety Code. §1250 (a) (b) (f).

11. *Jackson* v. *Power*, 743 P.2d 1376 (1987).

12. Dearborn M. Enterprise liability: reviewing and revitalizing liability for corporate groups. *California Law Rev*. 2009;97(1):1–69.

13. Restatement (Second) of Torts: Section 429 (1965).

14. *Simmons* v. *St Clair Memorial Hospital*, 332 Pa. Super. 444, 481 A.2d 870, 874 (1984).

15. *Gilbert* v. *Sycamore Municipal Hospital*, 622 N.E.2d 788 (1993).

16. *Pamperin* v. *Trinity Memorial*, 144 Wis. 2d 188 (1988).

17. *Baptist Memorial Hospital* v. *Sampson*, 969 S.W.2d 945 (1998).

18. *Ames* v. *Great S. Bank*, 672 S.W.2d 447 (1984).

19. *Simmons* v. *Tuoemy Regional Medical Center*, 330 S.C. 115, 498 S.E.2d 408 (Ct. App. 1998).

20. Restatement (Second) of Agency §250 (1958).

21. *Durkin* v. *Hansen*, 437 S.E.2d 550 (1993).

22. 57 C.J.S. Master and Servant, §591, at 365 (1948).

23. *Keitz* v. *National Paving*, 134 A.2d 296 (1957).

24. *Boren* v. *Weeks*, 251 S.W.3d 426 (2008).

25. *Thompson* v. *Nason Hospital*, 527 Pa. 330, 591 A.2d 703 (1991).

26. *Chandler General Hospital Inc.* v. *Purvis*, 123 Ga. App. 334, 181 S.E.2d 77 (1971).

27. *Johnson* v. *Misercordia Community Hospital*, 99 Wis.2d 708, 301 N.W.2d 156 (1981).

28. *Darling* v. *Charleston Memorial Hospital*, 211 N.E.2d 253 (1965).

29. *Wood* v. *Samaritan Institution*, 26 Cal. 2d 556 (Cal. Ct.App. 1945).

Chapter 101

Transfer

Case

The rescue squad called the emergency department (ED) to say they were bringing in a motorcyclist who had experienced a traumatic accident on a rural road. They had established intravenous lines and had the patient on high-flow oxygen, and they were concerned about a chest injury. The ED physician attempted to place the helicopter on standby for transfer to a regional trauma center, but the weather was too bad for the helicopter to fly, so the ground transport unit was dispatched.

The receiving hospital accepted the patient, but suggested he needed to be stabilized before transport. The chest radiograph revealed a small left-sided pneumothorax and the patient was on high flow to maintain oxygen saturation in the low 90s. The nurse asked if they were going to put a chest tube in, and the physician said no: the pneumothorax was small and since they weren't flying at altitude the patient would be OK for the transfer. The paramedics loaded the patient to go, continued to run fluid and administer oxygen, and took the records and chest radiograph with them to the receiving facility.

Later that year hospital counsel received a plaintiff pleading alleging medical malpractice. The receiving hospital felt the patient was unstable for transport. He had a pneumothorax that was not remedied, and had a long and complicated course in the intensive care unit (ICU) as a result.

The provider responded that the pneumothorax was small, the patient was oxygenating, and was able to be transferred in that condition; the requirement had been to get him to a trauma center rapidly.

Medical Approach

There is often uncertainty in the transfer process when patients are moved up a level of care. However, it is considered that the transferring facility takes responsibility and is required to institute and maintain stabilization maneuvers to ensure safe transport. The receiving facility does not take responsibility until the patient reaches its door. Often the transferring facility does not recognize this and feels that once the patient is transferred from their premises they have no further responsibility for the medical transfer. Aeromedical evacuation can minimize transfer problems. However, when that resource is not available, prolonged ground transport may make them worse.

A significant proportion of emergency medicine transfers involve the trauma population. Spain et al. evaluated transfers to a Level I academic trauma center after contact with their call center.[1] Of 821 patient transfer calls received, 6.3% (52) were for consultation only and 9.4% (77) were canceled by the referring hospital. This call incidence distilled down to 84.3% (692) transfer requests. The majority of patients (77%, 534) were accepted for transfer, 19% (134) were denied for no capacity, and 4% (24) were declined as not clinically indicated. The transferred patients were younger (32 ± 1.49 years vs. 38.9 ± 0.51 years, $P < 0.05$) and more likely to require an operation than directly admitted patients (58% vs. 51%, $P < 0.05$), but had similar injury severity scores and length of stay. The most commonly requested services were trauma (24%) and neurosurgery (24%), followed by orthopedics (20%). Surgical intervention occurred most commonly with orthopedics (60%), followed by neurosurgery (13%) and trauma (10%). The transferred patients, 20% of the admission volume, had an identical payer mix and similar operative needs to the local catchment area patients. The greatest impact was felt by orthopedics, neurosurgery, and the trauma service, as the reason for transfer was for specialty availability.

There has been an increase in both the number and nature of trauma patient transfers, as profiled by Esposito et al.[2] The trauma population increased by 6%, while the transfer population increased by 34%.

The prevalence of orthopedic injury increased by 25%, while the transfer rate increased by 48%. The incidence of head injury increased by 14%, while the transfer rate increased by 44%. The most common time for transfer was presentation between 3 p.m. and 7 a.m. at the outside facility. The mean malpractice premiums increased by 90% in the high-risk specialties: general, orthopedic, and neurosurgery. During the study period, waivers of regulatory compliance were requested by 28% of trauma centers (39%). There has been a disproportionate increase in trauma transfers.

Another area of focus is radiology imaging before transfer of trauma patients to a Level I trauma center from a rural ED. Lee et al. performed a questionnaire survey with a 68.3% (149/218) response rate.[3] Radiology imaging was obtained before transfer in one-third (33.1%) of cases because of the perception that it was desired by the trauma center independent of acuity. Likewise, 28% obtained imaging because of liability concerns, even if it delayed transfer. Overall, 45% obtained imaging for either a perceived requirement or concerns over liability. Those without Advanced Trauma Life Support training are more likely to use all available resources before transfer. There are numerous factors not related to patient acuity that may delay transfer.

The transfer rationale in most cases is to a higher level of patient care. Menchine performed an analysis of 347 ED directors with a 70% (243) response rate, soliciting opinions about specialty care capabilities.[4] The majority (80%) of respondents had internal medicine, obstetrics–gynecology, and pediatrics on call, but less than 60% of the EDs reported cardiac surgery, otolaryngology, neurosurgery, plastic surgery, or vascular surgery on call. The on-call coverage was rated to have worsened over the last 3 years for 10 of the 16 specialties surveyed. Rural EDs were likely to transfer at least one patient per day to a higher level of care. The longest delays, on average over 3 hours, were associated with ENT, orthopedics, plastic surgery, and mental health transfers. The use of pre-established specialty transfer protocols can improve the process.

Legal Analysis

In *Hastings* v. *Baton Rouge General Hospital*, the patient presented to the ED with multiple thoracic stab wounds and was resuscitated initially requiring a chest tube thoracostomy and blood transfusion.[5] The cardiothoracic surgeon was consulted, who allegedly asked the patient's insurance status and recommended transfer. The ED staff were uncomfortable with the transfer and offered to accompany the patient. Although initially stabilized, he decompensated in the ambulance, was returned to the ED, and succumbed to his injury. The cardiothoracic surgeon who was consulted for care opined that even if the patient had survived the transfer, the outcome would likely have been unchanged. The trial court granted a directed verdict in favor of the defendant physicians and hospital, which was affirmed by the appeal court holding that there was no surgical negligence or deviation from the standard of care. The directed verdict is granted when, "the facts and inferences point so strongly in favor of one party that reasonable people could not reach a contrary verdict." It is appropriate not when there is a preponderance of evidence, but only when the evidence overwhelmingly points to one conclusion.[6] The Supreme Court of Louisiana held that reasonable people could disagree as to whether there was negligence. The appeal court verdict was reversed and remanded to trial court for decision on case merits.

In *Power* v. *Arlington Hospital Association*, the patient presented to the ED with hip, back and abdominal pain, difficulty walking, and chills.[7] She was evaluated by two physicians, and discharged with pain medication and orthopedic follow-up. She returned, was diagnosed with septic shock, and ultimately transferred to a hospital closer to home after a 4-month stay. The patient filed suit alleging as one issue in addition to medical screening, that the transfer was improper, as she was unstable, violating Emergency Medical Treatment and Labor Act (EMTALA) requirements.[8] The trial court jury awarded damages to the plaintiff on the medical screening issue. They denied the hospital's summary judgment motion, but jury found in favor of the hospital on the transfer count. The United States Court of Appeals, Fourth District affirmed this verdict on the transfer issue, and vacated the damage award and remanded to district court to conform verdicts to Virginia statutory caps on medical malpractice damages.[9,10] The trial court was ultimately persuaded that the transfer matter pertained to ED transfers, thus by accepting this as factual the decision of whether it was appropriate was avoided.

In *Roberts* v. *Galen of Virginia, Inc.*, the patient presented to the ED with severe injury after a truck versus pedestrian accident.[11] After a 6-week hospital stay, she was transferred to a health-care facility across state lines, where she did not qualify for financial assistance because of the residency criteria. The petitioner filed a federal action alleging violation of the EMTALA stabilization and transfer requirement.[8] The district court granted summary judgment to the respondent on the grounds that the petitioner failed to show either she was stable, or the decision to authorize transfer was made for an improper motive. The appeal court affirmed, stating that to prove the stabilization requirement, an "improper motive" was required by EMTALA. The Supreme Court of the United States granted certiorari and reversed, reinstating the trial court summary judgment verdict for the facility respondent. They held that the "improper motive" contention does not have basis in any statutory construction.

In *Coleman* v. *Deno*, the patient made two visits to the hospital ED, first with chest pain and then with arm swelling, bullae, and fever.[12] He was about to be discharged again with a diagnosis of cellulitis and outpatient antibiotics, but his white blood cell count was found to be elevated and a transfer was sought. The decision was made allegedly on the basis of insurance status and greater experience with complicated infection. An evidentiary ruling by the trial judge precluded the jury from being informed of the alleged insurance rationale for transfer. The patient was transferred to the tertiary care referral center and underwent lifesaving surgery requiring left arm amputation. The plaintiff sued the ED physician for "improper transfer" of the patient under general tort law. The Supreme Court of Louisiana concluded the cause of action was based solely on medical malpractice, based on the Medical Malpractice Act.[13] Thus, the appeal court finding of intentional tort, based on "patient dumping," was in error. The case was remanded for meaningful review of the malpractice issue.

Conclusion

Clearly, every patient transfer undergoes a significant amount of scrutiny so proper care is required in all aspects of the transfer process. Most institutions have protocolized the process, allowing the staff to utilize simple checklists to ensure proper procedural compliance.

References

1. Spain D, Bellino M, Kopelman A, Chang J, Park J, Gregg D, Brundage SI. Requests for 692 transfers to an academic Level 1 trauma center: implications of the Emergency Medical Treatment and Active Labor Act. *J Trauma*. 2007;62(1):63–68.

2. Esposito TJ, Crandall M, Reed LR, Gamelli RL, Luchette FA. Socioeconomic factors, medicolegal issues, and trauma patient transfer trends: is there a connection? *J Trauma*. 2006;61(6):1380–1388. DOI:10.1097/01.ta.0000242862.68899.04.

3. Lee CY, Bernard AC, Fryman L, Coughenour J, Costich J, Boulanger B, et al. Imaging may delay transfer of rural trauma victims: a survey of referring physicians. *J Trauma*. 2008;65(6):1359–1363. DOI:10.1097/TA.0b013e31818c10fc.

4. Menchine MD. On-call specialists and higher level of care transfers in California emergency departments. *Acad Emerg Med*. 2008;15(4):329–336. DOI:10.1111/j.1553-2712.2008.00071.x.

5. *Hastings* v. *Baton Rouge General Hospital*, 498 So. 2d 713 (1986).

6. *Breithaupt* v. *Sellers*, 390 So. 2d 870 (La.1980).

7. 751. *Power* v. *Arlington Hospital Association*, 42 F.3d 851 (1994).

8. EMTALA 42 USCA §1395dd.

9. Virginia Code Annotated §8.01–581.15. Limitation on Recovery in Certain Medical Malpractice Actions.

10. Virginia Code Annotated §8.01–38. Tort Liability of Hospitals.

11. *Roberts* v. *Galen of Virginia, Inc.*, 525 U.S. 249 (1999).

12. *Coleman* v. *Deno*, 813 So. 2d 303 (2002).

13. Louisiana Revised Statutes 40:1299.41: Medical Malpractice Act.

Chapter 102

Translation, Interpreting, and Language Issues

Case

The nurse came to get the physician and said they were having trouble because the patient didn't speak English. She couldn't get a history from him, or any information about medications or allergies. There was no one accompanying the patient, who had apparently been staying at a local shelter. It was hard even to figure out a chief complaint, but he seemed to be motioning to his legs. The physician went to talk to the patient, but did not do any better. They had a hard time even finding out what country he was from, but he was able to point out a general region on a world map. There were no family or friends to translate for him. One of the residents from the shelter was invited to the emergency department (ED) to help, and eventually they were able to determine the patient's country of origin. This made it possible to use the standard commercial language line to help facilitate the discussion. His problem was that his feet hurt, and his medical issues were resolved relatively quickly. The ED staff were able to find a social media page offering cultural support from a local group of established residents who had previously immigrated from this area of the world, and someone from the group came to help with the patient's discharge when the care was done.

Medical Approach

The ED is a difficult environment to work in at any time, and language difficulties can make matters even worse. How easy it is to resolve this problem depends on the origin and rarity of the language. Most programs have an informal approach that begins with a staff language databank involving both employees and physician health-care providers.

We make use of family members if we can, but a common scenario in which the child of an immigrant has a good command of the English language leaves us with the ethical quandary of asking a child to translate

for an adult, which is not a proper intervention unless there are exigent circumstances. We typically cannot rely on a history obtained in this way as it may be modified to facilitate the third-party discussion. Also, requiring a minor to take medical responsibility for an adult parent is not morally or legally sound.

The physician–patient relationship is built through communication promoted by the effective use of a common language.[1] Not only is this essential to the diagnostic process, it establishes an empathetic baseline as well. Language barriers deprive the patient and physician of this valuable connection.

"Limited English proficient" (LEP) is the term used by the US Department of Health and Human Services (DHHS) Office for Civil Rights to define that portion of the US population that has little or no English-speaking ability. The DHHS views inadequate language interpretation as a form of discrimination.[1] The Civil Rights Act of 1964 states that "no person in the United States shall on the ground of race, color, or national origin be excluded from participation in, be denied the benefits of or be otherwise subjected to discrimination" under any federally supported program.[2] In 2000, President Clinton signed Executive Order 13166, Improving Access to Services for Persons with Limited English Proficiency.[3] This order required federal agencies to examine the services they provide, identify any need for services to those with LEP, and develop and implement a system to provide those services and provide meaningful access to them (Table 102.1).

The DHHS Office of Minority Health issued the National Standards for Culturally and Linguistically Appropriate Services (CLAS) in Health Care: Final Report in 2001 (Table 102.2).[4] These standards recommend that all patients receive culturally appropriate care in their preferred language. Bilingual staff or interpretation services should be available during all hours of operation. The preferred language should

Table 102.1 Improving access to services for those with limited English proficiency (LEP)

1. Examine the services provided
2. Identify needs for services
3. Develop and implement system
4. Provide meaningful access

Reference: Clinton.[3]

Table 102.2 Culturally and linguistically appropriate services (CLAS) in health care

1. Care culturally consistent and in preferred language
2. Diverse staff characteristic of the service area
3. Education in culturally and linguistically appropriate care
4. Provide language assistive services, bilingual staff, and interpreters
5. Verbal and written notice of language assistive service
6. Family and friends should not provide service (except at patient's request)
7. Easily understood patient materials and signage
8. Written strategic plan, accountability, and oversight
9. Organizational self-assessment of CLAS-related activity
10. Patient communication information incorporated in record
11. Maintain demographic, cultural, and epidemiological community profile
12. Develop and maintain community collaborative partnerships
13. Conflict and grievance procedures should be culturally sensitive
14. Public notices and information include standards

Reference: CLAS.[4]

Table 102.3 Guidance regarding Title VI prohibition against national origin discrimination affecting people with limited English proficiency

Interpretation: oral language service

1. Hiring bilingual staff
2. Hiring staff interpreters
3. Contracting for interpreters
4. Using telephone interpreter lines
5. Using community volunteers
6. Using family members or friends

Translation: written language service

1. Safe harbor
   a. 5%, 1000 persons: Translated materials
   b. 5%, 50 persons: Translated availability notice
2. Maintain competence of translators

Effective language assistance plan

1. Identify those in need of LEP services
2. Specify the language assistive measures provided
3. Train staff effectively
4. Provide notice to those with LEP needs
5. Monitor and update the LEP Plan

Reference: DOJ.[5]

be available in verbal or written format. Family and friends should not be used to interpret unless the patient requests it. There should be ongoing staff education, program assessment, and community orientation to the CLAS program.

The Department of Justice regulations, implementing Title VI of the Civil Rights Act of 1964, state that recipients of federal financial assistance have a responsibility to ensure meaningful access to their programs and activities by persons with LEP (Table 102.3).[2,5] They recommend providing language assistance services. First, interpretation, or oral language services include: (1) hiring bilingual staff,;(2) hiring staff interpreters; (3) contracting for interpreters; (4) using telephone interpreter lines; (5) using community volunteers; (6) use of family members or friends.

Second, translation, or a written language service. The facility should comply with safe harbor requirements. The need for translated documents is triggered at the 5% or 1000 population served level, whichever is less. The need for a written notice in the primary language discussing availability of materials is triggered if there are less than 50 persons at the 5% level. The facility must ensure the competence of translators.

Third, the regulations describe the elements of an effective language assistance plan to include: (1) identifying those in need of LEP services; (2) specifying the language assistive measures provided; (3) training staff effectively; (4) providing notice to those with LEP needs; (5) monitoring and updating the LEP plan.

The Americans with Disabilities Act of 1990 (ADA) requires that the needs for people with communication disabilities involving vision, hearing and speech be met.[6] Those with hearing impairment typically require the use of an American Sign Language interpreter, or communication in writing. Those with visual impairment often require auditory or tactile communication materials.

The facility is required to provide "auxiliary aids and services" to assist. Those with vision loss can be provided with (1) a qualified reader, (2) large print materials, (3) Braille materials, (4) computer screen-reading software, or (5) an audio recording of printed material. Those with hearing impairment may be provided with (1) a qualified notetaker, (2) a sign language interpreter, (3) an oral interpreter, (4) a cued speech interpreter, (5) a tactile interpreter, or (6) real-time captioning. Those with speech impairment could be provided with (1) a transliterator, a person trained to recognize unclear speech or (2) a communications board.[7] Newer technology includes real-time captioning, telecommunications relay service, video relay services, and video remote interpreting.

Health-care providers in the United States are encountering a rising number of LEP patients, currently 26 million. The number has increased by 30% over the past decade, triple the growth rate of the total population.[8] The average US hospital spends nearly $1 million a year on language services. This must be balanced against the medicolegal risk associated with an unresolved language barrier. The legal risks of ineffective communication are manifest in all aspects of medical practice.[9] First, there is increased risk of malpractice litigation as a result of obtaining an inadequate medical history. Second, there is legal vulnerability concerning the lack of informed consent. Third, there can be a breach of the duty to warn of the risks associated with treatment methods and medications. Fourth, there can be a breach of the patient's privacy rights (Table 102.4).

Language barriers may have significant impact on patient interactions in the ED. Timmins studied a group of systematic reviews of language barriers in health care for Latino populations.[10] They evaluated access to care, quality of care and health status, and outcomes. First, they found that 55% (5/9) experienced a significant adverse effect on access to care

based on language issues, while 33% (3) found weak or mixed evidence. Second, 86% (6/7) of studies evaluating quality of care found an adverse effect. Third, 66% (2/3) found language barriers a risk factor for adverse outcome. They concluded that non-English-speaking populations were at risk for decreased health-care access.

The interface and language barrier between resource availability and utilization has come into question. Waxman and Levitt evaluated whether non-English-speaking patients presenting to the ED had more diagnostic tests, higher admission rates, and longer length of stay.[11] They evaluated 324 patients, of whom 172 were non-English-speaking. The language distribution was Spanish (31.0%), Cantonese (5.9%), Hindi (2.5%), Arabic (1.9%), Mien (1.5%), Russian (0.9%), Mandarin (0.6%), Korean (0.3%), and other (9.0%). Non-English-speaking patients had more tests ordered, including three times as many CT scans for abdominal pain, but there was no difference with chest pain test ordering, admission rates, or ED length of stay.

Language barriers can impact patient satisfaction as well. Carrasquillo et al. surveyed 2333 patients presenting to the ED, in which 15% (354) reported English was not their primary language.[12] There was significant difference in overall satisfaction between English-speaking (71%) and non-English-speaking (52%) patients ($P < 0.01$): 9.5% of the English-speaking and 14% of the non-English-speaking patients would not return to the same ED if they had an emergency condition ($P < 0.05$). Multivariate analysis found non-English-speakers were less likely to be satisfied with their care, or return to the same ED. They were more likely to report problems with care, communication, and testing (Table 102.5). Targeted strategies are

Table 102.4 Legal risks of ineffective communication

1.	Increased risk of malpractice litigation
2.	Lack of informed consent
3.	Breach of the duty to warn
4.	Breach of patient's right to privacy

Reference: Kempen[9]

Table 102.5 Impact of language barriers on patient satisfaction

Parameter	Significance OR, 95% CI
Less Likely	
1. Less likely to be satisfied	0.59, 0.39–0.90
2. Less likely to return	0.57, 0.34–0.95
More likely	
3. Report care problems	1.70, 1.05–2.74
4. Communication issues	1.71, 1.18–2.47
5. Testing issues	1.77, 1.19–2.64

Reference: Carrasquillo et al.[12]

needed to address satisfaction in this group, although most facilities have language translation software such as AT&T Language Line or Google Translate available in their ED.

Ramirez et al. performed a literature review of studies comparing outcome of those with LEP presenting to the ED.[13] This group was associated with less satisfaction with medical encounter, having different rates of diagnostic testing, and receiving less information on follow-up. The use of professional interpretation services has been associated with improved satisfaction and access to health care. These services are often underutilized due to the perceived time, labor, and cost required, and facilities often rely on ad hoc interpreters.

Karliner et al. evaluated the effect of professional interpreters measured in a review of 3698 references, in which 21 studies that used professional interpreters were identified.[14] They studied communication (errors and comprehension), utilization, clinical outcome, and satisfaction. The use of a professional interpreter was associated with improved clinical care comparable to patients without language limitations.

Legal Analysis

In *Gerena* v. *Fogari*, the patient saw an office-based physician monthly for an ongoing chronic condition.[15] The patient requested a sign language interpreter for her visits, and the physician allegedly declined because the cost of the translation service would exceed visit billing. Patient and physician communicated with an ad hoc repertoire of gestures, family assistance, and writing. The patient was concerned, but continued with the physician. The trial court awarded both compensatory and punitive damages for the plaintiff. Afterwards, there was an appeal by the physician, and pretrial settlement.

In *Quintero* v. *Encarnacion*, the patient was involuntarily committed to a state hospital, after being found wandering, and diagnosed with schizophrenia.[16] She was a member of an indigenous group and did not speak English. Suit was filed by the plaintiff in conjunction with an advocacy group alleging violation of federal law, 42 U.S.C. §1983, and the defendants moved to dismiss on qualified immunity grounds.[17] The district court dismissed social workers and psychologists, but denied immunity for administrators and physicians. Qualified immunity shields government officials performing discretionary functions from individual liability unless their conduct violates "clearly established statutory or constitutional rights of which a reasonable person would have known."[18,19]

The United States Court of Appeals, Tenth Circuit ruled on the interlocutory appeal of denial of qualified immunity, and affirmed. They rejected any claim that discussion of new medications could be fulfilled by conducting explanation in a language the patient could not understand.

Conclusion

Medical decision-making requires a significant amount of question-and-answer between provider and patient, especially for more complex points of discussion. It is essential for the two to be able to communicate. The current endorsed interpretation standard is a commercial language line, a paid service which is extremely helpful. The cost is a significant factor, but the language line remains the standard of care, as we are obligated to provide interpretation services to establish proper communication approaches for all patients.

References

1. Woloshin S, Bickell NA, Schwartz LM, Gany F, Welch G. Language barriers in medicine in the United States. *JAMA*. 1995;273(9):724–728.

2. Civil Rights Act of 1964, Pub.L. 88–352, 78 Stat. 24, Employment Discrimination.

3. Executive Order 13166: Improving Access to Services for Persons with Limited English Proficiency, US Department of Justice, 2000.

4. U.S. Department of Health and Human Services, OPHS Office of Minority Health. National Standards for Culturally and Linguistically Appropriate Services in Health Care. Final Report. Washington, D.C., March 2001.

5. US Department of Justice. Guidance to federal financial assistance recipients regarding Title VI prohibition against national origin discrimination affecting limited English proficient persons. *Fed. Reg.* 2002;67(117):41455–41472.

6. Americans with Disabilities Act of 1990, Pub. L. No. 101–336, §1, 104 Stat. 328 (1990).

7. US Department of Justice. Civil Rights Division. Disability Rights Section. Effective communication. www.ada.gov/effective-comm.htm. Accessed April 15, 2016.

8. Interpreting service: average US hospital spends $1 million per year on translations. True Blue Tribune. June 3, 2014.

9. Kempen AV. Legal risks of ineffective communication. *AMA J Ethics Virtual Mentor*. 2007;9(8):555–558.

10. Timmins CL. The impact of language barriers on the health care of Latinos in the United States: a review of the literature and guidelines for practice. *J Midwifery Womens Health*. 2002;47(2):80–96. DOI:10.1016/S1526-9523(02)00218-0.

11. Waxman MA, Levitt MA. Are diagnostic testing and admission rates higher in non-English-speaking versus English-speaking patients in the emergency department? *Ann Emerg Med*. 2000;36(5):456–461. DOI:10.1067/mem.2000.108315.

12. Carrasquillo O, Orav EJ, Brennan TA, Burstin HR. Impact of language barriers on patient satisfaction in an emergency department. *J Gen Int Med*. 1999;14(2):82–87.

13. Ramirez D, Engel KG, Tang TS. Language interpreter utilization in the emergency department setting: a clinical review. *J Health Care Poor Underserved*. 2008;19(2):352–362. DOI.10.1353/hpu.0.0019.

14. Karliner LS, Jacobs EA, Chen AH, Mutha S. Do professional interpreters improve clinical care for patients with limited proficiency? A systematic review of the literature. *Health Serv Res*. 2006;42(2):727–754. DOI:10.1111/j.1475-6773.2006.00629.x.

15. *Gerena* v. *Fogari*, N.J. Sup. Ct., App-Div.

16. *Quintero* v. *Escarcnacion*, 98–3129 (10th Circ. 1999).

17. 42 U.S. Code §1983, Civil Action for Deprivation of Rights.

18. *Baptiste* v. *J.C. Penney Co.*, 147 F.3d 1252 (10th Circ. 1998).

19. *Harlow* v. *Fritzgerald*, 457 U.S. 800 (1982).

Chapter 103

Triage

Case

The hospital facility had recently undergone a new initiative to address the triage process in the emergency department (ED). This began with additional education and instituted a new triage system, in which the nurses were reoriented as the system began. The nurses had concerns that the system was prone to overtriage, often overutilizing scarce resources, but on occasion that had been noted under the previous triage process as well. Gradually the personnel adapted and the program continued without apparent concern.

About a year later a subpoena was delivered to the ED alleging a medical malpractice event. The agent was directed to take the subpoena to the hospital risk management department, but they declined and instead handed the subpoena directly to the physician, who immediately forwarded it to the Risk Management department. Risk Management contacted the ED director about a week later and reviewed the complaint which concerned an allegedly missed chest pain, clearly an atypical presentation. One of the allegations was that the patient was mistriaged in the process; it was suggested this had a significant adverse impact on the patient. The director's response was that he was happy to comment on the medical issues involved, but the physicians may have had little to do with the triage process, which is often a hospital nursing-based initiative although the physician typically assists with the implementation. The ED director recommended a discussion with the nursing department director as well, with concerns about the triage process.

Medical Approach

Most medical malpractice allegations are all-encompassing, typically working from a template invoking every conceivable portion of the healthcare process as a potential area of deviation from the standard of care. One of those areas is often the triage process, alleging the patient was undertriaged, resulting in some additional or compound injury.

The typical triage process distinguishes anything from three to five ED triage categories, with the five being the most common. A simplistic analysis estimates that 10% of patients are critically ill or injured, 30% are seriously ill or injured, and 60% have minor injury or illness. Historically, the triage process was used to allocate scarce resources. This has largely been supplanted by a "demand triage" process when the ED gets busy. Some facilities have moved to a "bedside triage" process in which the screening function is transitioned to more of a documentation function.

Perhaps the most crucial question involves the ethics of the triage process itself. Aacharya questioned the ethical basis of the "routine triage" process based on the four principles of biomedical ethics (Table 103.1).[1] First, the respect for autonomy establishes that competent patients have the right to make their own medical decisions. This complicates the triage process, as most believe their complaint is a "true emergency." Second, the principle of nonmaleficence or "do no harm," with its Hippocratic origin. Undertriage may manifest as a patient's prolonged wait for care. Third, beneficence is the moral obligation to perform good acts for the patient. Overtriage may make valuable resources less available for others. Fourth, the concept of distributive justice requires fair allocation of resources, if they are limited. This manifests as a fair, but not equitable,

Table 103.1 Ethical basis of triage

1.	Respect for autonomy
2.	Nonmaleficence: "do no harm"
3.	Beneficence: "good acts"
4.	Justice: "proper balance"

Reference: Aacharya et al.[1]

distribution of resources. This is the basis of acuity-based triage, rather then temporal-based triage.

The obvious question is, how reliable is the triage process? Fernandez et al. utilized scripted encounters twice in a 6-week period with triage nurses using a five-tier system.[2] The nurses estimated severity, probability of admission, timeframe to physician evaluation, need for monitored bed, and need for diagnostic services. There were 37 participants in which 33% (4) of the nurses assigned the same severity. The nursing interrater agreement was 0.757 for triage severity. The nursing–physician agreement in need for monitoring was substantial.

The same research group headed by Wuerz revisited this issue in a larger study with 87 participants.[3] Interrater agreement on triage category was now poor (Kendall correlation $(K) = 0.347$). Only 24% (13/25) of participants rated the five scripted scenarios at the same severity in both phases, with K ranging from 0.145 to 0.554. There was wide variation in estimates of admission probability and time to physician evaluation. However, there was good correlation over diagnostic studies or need for a monitored bed. The conclusion is that there is significant variability in intrarater and interrater liability.

Another question is whether triage can be used to refer patients outside of the ED for care. Lowe et al. performed a historical cohort study in which two ED nurses reviewed triage sheets to determine whether cases met published triage guidelines to refuse care.[4] They identified 106 patients who could have been potentially refused care according to published triage guidelines, where 33% (35) actually had appropriate visits and 3.7% (4) would have required admission. The triage guidelines were not sufficiently sensitive to identify those who needed or did not need ED care.

Legal Analysis

In *Phillips* v. *Hillcrest Medical Center*, the patient presented to the ED with chest pain and pneumonia-like symptoms, with some uncertainty over his insurance status.[5] He was registered, "triaged" by a registered nurse, seen by a physician on the minor care side, and discharged with prescriptions and follow-up care with a clinic. He presented to another facility, there were some historical inconsistencies, and he eventually died allegedly due to endocarditis. The family filed a claim alleging medical malpractice and an Emergency Medical Treatment and Labor Act

(EMTALA) violation.[6] The district court dismissed the EMTALA claim, the jury found for the medical center, and plaintiffs appealed. As one issue, the appellants alleged disparate treatment, as they were not allowed to cross-examine the triage nurse, but allowed to review records. They specifically asked if chest pain patients were more commonly sent to the emergency side or the minor side. The nurse later responded that she could make no categorical statement. The United States Court of Appeals, Tenth Circuit affirmed the ruling. They held the district court did not abuse its discretion in deciding the presentation of evidence by alternative means.

In *Costello* v. *Christus Santa Rosa Health Care Corp.* the patient presented to the ED with a complaint of chest pain.[7] She was "triaged" by the nursing staff, returned to the waiting room, and suffered a cardiac arrest there, from which she could not be resuscitated. The family filed suit, alleging that patients presenting with chest pain, especially in this patient's age group, "require immediate triage to an examination room, placement on a telemetry monitor, and a 'stat' EKG followed by prompt physician evaluation." The trial court dismissed the plaintiff medical malpractice claim, holding the expert reports did not satisfy the Texas Medical Liability and Insurance Improvement Act, and affirmed by the Court of Appeals of Texas, San Antonio.[8] The appeal contended that the trial court abused its discretion in holding that the expert reports did not make a good-faith effort to meet the requirements of the Act. The expert report must provide enough information to fulfill two purposes: (1) inform the defendant of the specific conduct called into question and (2) provide a basis for the trial court to conclude the claims have merit.[9,10] The court held that the nurse expert did not establish her qualifications to express an expert opinion on causation of someone's death, or render a medical diagnosis. A nursing license does not automatically qualify the registered nurse as an expert on any medical subject, nor is a licensed medical doctor qualified on all issues. "Those who purport to be experts truly have expertise concerning the actual subject about which they are offering an opinion."[11] Likewise, they determined the physician expert opinion was conclusive on the issue of causation. Once it was felt that neither expert testimony complied with the statutory requirements of the Act, the court had no discretion and dismissed with prejudice, which was affirmed.

In *Howland* v. *Wadsworth*, the patient presented to the ED with bilateral foot pain and coldness.[12] Emergency medical services (EMS) personnel found normal vital signs and physical exam. The triage nurse assigned the patient a Level IV status, designating her condition "non-urgent." She was evaluated by the physician assistant, care was discussed with the supervising physician, and she was discharged with a cellulitis diagnosis. Twelve hours after discharge, EMS was again summoned, cardiopulmonary resuscitation (CPR) was begun, she was resuscitated, and required bilateral below-knee amputations. The family filed a claim for ordinary and gross negligence, alleging failure to provide the necessary medical treatment. The defendants moved for a directed verdict because the action arose from the delivery of "emergency medical care" and they failed to prove gross negligence as required by "clear and convincing" evidence as required by the Georgia Code.[13] The trial court denied the motion, the jury applied the ordinary negligence standard, and awarded the plaintiff financial damages. The defendants appealed and the Court of Appeals of Georgia affirmed the trial court decision. They held there was no undue influence or misleading instructions to the jury, who made their determination of the negligence standard applied.

The jury instruction recommended that if the care provided to the defendant was "emergency medical services" the gross negligence standard applied; if not, then the ordinary negligence standard applied. As the patient was assigned a non-urgent severity classification, there was not a compelling argument from the defendant on this matter.

Conclusion

The important point is that responsibility for decision-making in the triage process is routinely hospital-based, involving nursing service education. It typically does not involve physicians, except at the administrative level in a conjoint oversight process. It is thus important to direct any concerns to the appropriate area, while presenting a unified strategy as a departmental initiative.

References

1. Aacharya RP, Gastmans C, Denier Y. Emergency department triage: an ethical analysis. *BMC Emerg Med*. 2011;11:16. DOI:10.1186/1471-227X-11-16.

2. Fernandes CMB, Wuerz R, Clark S, Djurdjev O. How reliable is emergency department triage? *Ann Emerg Med*. 1999;34(2):141–147. DOI:10.1016/S0196-0644(99)70248-9.

3. Wuerz R, Fernandes CMB, Alarcon J. Inconsistency of emergency department triage. *Ann Emerg Med*. 1998;32(4):431–435. DOI:10.1016/S0196-0644(98)70171-4.

4. Lowe RA, Bindman AB, Ulrich SK, Norman G, Scaletta TA, Keane D, et al. Refusing care to emergency department patients: evaluation of published triage guidelines. *Ann Emerg Med*. 1994;23(2):286–293. DOI:10.1016/S0196-0644(94)70042-7.

5. *Phillips* v. *Hillcrest Medical Center*, 244 F.3d 790 (2001).

6. EMTALA 42 USCA §1395dd.

7. *Costello* v. *Christus Santa Rosa Health Care Corporation*, 141 S.W.3d 245 (2004).

8. Texas Medical Liability and Insurance Improvement Act: Tex.Rev.Civ.Stat.Ann. art 4590i, §13.01 (l).

9. *Bowie Memorial Hospital* v. *Wright*, 79 S.W.3d 48 (Tex. 2002).

10. *American Transitional Care Ctrs. of Tex, Inc.* v. *Palacios*, 46 S.W.3d 873 (Tex. 2001).

11. *Borders* v. *Heise*, 924 S.W.2d 148 (Tex. 1996).

12. *Howland* v. *Wadsworth*, 749 S.E.2d 762 (2013).

13. 2010 Georgia Code, Title 51-Torts §51-1-29.5. Definitions; limitation on health care liability claim to gross negligence in emergency medical care; factors for jury consideration.

Unanticipated Death

Case

The patient had come in to the emergency department (ED) with gastroenteritis-type symptoms, including nausea, vomiting, and a slight fever. She had children at home who were also sick, and felt she had improved a little over the last day. The ED physician had done the standard laboratory evaluation, including blood work, urinalysis, and a chest radiograph, all of which were normal. The patient was discharged home with supportive therapy after the physician had a discussion with her primary care physician (PCP), who stated he would see her in his office tomorrow.

On his return to the ED for his next scheduled shift, 4 days later, one of the nurses told him the patient they had seen that day had apparently succumbed at home to an uncertain illness. The physician checked the record to confirm his memory that all her testing was normal, she looked fine, and she had arranged to see her PCP. The nurse confirmed this and said the PCP had called the ED to say everything had seemed OK to him as well.

Medical Approach

It is an adage in emergency medicine that nothing good is coming when you hear the words, "Do you remember that patient you saw?" Even with the most comprehensive workup and evaluation, patients may have an untoward outcome. It may or may not have anything to do with a recent evaluation, but the allegation is usually that it was related.

A mortality benchmark or comparison is always useful. Forster et al. investigated the incidence and severity of adverse events after hospital discharge.[1] They evaluated 400 consecutive discharges from a tertiary care academic hospital, in which 19% (76) had an adverse event after discharge (Table 104.1). Of these events, one-third were preventable and one-third were felt to be ameliorable. The adverse events were

symptoms in 65%, 30% involved a non-permanent disability, 3% were laboratory abnormalities, and 3% were permanent disabilities. The most common type of event was an adverse drug reaction (66%) followed by procedural injuries (17%). The 25 adverse events associated with at least a non-permanent disability were felt to be preventable in about half the cases (48%, 12) and ameliorable in one-quarter (24%, 6). They concluded adverse events occur frequently after hospital discharge and can be addressed with simple strategies.

Focusing on terminal events in the intensive care unit (ICU), Vincent et al. analyzed 258 patients who died in a single ICU.[2] The most common preterminal events were worsening coma in 40.3% (104) and acute circulatory failure in 34.8% (90). Only a minority (12%) of deaths occurred in a sudden, catastrophic way. In the majority (65%, 168) of patients, death was considered inevitable, while 9% (22) of patients were allowed to die after support was withdrawn.

Table 104.1 Adverse events after hospital discharge

Adverse events (AE)	Comparison
	95% CI, %
1. Total AE	19, 15–23
2. Preventable AE	6, 4–9
3. Ameliorable AE	6, 4–9
Type	
4. Adverse drug events	66, 55–76
5. Procedure-related injury	17, 8–26
Disability	
7. All disability	6.2
8. Preventable	48, 28–68
9. Ameliorable	24, 7–41

Reference: Forster et al.[1]

Table 104.2 Death after ED discharge

Death	Outcome	
N = 42	Expected	Unexpected
Related	14% (6)	21% (9)
Unrelated	7% (3)	57% (24)

Reference: Kefer et al.[3]

Table 104.3 High-risk conditions for death after ED discharge

1. Atypical presentation of an unusual problem
2. Established chronic illness with clinical decompensation
3. Abnormal vital signs at discharge
4. Mental disability, psychiatric illness, substance abuse
5. Prone to not return with symptom worsening

Reference: Sklar et al.[4]

Table 104.4 High-risk predictors of death after ED discharge

Risk factors	
1. Increasing age	
2. Male sex	
3. Number of pre-existing comorbidities	
Primary discharge diagnosis	**Significance**
	OR, 95% CI
4. Non-infectious lung disease	7.1, 2.9–17.4
5. Renal disease	5.6, 2.2–14.2
6. Ischemic heart disease	3.8, 1.0–13.6

Reference: Gabayan et al.[5]

Circulatory shock is the most common reversible condition and should be monitored with quick intervention. Most ICU deaths when they occur are expected, and Do Not Resuscitate (DNR) orders or complete support withdrawal may be appropriate in selected cases.

Focusing on unanticipated death after ED discharge, Kefer et al. evaluated 13 facilities with 383,416 ED visits, with an 85% discharge rate.[3] The medical examiner evaluated patients seen in an ED within 8 days of their time of death: 15.7% (42/2665) of cases met inclusion criteria. The outcome measure monitored was whether the death was expected and directly related to the ED visit, after review of the death certificate. The majority of the deaths (57%, 24) were considered unexpected and not related to the ED visit (Table 104.2), 21% (9) deaths were unexpected but directly related, 14% (6) of deaths were considered expected and were directly related, and 7% (3) deaths were considered expected but not directly related to the visit. The death rate was 13 per 100,000 discharged patients. The most common cause of unexpected death presumably related to the ED visit was ruptured aortic aneurysm. Kefer et al. concluded that death after an ED visit was uncommon, but being vigilant for vascular catastrophe is essential.

Sklar et al. evaluated a retrospective cohort of ED patients discharged home from an urban tertiary care facility over a 10-year period.[4] The study population was those aged 10 years and over, amounting to 186,859 patients accounting for 387,334 visits. They identified 117 patients who died within 7 days of discharge, an incidence of 30.2 deaths per 100,000 ED discharges home (95% CI, 25.2–36.2). Half of the cases (50%, 58) were in the target group – unexpected death, but related to the ED visit – and in the majority of these (60%, 35) a possible error was identified. Four themes were identified in this high-risk group (Table 104.3): first, an atypical presentation of a common problem; second, an established chronic disease with clinical decompensation; third, patients discharged with abnormal vital signs; fourth, patients with mental disability, psychiatric problem, or substance abuse. The unifying factor is that this group may be less likely to return to the ED if their symptoms worsen.

The key is to try to define patterns and predictors of short-term death after ED discharge. Gabayan et al. evaluated a group of 475,829 insurance plan patients with 728,312 discharges in a 1-year period (Table 104.4).[5] The incidence of death within 7 days of discharge was 0.05% (357). There was a higher risk of death with (1) increasing age, (2) male sex, and (3) number of pre-existing comorbidities. The top three primary discharge diagnoses predictive of 7-day post-discharge death are (1) non-infectious lung disease (OR 7.1, 95% 2.9–17.4), (2) renal disease (OR 5.6, 95% 2.2–14.2), and (3) ischemic heart disease (OR 3.8, 95% 1.0–13.6). They identified that 50 in 100,000 patients die within 7 days of ED discharge. High-risk conditions should be sought and monitored to address this post-discharge mortality.

The most important intervention is to start the analysis at an earlier point, such as monitoring unplanned

Table 104.5 Predictors of unscheduled return visit admission

Independent predictors	Significance
	OR, 95% CI
1. Doctor-based factors	3.5, 2.0–6.1
2. Age >65 years	2.2, 1.4–3.5
3. High triage grade	2.1, 1.3–3.2

Reference: Hu et al.[7]

72-hour revisits, in an attempt to prevent the issue entirely. Wu et al. profiled the ED 72-hour revisit rate of a sample of 34,714 patients over a - year period to a secondary referral teaching hospital.[6] They identified a 5.47% 72-hour return rate, with a monthly variability range of 2.85–6.25%. The return etiology was attributed to patient illness in 80.9%, patient issues in 10.9%, and physician issues in 8.2% of returns. The physician misdiagnosis rate was 3.7% (70) with the most common complaint being abdominal pain identified in over half (55.7%, 39) of the cases. The most common initial ED presentations were for abdominal pain (12.9%), fever (12.6%), vertigo (4.5%), headache (2.1%), and upper respiratory infection (2.1%). Unplanned ED revisits are associated with medical error in prognosis, treatment, follow-up care, and information provided, with most revisits being illness related. It is difficult to differentiate between natural disease course, suboptimal therapy, medical error, and patient or family anxiety.

The unscheduled visit 72-hour return rate was also studied by Hu et al., reporting on 413 return visits with a 3.1% incidence (Table 104.5).[7] One-third (36%, 147) of the return visit patients required admission, with an associated mortality rate of 4.1%. These patients had a higher prevalence of old age, non-ambulatory status, high-grade triage, and chronic underlying disease – malignancy, diabetes mellitus, hypertension, coronary artery disease, heart failure, and chronic obstructive pulmonary disease. Independent predictors were identified as age, high triage grade, and physician factors. Interestingly, there was no correlation with staff experience or ED crowding.

Legal Analysis

In *Cleland* v. *Bronson Health Care Group*, a 15-year-old patient presented to the ED with cramps and vomiting.[8] He was treated for 4 hours, diagnosed with influenza, and discharged home. He later returned to the ED, suffered cardiac arrest, and died. The actual diagnosis was intussusception. The family filed suit alleging an Emergency Medical Treatment and Labor Act (EMTALA) claim for failure to provide proper medical screening.[9] The trial court offered a literal interpretation of the EMTALA statute, as it was unlikely Congress intended this to be a theory to support general malpractice litigation. There was no indication the discharge decision was related to any rationale other than the medical judgment of the hospital. They dismissed the case on failure to state a claim rationale, and appeal followed. The United States Court of Appeals (USCA), Sixth Circuit affirmed the trial court ruling for the defense. They held Congress intended an "any and all patient" standard applied to all patients, regardless of payment, for "appropriate medical screening" and "emergency medical condition." However, these conditions – screening, stabilization, or transfer – are actionable if they give the appearance of a backdoor means of limiting coverage for the indigent or uninsured.

In *Del Carmen Guadalupe* v. *Negron Agosto*, the patient was brought to the medical office by his wife with complaints of urinary retention, edema, high blood pressure, and pain and was referred to the ED now with respiratory difficulty, dry cough, and fever.[10] They were met by a family member, a nurse, who worked at the hospital. The patient was brought back immediately for blood work and a chest radiograph and was diagnosed with bronchopneumonia. He was discharged at 3 a.m. with medications for home and allegedly misplaced the medicine, but decided to rest at home rather than making a return visit to the ED. He deteriorated and returned to another hospital that afternoon and died there, with pneumonia as the cause of death.

The family filed suit, again alleging an EMTALA claim citing failure to provide an appropriate medical screening exam to identify emergency conditions.[9] The district court awarded the summary judgment motion to the hospital, and this decision was affirmed by the USCA, First Circuit. First, they held that the "medical screening standard" should be "reasonably calculated to identify critical medical conditions."[11] The claim would have required that the desired test of intervention was available at the facility and not offered to the patient, which was not substantiated here. Second, the "disparate treatment" allegation was not substantiated by the plaintiff, by a failure to submit any policies on the initial screening standards. Third, the "stabilization requirement" was invoked and district court held that if no emergency medical condition was found, the stabilization requirement was not applicable.

In *Vickers* v. *Nash General Hospital*, the patient presented to the ED after alleged involvement in an altercation where he fell, struck his head, and received multiple head lacerations.[12] He had laceration repair and normal cervical spine radiograph and was discharged after an 11-hour stay. Four days later emergency medical services were summoned, the patient returned to the ED, and died as a result of a parietal skull fracture and epidural hematoma. The family filed an EMTALA claim alleging failed screening and stabilization concerning the association of head laceration and skull fracture.[9] The district court dismissed the EMTALA claim under the Federal Rules of Civil Procedure for failure to state a claim on which relief can be granted.[13] The USCA, Fourth Circuit reversed the district court dismissal and remanded for further proceeding. They recognized that disparate treatment is the cornerstone of the EMTALA claim. However, the facts supporting this claim need be stated, and the plaintiff should be allowed to undertake discovery.

Conclusion

There are numerous surveys and evaluations of unanticipated post-discharge death as it applies to the emergency medicine patient. Often the goal is to develop a demographic profile for other parameters that may allow prediction of an untoward event after discharge.

It is critically important for facilities to have a protocol to deal with this unfortunate and sometimes unavoidable scenario, so that all staff have a working plan to further process and evaluate the situation if it occurs. Proper communication with the appropriate individuals by designated personnel within the system in a supportive way is most important.

References

1. Forster AJ, Murff HJ, Peterson JF, Gandhi TK, Bates DW. The incidence and severity of adverse events affecting patients after discharge from hospital. *Ann Int Med*. 2003;138(3):161–167.

2. Vincent JL, Parquier JN, Preiser JC, Brimioulle S, Kahn RJ. Terminal events in the intensive care unit: reviews of 258 fatal cases in one year. *CCM*. 1989;17(6):530–533.

3. Kefer MP, Hargarten SW, Jentzen J. Death after discharge from the emergency department. *Ann Emerg Med*. 1994;24(6):1102–1107. DOI:10.1016/S0196-0644(94)70239-X.

4. Sklar DP, Crandall CS, Loeliger E, Edmunds K, Paul I, Helitzer DL. Unanticipated death after discharge home from the emergency department. *Ann Emerg Med*. 2007;49(6):735–745. DOI:10.1016/j.annemergmed.2006.11.018.

5. Gabayan GZ, Derose SF, Asch SM, Yiu S, Lancaster EM, Poon T, et al. Patterns and predictors of short-term death after emergency department discharge. *Ann Emerg Med*. 2011;58(6):551–558. DOI:10.1016/j.annemergmed.2011.07.001.

6. Wu CL, Wang FT, Chiang YC, Chiu YF, Lin TG, Fu LF, Tsai TL. Unplanned emergency department revisits within 72 hours to a secondary teaching referral hospital in Taiwan. *J Emerg Med*. 2010;38(4):512–517. DOI:10.1017//j.jemermed.2008.03.039.

7. Hu KW, Lu YH, Lin HJ, Guo HR, Foo NP. Unscheduled return visits with and without admission post emergency department discharge. *J Emerg Med*. 2012;43(6):1110–1118. DOI:1016/j.jemermed.2012.01.062.

8. *Cleland* v. *Bronson Health Care Group, Inc.*, 917 F.2d 266 (1990).

9. EMTALA, 42 U.S.C. §1395dd.

10. *Del Carmen Guadalupe* v. *Negron Agosto*, 299 F.3d 15 (2002).

11. *Correa* v. *Hospital San Francisco*, 69 F.3d 1184 (1995) at 1192.

12. *Vickers* v. *Nash General Hospital, Inc.*, 78 F.3d 139 (1996).

13. Federal Rules of Civil Procedure Rule12 (b) (6): Motion for Failure to State a Claim.

Chapter 105

Urgent Care

Case

The physician had logged a good number of hours in the emergency department (ED), working there for almost 30 years. It was a busy department, and she wanted to slow down a bit. She made the transition to working urgent care as there was a freestanding urgent care center (UCC) near her home and one of her work colleagues had recommended it to her. One of the first things she noticed was that the UCC was busier than described and she was often required to see three or four patients an hour. Even though there was an advanced practice provider (APP) there, they both worked very hard. The nurses were good and did the best they could, but this was often a busy environment.

On one very busy night, a young female patient presented to the UCC with non-specific chest pain and some shortness of breath. She was generally healthy, but had recently taken a long trip which always raises a concern of a pulmonary embolism. The urgent care physician suggested the patient be evaluated in the hospital ED, which had the capability of dealing with this type of complaint. The patient declined and said that she had to go home first. The physician offered to arrange ambulance transport to get her to the hospital facility and call the ED to make sure they knew she was coming, so there would be no time lost. Once again, the patient and her husband refused, saying they appreciated the offer, but they had to go home first and then they would go to the hospital. Once again, the physician expressed her concerns and said that if there was any issue they should call her back and she would contact the ED to let them know to expect the patient.

On the physician's next shift, 2 days later, the director of the UCC called her into the office to inform her that the patient had a pulmonary embolism. She was still hospitalized and was threatening legal action.

It was alleged that she should have been transferred by ambulance and her husband, who worked in health care, stated that it was an Emergency Medical Treatment and Labor Act (EMTALA) violation. The physician pointed out that she had discussed the risk of pulmonary embolism with the patient, and she had offered to arrange transport to the hospital ED and call to let them know that she was coming, but they had declined the offer.

Medical Approach

The urgent care system is an efficient and effective part of the health-care delivery system in the US. Here, lower-acuity patients are seen in higher volume, recognizing that sophisticated care resources may not be available. Unfortunately, patients often present to the UCC with complaints that are more emergent than they realize. It is important to recognize that the average UCC has a high-efficiency benchmark. On average a physician might be seeing two patients per hour in the ED, and three patients per hour in a UCC, which is one patient every 20 minutes.

The development of UCCs or minor injury departments has been discussed since the early 1980s.[1] A UCC is a freestanding or integrated facility that evaluates patients without life-threatening or significant illness or injury on a walk-in basis. The typical staffing pattern for an integrated fast-track unit involves APPs, either nurse practitioners (NP) or physician assistants (PA). Current sites may see one-third of ED patients on average. Freestanding UCCs are typically staffed by physicians often with primary care training. Buchanan performed an early evaluation, in which 21% of patients were evaluated by an NP-staffed minor emergency area.[2]

The characteristics of the urgent care patient have been profiled as well, finding that the UCC volume is inversely proportional to primary care physician

Table 105.1 Non-urgent ED use

		Non-urgent	Semi-urgent
		%	%
1.	Age (years)	43 ± 18.1	49± 20.1
2.	Proportion	25.4 (454)	74.6 (1329)
3.	Health conditions (no.)	3.1	3.9
4.	Ambulance arrival	5	22
5.	Admitted	4	24
6.	PCP follow-up	70	75
7.	PCP care prior	22	27

Reference: Afilalo et al.[4]

Table 105.2 Non-urgent patients not seeking PCP care

	Reason	Incidence (%)
1.	Accessibility	32
2.	Perception of need	22
3.	Referral/follow-up ED	20
4.	Familiarity with ED	11
5.	Trust in the ED	7
6.	No reason	7

Reference: Afilalo et al.[4]

Table 105.3 Presenting complaint vs. discharge diagnosis

	Prediction	Significance
		95% CI, %
1.	Primary care treatable diagnosis	6.3, 5.8–6.7
2.	Chief complaint reported	88.7, 88.1–89.4
ED triage prediction		
3.	Immediate or emergency care	11.1, 9.3–13.0
4.	Hospital admission	12.5, 11.8–14.3
5.	Operating room	3.4, 2.5–4.3

Reference: Raven et al.[7]

(PCP) availability. Gill and Diamond described a program in which Medicaid patients were referred to PCPs.[3] After institution of the referral program, ED use decreased compared to controls (24 vs. 4%).

The use of the ED for non-urgent complaints is a difficult operational question. Afilalo et al. evaluated non-urgent, semi-urgent, and urgent care requirements, contacting 2348 patients of whom 77% (1783) participated.[4] Those with non-urgent complaints were in the minority (25.5%, 454) compared to those with more urgent complaints (74.5%, 1329). The patients with non-urgent conditions tended to be younger, in better health, less likely to arrive by ambulance, less often admitted, and less likely to have PCP care before the visit or in follow-up (Table 105.1). The reasons cited to not seek PCP care and present to the ED for minor complaints included accessibility (32%), perception of need (22%), referral or follow-up from the ED (20%), familiarity with the ED (11%), trust in the ED (7%), and no reason offered (7%) (Table 105.2). A positive focus on these attributes allows the urgent care system to be successfully tailored.

The usual source of medical care was correlated to subsequent non-urgent ED use. Sarver et al. evaluated 9146 patients who had a usual source of care other than the ED, but were dissatisfied with that care.[5] The reasons to present to the ED with a minor complaint include dissatisfaction with their usual source of care, citing issues with the staff, lack of confidence in staff ability, scheduling difficulty, difficulty in phone contact, and prolonged waiting times ($P < 0.05$). These positive associations persisted even after controlling with a multiple logistic regression analysis and being more likely to visit an ED with a non-urgent complaint.

There is disagreement among health-care professionals about the distinction between urgent care and the ED. Gill et al. reported on a chart review of 266 ED patients reviewed by ED and family physicians and nurses.[6] The proportion of patients rated as meeting urgent care criteria retrospectively ranged from 11% to 63%. The agreement rating was only fair (Kendall correlation $(K) = 0.38$, 95% CI 0.30–0.46), and no better among those of the same specialty. The agreement was even less between the triage nurse prospective assessment and that of the retrospective study nurse ($K = 0.19$, 95% CI 0.07–0.31). Clearly there is an issue with acuity prediction, because of its subjective nature.

Another analysis involves comparing the presenting complaint to the final discharge diagnosis to identify "non-emergency" ED visits. Raven et al. applied a predictive algorithm to a 34,942 visit dataset to identify 6.4% (95% CI 5.8–6.7%) of the patients determined to have a diagnosis that was primary-care treatable (Table 105.3).[7] The initial and final primary care diagnoses were consistent in 88.7% of ED visits. However, one-quarter had a concerning course in which 11.1% needed immediate or emergency care, 12.5% required admission, and 3.4% went directly to the operating room. There is clearly limited concordance between presenting complaint and discharge diagnosis. The ability to accurately predict non-emergency ED visits is suspect.

Another medicolegal concern relates to APP supervision. Gifford et al. sent a questionnaire to 1000 emergency physicians in 2004 and again in 2009.[8] The majority (70%) of the physicians believed that when the PAs were "adequately supervised" there was no greater risk of malpractice than for any other clinician. Likewise, in both surveys 80% of the clinicians did not believe PAs were more likely to be sued. This perceived PA lawsuit risk is inversely proportional to time spent in emergency medicine or supervising PAs. The number of physicians practicing with PAs increased by 26% and the number working directly with patients by 19% between the two studies. The number who thought patient waiting times were shorter increased by 13%, and 10% thought patient satisfaction increased as well. This finding appears to be related to physicians' familiarity in working with and supervising PAs.

Legal Analysis

In *Parris* v. *Sands*, a patient who presented to the UCC with upper respiratory symptoms was diagnosed with malignancy.[9] She was known to have a splenectomy, was febrile, with no cough, "dull" eardrum, no lymphadenopathy, and a borderline elevated white blood cell count, and was discharged without antibiotic therapy. She presented to another facility 3 days later, and was hospitalized for 6 weeks with bacterial pneumonia. The patient filed suit and the trial court jury favored the physician defendant. The Court of Appeals of California, Second District affirmed, holding the physician had no duty to inform the patient of the various "schools of thought" regarding the use of antibiotics in asplenic patients. When there is a difference of opinion among medical experts, or different medical approaches to a problem, the "schools of thought" approach is a valid defense.

In *Matsuyama* v. *Birnbaum*, the patient presented to a UCC with a complaint of a skin lesion and severe abdominal pain, in which gastritis was diagnosed.[10]

There was a follow-up visit with his PCP with some additional testing including a positive *H. pylori* test, which was treated. The patient succumbed to a cancer. Medical malpractice was alleged, invoking the "loss of chance" doctrine. Here, the alleged negligence reduces or eliminates the patient's prospects for a more favorable recovery, and any survival is a thing of value to the aggrieved. The superior court jury trial found the defendant PCP liable for misdiagnosis, and a "substantial contributing factor" in the outcome. The Supreme Judicial Court of Massachusetts, Norfolk held that recognizing the loss of chance of survival in the limited domain of medical negligence advances the goals of tort law and affirmed the judgment.

In *Cox* v. *Primary and Urgent Care Clinic*, the patient had made multiple visits to the UCC for various ailments.[11] She made four visits with respiratory complaints and fatigue, and was evaluated by the PA in phone contact with the clinic director. While on a trip, she sought care at two different EDs and was eventually diagnosed with a cardiac condition requiring surgery. The plaintiff filed suit alleging misdiagnosis by the PA and by the oversight physician, and sued the physician and the clinic but not the PA. The trial court granted the defendant's motion for summary judgment. They failed to establish a breach of the standard of care for the care provided by the PA. The appeal court reversed, holding that the standard of care for the PA was the same as for the physician. The Supreme Court of Tennessee at Nashville reversed again, concluding the standard of care for the PA is separate and distinct from that of the physician.[12,13]

In *Wilson* v. *Southampton Urgent Medical Care*, the patient made 11 visits to the UCC over a 2-year period for various complaints including headache.[14] The patient died of cancer and the family filed suit against the clinic owner, eventually adding the treating physician, alleging failure to diagnose her condition in a timely way. The defendants moved to dismiss all claims based on the statute of limitations. The court recognized that not all the UCC visits were related to to the medical issue in question. As well, there was intermittent follow-up to address these issues. The Appellate Division of the Supreme Court of New York ruled that the physician defendant added later should be afforded the right to have her summary judgment dismissal motion heard that did not apply to the other defendants.

Conclusion

It is important to realize that the UCC should have a transfer capability for emergency patients. Freestanding departments should have an established arrangement with an ED for transfers to be done routinely. However, a freestanding UCC is not an ED and does not have an EMTALA obligation to stabilize and transfer patients. Facilities that are affiliated with an established hospital health-care system, or that are physically adjacent, typically do have a de facto EMTALA requirement. This requires a stabilization protocol and procedure to transfer unstable patients to a higher level of care if necessary.

References

1. Zasa R. The development of urgent care centers. *J Ambul Care Manage*. 1986;9(2):1–12.

2. Buchanan L, Powers RD. Establishing an NP-staffed minor emergency area. *Nurse Prac*. 1997:22(4):175–178.

3. Gill JM, Diamond JJ. Effect of a primary care referral on emergency department use: evaluation of a statewide Medicaid program. *Family Med*. 1996;28(3):178–182.

4. Afilalo J, Marinovich A, Afilalo M, Colacone A, Leger R, Unger B, Gigure C. Nonurgent emergency department patient charactersitics and barriers to primary care. *Acad Emerg Med*. 2004:11(12):1302–1310. DOI:1197/j.aem.2004.08.032.

5. Sarver JH, Cydulka RK, Baker DW. Usual source of care and nonurgent emergency department use. *Acad Emerg Med*. 2002;9(9):916–923. DOI:10.1197/aemj.9.9.916.

6. Gill JM, Reese CL, Diamond JJ. Disagreement among health care professionals about the urgent care needs of emergency department patients. *Ann Emerg Med*. 1996;28(5):474–479. DOI:10.1016/S0196-0644(96)70108-7.

7. Raven MC, Lowe RA, Maselli J, Hsia RY. Comparison of presenting complaint vs discharge diagnosis for identifying "nonemergency" emergency department visits. *JAMA*. 2013;309(11):1145–1153. DOI:10.1001/jama.2013.1948.

8. Gifford A, Hyde M, Stoehr JD. PAs in the ED: do physicians think they increase the malpractice risk? *J Am Acad Phys Asst*. 2011;24(6):34–38.

9. *Parris* v. *Sands*, 25 Cal. Rptr.2d 800 (1993).

10. *Matsuyama* v. *Birnbaum*, 452 Mass. 1 (2008).

11. *Cox* v. *Primary and Urgent Care Clinic*, 313 S.W.3d 240 (2010).

12. Tennessee Comprehensive Rules and Regulations, 0880-03.01–24. Physician Assistant Practice (2009).

13. Tennessee Code Annotated §§63-19-105, 6: Physicians Assistants Act.

14. *Wilson* v. *Southampton Urgent Care*, 977 N.Y.S.2d 224 (2013).

Violence

Case

The patient was brought in to the emergency department (ED) by the police after they received a call that he was in the community, visibly agitated and threatening violence in his neighborhood. When the police officers entered his apartment he became combative and required physical restraint, as well as some sedation. The ED physician was able to get a history to the effect that the patient was drinking and the patient thought somebody had put something in the marijuana that he smoked. He had been depressed recently, and had a couple of previous psychiatric hospitalization events. He had now threatened his neighbor over a property dispute. In light of the circumstances – drug and alcohol intoxication, physical violence, and a threat to his community – the plan was to involuntarily commit the patient. After the chemical intoxicants had worn off, a psychiatric professional agreed and he was transferred later that evening for a hospital stay to evaluate and treat his mental illness.

Later that month a complaint was filed with the state health department alleging the patient was deprived of his rights and a family member alleged his confidentiality was breached with regard to the psychiatric hospitalization.

Medical Approach

There is a societal duty to protect the public against violent threats that emanate from patients who are in one's care. There is an affirmative obligation to report this behavior to the appropriate law enforcement authorities while still protecting the patient's confidentiality throughout the evaluation and treatment process.

Ideally, two health-care professionals, including a psychiatric professional, are involved in the involuntary commitment procedure, and sometimes other public service personnel, including police, fire, and emergency medical services (EMS) to define potentially dangerous behavior and isolate and protect the patient as well as the public.

The ED can be the focus of a workplace violence rubric. Taylor and Rew attempted to define the understanding of workplace violence in the ED.[1] There are a host of studies that examine the incidence of ED violence, but few studies of the framework for accurate information gathering. The limitations cited include: (1) underreporting of violence; (2) barriers and attitudes toward reporting; (3) description and characterization of incidents of violence; (4) predisposing factors; (5) lack of fear (Table 106.1). Formalizing the review process will result in improved implications for practice guidance.

Violence in the ED is a worldwide problem. Jenkins et al. sent questionnaires to 273 consultants responsible for 310 EDs with 85% (233) reporting verbal abuse and physical violence.[2] Patients were the most common perpetrators, and nurses the most common victims. The most common precipitating factors included alcohol use, prolonged waiting times, recreational drug use, and unmet patient expectations. There were 557 staff injuries with the majority (90.6%, 505) soft tissue injuries, 7.5% (42) lacerations, and 1.8% (10) fractures. There were 399 legal interventions, in which the majority (74.6%, 298) of alleged

Table 106.1 Workplace violence in the emergency department

1.	Underreporting of violence
2.	Barriers and attitudes toward reporting
3.	Description and characterization of incidents of violence
4.	Predisposing factors
5.	Lack of fear

Reference: Taylor and Rew.[1]

Table 106.2 Improving emergency department security

1. Training staff in breakaway techniques
2. Increasing availability of security officers
3. Issuing personal alarms
4. Encouraging staff to report all incidents

Reference: Rose.[3]

perpetrators were arrested, 25.3% (101) appeared in court, and 19.0% (76) were convicted. Most departments have conventional security measures including panic buttons and video monitoring systems. There appears to be a systemic pattern of verbal and physical abuse with inner city departments the most affected, and only a minority of perpetrators convicted.

Nurses are more commonly involved in these events than physicians typically because of closer contact with the patients in day-to-day operations. Rose performed a questionnaire survey of 36 nurses with a 75% response rate and 69% (9/13) of patient care assistants.[3] The survey found that half of the nurses reported physical or verbal assault, with one-third within the past 12 months. Only a small fraction (7.4%, 2/27) of nurses were not concerned about physical assault. These two were both male, trained as psychiatric nurses, and had never been assaulted. Most verbal abuse was not reported, and 29% had not reported their last episode of physical abuse. However, the likelihood of verbal violence being reported increased with age and experience. Respondents believed assaults on nurses were treated less seriously than similar incidents involving private citizens, and there was less institutional support available to them. Suggestions to improve staff security include: (1) teaching staff breakaway techniques; (2) increasing the number of security officers on duty; (3) issuing personal alarms to staff members; (4) encouraging staff to officially report all incidents (Table 106.2).

Violence against ED workers can involve both patients and visitors as well. Gates et al. surveyed 242 employees with direct patient contact working at five different hospitals, where most workers had been verbally harassed at least once by a patient or visitor.[4] There were 329 assaults with the great majority (96.9%, 319) committed by patients, but 3.1% (10) were committed by visitors. However, the majority (65%) of those assaulted never reported the incident to hospital authorities. As well, the majority (64%) had not had any violence training in the previous year.

There is significant correlation between employee exposure to violence, feelings of safety, job satisfaction, and employee retention. The major concern is that verbal abuse, if left unchecked, can create a hazardous work environment. The next step would be assaultive behavior, with a verbal threat of physical harm by someone with capacity to create a feeling of dread. This can be followed by battery, in which a physical act follows the threat, described as an "unlawful touching."

The incidence of battery in the ED was investigated by Foust and Rhee in a prospective study over 9 months of a metropolitan Level I trauma center with a 64,000 annual volume.[5] There were 19 episodes of violence directed against the staff where they were kicked (7), punched (6), grabbed (3), spat on (2), and pushed (1). The blows were equally split between the face or head (7) and the extremities (7). Hospital incident reports were completed in only 21% (4/19) of the battery events, and there were no cases requiring ED treatment or disability leave. The assailant was typically male (79%) and in the ED on a psychiatric or substance abuse detainment (79%). Although these events are often minor, monitoring high-risk scenarios is crucial for success.

The other area of concern is the violent patient, with resultant obligations to both the patient and society. The high incidence of gun crime has created the obligation for the ED personnel to report gunshot wounds to law enforcement. Frampton describes the legal and ethical issues surrounding the relinquishment of confidentiality in the setting of a gunshot wound.[6] There is an obvious duty of patient confidentiality. In reality, however, the duty of confidentiality owed is not absolute, and may depend on the circumstances. There is a balance between individual and societal rights. There is a clear duty to disclose for issues in which the public interest in knowing outweighs the right of the individual to consent to disclosure of select health information.

There are legal obligations both to the dangerous patient and to society (Table 106.3).[7] First, a limited breach of confidentiality is allowed, involving third-party disclosure without consent involving law enforcement or judicial intervention. Second, there is a duty to warn third parties in light of those who are a known danger. Third, the duty to report involves specific conditions such as child abuse, elderly abuse, or domestic violence. Fourth, for those presenting imminent danger to themselves or others, the authority to

Table 106.3 Legal obligations with the dangerous patient

1. Breach of confidentiality
2. Duty to warn
3. Duty to report
4. Authority to detain

Reference: Buppert.[7]

detain exists through an involuntary commitment procedure.

Ideally, the goal is to be able to accurately predict a patient's propensity to violence. Lidz et al. studied two matched consecutive samples of patients presenting to a psychiatric ED and then followed for a 6-month period.[8] Of the initial cohort of 2452 patients, 79.4% (1948) consented to participate and 14.5% (352) were felt to be likely violent. Violence occurred during the follow-up period on average in 45% of the ED population. The incidence in the predicted group was 53% compared to 36% in the control group. Overall predictive capability was modest, and for women it was no better than chance.

Legal Analysis

In *Capan* v. *Divine Providence Hospital*, the patient presented with a severe nosebleed, developed delerium tremens, and became violent.[9] The on-call physician was summoned to answer emergencies, and the patient was medicated with a series of drugs for combative behavior. The patient was alleged to have suffered a cardiac arrest that evening. The patient's family brought suit, and all physicians were non-suited except the treating ED physician. A jury trial awarded the verdict to the hospital and treating physician. The Superior Court of Pennsylvania vacated the judgment, remanding for a new trial based on a jury instruction concerning the physician's employment relationship as an independent contractor rather than an employee.

In *Isaacs* v. *Huntington Memorial Hospital*, the physician parked in a hospital lot, his wife went to visit a friend, and he attended to some patients.[10] When they left the hospital building at 10 p.m., the physician was accosted in the parking lot and was shot by an assailant, surviving with sequelae. They sued the hospital and insurance company alleging failure to provide adequate security measures to protect invitees and licensees against the criminal acts of third parties on the premises, related to a decision to disarm the security guards. The trial court denied the hospital's summary judgment motion to dismiss, and trial began. It was acknowledged that the facility was located in a high crime neighborhood, with unarmed security and video monitoring. Foreseeability of harm is typically a question for the jury considering what is reasonable. The defendant contended that proof of foreseeability required evidence of prior similar events. The Supreme Court of California held that limiting to the "prior similar events" standard of foreseeability is inherently unfair and contradictory to public policy. The non-suit judgment was reversed and case remanded to trial court for further consideration.

In *Wilson N. Jones Memorial Hospital* v. *Ammons*, a visitor who accompanied her husband to the ED was assaulted by a psychiatric patient who was being detained as a danger to himself but not to others.[11] The injured visitor filed suit, alleging the patient had numerous previous visits, with a history of violent and irrational behavior requiring physical restraint and sedation. The trial court denied the defendant's motion to dismiss as a non-patient filing a "health care liability claim" pursuant to Section 74.001 (a) (13), 74.351 (a) of the Texas Civil Practice and Remedies Code, which required the filing of an expert report.[12] The Court of Appeals of Texas, Dallas concluded the trial court abused its discretion by declining to dismiss the facility's motion for dismissal with prejudice as a health care liability claim, and remanded for hospital's claim for attorney's fees.

Conclusion

The key is to recognize that the ED can be a high-risk environment, and it is essential to protect patients, visitors, and staff from potential violence. Integrated security plans involving staff awareness, hospital-based security, and law enforcement personnel should be instituted to minimize risk to patients, their families, and staff.

References

1. Taylor JL, Rew L. A systematic review of the literature: workplace violence in the emergency department. *J Clin Nurs*. 2011;20(7–8):1072–1085. DOI:10.1111/j.1365–2792.210.03342.x.

2. Jenkins MG, Rocke LG, McNicholl BP, Hughes DM. Violence and verbal abuse against staff in accident and emergency departments: a survey of consultants in the

UK and the Republic of Ireland. *J Accid Emerg Med* 1998;15:262–265. DOI:10.1136/emj.15.4.262.

3. Rose M. A survey of violence toward nursing staff in one large Irish accident and emergency department. *J Emerg Nurs*. 1997;23(3):214–219. DOI:10.1016/S0099-1767(97)9001–6.

4. Gates DM, Ross CS, McQueen L. Violence against emergency department workers. *J Emerg Med*. 2006;31(3):331–337. DOI:10.1016/j.jemermed.2005.12.028.

5. Foust D, Rhee KJ. The incidence of battery in an urban emergency department. *Ann Emerg Med*. 1993;22(3):583–585. DOI:10.1016/S0196-0644(05)81946–8.

6. Frampton A. Reporting of gunshot wounds by doctors in emergency departments: a duty or a right? Some legal and ethical issues surrounding breaking patient confidentiality. *Emerg Med J*. 2005;22(2):84–86. DOI:10.1136/emj.2004.016733.

7. Buppert C. Legal obligations to the dangerous patient. *Topics in Advanced Practice Nursing eJournal* 2009;9(3). Medscape, August 18, 2009.

8. Lidz CW, Mulvey EP, Gardner W. The accuracy of predictions of violence to others. *JAMA*. 1993;269(8):1007–1011. DOI:10.1001/jama.1993.03500080055032.

9. *Capan* v. *Divine Providence Hospital*, 430 A.2d 647.

10. *Isaacs* v. *Huntington Memorial Hospital*, 695 P.2d 653 (1985).

11. *Wilson N. Jones Memorial Hospital* v. *Ammons*, 266 S.W.3d 51 (2008).

12. Texas Civil Practice and Remedies Code. §§74.001 (a) (13), 74.351 (a) (2008).

Glossary

Medical

Aminoglycoside antibiotic active against Gram-negative rods

Axis I major disorder highest level of psychiatric involvement according to the *Diagnostic and Statistical Manual* (DSM) classification system

Basic metabolic panel (BMP) measure of electrolytes, renal function, and blood glucose

Called typically to end resuscitative efforts

Cardiac enzyme measure of cardiac injury

Cath lab area where cardiac catheterization and other intervention is performed

Chem-7 measure of electrolytes, renal function and blood glucose

Clindamycin macrolide antibiotic active against Gram-positive cocci and rods

Code Blue a hospital-sponsored resuscitation team intervention for a patient with a life-threatening event

C-reactive protein (CRP) measure of inflammatory state

Curbside consulting unofficial consult to a physician colleague for a patient care opinion

Deferred consent solicited after care has been administered in emergency setting

Dextran polysaccharide-based fluid expander used in trauma resuscitation

Diuretic medication that induces fluid loss by increasing urine production

Diversion referral of patients to other hospitals when capacity is reached

Electrocardiogram (EKG) a test sensing electrical activity of the heart

Emergency consent health-care provider consents for patient in exigent circumstances

End-tidal carbon dioxide (CO_2) measure of exhaled CO_2 defining the efficiency of ventilation, often used to confirm endotracheal tube placement

Epoetin alfa recombinant protein stimulating bone marrow production of red blood cells (RBC)

External fixator exterior stabilizing device for a complex fracture

Fecal occult blood (FOB) blood in stool not apparent without special testing

Hetastarch starch-based blood volume expander used in trauma

Hypoxemia decrease in blood circulating oxygen

Implied consent more formalized balancing of factors in which the health-care provider consents

Intensivist specialist in critical care medicine

Non-STEMI coronary ischemic event without ST elevation

Oxygen saturation (SO_2) proportion of hemoglobin binding sites occupied by oxygen

Partial pressure of carbon dioxide (PCO_2) measure of ventilatory efficiency

Percutaneous coronary intervention (PCI) invasive cardiology procedure to remedy vascular insufficiency

Placenta previa low-lying placenta over the cervix, prone to bleeding and possibly endangering the fetus

Pyelonephritis urinary tract infection involving the upper tract or kidney

STEMI coronary ischemic event with ST elevation

Stridor high-pitched, often musical breath sounds during inspiration, indicative of airway obstruction

Sympathomimetic drug that stimulates the sympathetic nervous system

Toxic appearance that implies significant illness

Transient ischemic attack (TIA) neurologic deficit of brief duration, typically a few minutes

Troponin cardiac-specific protein indicative of injury to the heart

Legal

Affirm assert validity as a judicial decree

Alternative jury instruction a stipulation that multiple interpretations of the same information are plausible

Best interest test decision-making that includes historical patient factors and preferences

Bright-line rule test that produces an unequivocal, predictable outcome

Common law decisions based on previous judicial precedent rather than statute

Capacity ability to accomplish a task

Certiorari superior court request for information from lower court or judicial agency

Competence ability to comprehend relevance of decision-making

Contributory negligence legal defense that alleges the plaintiff's conduct was responsible in whole or in part for damage incurred

Corporate liability doctrine hospital may be liable for the acts of an independent physician

Declaratory judgment court makes non-binding recommendation in legal proceeding

De facto as a fact

Demurrer written legal objection to a claim suggesting legal insufficiency in the filing to prevail

Demurrer without leave to amend judicial disposition of cause of action by sustaining motion for dismissal alleging facts do not support a legal cause of action, without the ability to refile the complaint

Discovery pretrial formal request for evidence production

Dismissed with prejudice a merit-based disposition that precludes further judicial consideration

Dismissed without prejudice judicial disposition that permits refiling by the party

Emancipated minor responsible for their own care as they are making adult decisions, although below the normal age of majority

En banc decision by all judges that comprise the court

Estoppel prevent assertion contradictory to position previously held by party or judicial determination

Ex parte discussion involving only one of the parties

First impression legal question that may not have been encountered before

Grandfathered pre-existing rule will apply to old cases, although a new rule applies to future issues

Guardian ad litem court-appointed volunteer to protect the interests of one who is not competent to do so

Indictment formal charge of criminal allegation

Interlocutory provisional decision in the legal process

Interlocutory order offered at an intermediate stage of the legal process

Locality rule expert testimony must be based on similar means of practice

Justiciable able to be decided in a judicial setting

Last chance doctrine defendant is liable if they had the final opportunity to avert the issue

Loco parentis standing in place of parents for decision-making

Loss of consortium damage claim by family member for death or significant injury in a legal action

Mandamus performance of a specified act compelled by a superior court writ

Minor before the age of majority, typically 18

Miranda rights suspect's right to decline interrogation if they desire, and their right to an attorney

Motion to dismiss challenge of legal sufficiency of stated claim

Motion in limine petition filed with the court to limit specific evidence from trial consideration

Motion to suppress defendant request to exclude evidence at trial

Non-delegable duty doctrine an employer may not defer complete responsibility to a third party for an essential duty, such as safety

Non-precedential does not establish a case example for future legal guidance

Parens patriae governmental agency has the right to assume essential care responsibilities if required

Petition of mandate higher to lower court compunction of performance

Prima facie premise is accepted as factual until rebutted

Quid pro quo transfer of goods or services as an exchange

Rational basis test unless a constitutionally based interest, the law is upheld if logically related to any legitimate governmental interest

Remanded case referred back to the originating court for reconsideration

Res ipsa loquitur doctrine the occurrence of an event in itself implies negligence

Respondeat superior supervising party is responsible for their agents

Safe harbor action specifically identified as permitted in a more comprehensive law or statute

Statutory law decisions based on voted legislative initiatives

Strict liability applies to inherently dangerous conditions in which proving blameworthiness or intent is not required

Subpoena duces tecum order compelling production of documents for court appearance

Total mix standard all relevant information included in the decision-making, rather than a definite limiting standard

Writ of mandate (mandamus) court order to another agency or court to co\mply with the law

Index